ALSO BY MELANIE THERNSTROM

Halfway Heaven: Diary of a Harvard Murder

The Dead Girl

THE PAIN CHRONICLES

THE
PAIN
CHRONICLES

Cures, Myths, Mysteries,

Prayers, Diaries, Brain Scans,

Healing,

and the Science of Suffering

MELANIE THERNSTROM

Farrar, Straus and Giroux   New York

FARRAR, STRAUS AND GIROUX
18 West 18th Street, New York 10011

Grateful acknowledgment is made for permission to reprint the following
previously published material:
"Final Soliloquy of the Interior Paramour," from *The Collected Poems of Wallace Stevens*
by Wallace Stevens, copyright © 1954 by Wallace Stevens, renewed © 1982 by Holly
Stevens. Used by permission of Alfred A. Knopf, a division of Random House, Inc.
Excerpts from "The Poem of the Righteous Sufferer," translated by
Benjamin R. Foster, from *Before the Muses: An Anthology of Akkadian
Literature.* Used by permission of CDL Press.

Library of Congress Cataloging-in-Publication Data
Thernstrom, Melanie, 1964–
    The pain chronicles : cures, myths, mysteries, prayers, diaries, brain scans, healing,
and the science of suffering / Melanie Thernstrom.— 1st ed.
        p. ; cm.
    Includes bibliographical references and index.
    ISBN 978-0-86547-681-3 (hardcover : alk. paper)
    1. Pain—Popular works. I. Title.
    [DNLM: 1. Pain—etiology—Personal Narratives.   2. Chronic Disease—
psychology—Personal Narratives.   3. Chronic Disease—therapy—Personal
Narratives.   4. Pain—psychology—Personal Narratives.   5. Pain—therapy—
Personal Narratives. WL 704 T411p 2010]
    RB127.T485 2010
    616'.0472—dc22

                                                                    2010002390

Designed by Abby Kagan

www.fsgbooks.com

1   3   5   7   9   10   8   6   4   2

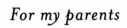

For my parents

Dolor dictat

CONTENTS

THE PAIN CHRONICLES

INTRODUCTION: THE TELEGRAM

I magine, as I imagine, a community of consumptives, coughing blood in a progressive nineteenth-century mountain sanatorium. Their well-regulated hospital life includes the most modern of treatment protocols: antiquated purging and bloodletting have been replaced by mineral baths, good nutrition, mountain air, and heliotherapy—sunbathing. Yet attitudes have not evolved very far from those of Hippocrates, who, in the fifth century B.C.E., warned colleagues against visiting patients who had advanced consumption (the most prevalent disease of the time), because their inevitable deaths might damage the physicians' reputations.

Through the centuries, there were many theories about consumption's causes—heredity, evil spirits, vampirism, vapors, sewage, swampland odors, and corruption within the body. In the nineteenth century a fashionable conception of the disease was as a spiritualizing struggle between the body and the soul, in which the mortal flesh was slowly consumed in a way that heightened both beauty and creativity. But in the spring of 1882, a German physician identified *Mycobacterium tuberculosis*. Four thousand years of myth vanished in a moment as the bacterium materialized under the microscope. Although everything about the presentation of the disease, from sufferers' glittering eyes to their disappearing flesh, had lent itself to metaphor, science abruptly dissented. Consumption became tuberculosis—a disease, not a state of being. Although the cure—antibiotics—was still half a century away, there was a diagnosis.

In *Illness as Metaphor*, Susan Sontag describes the transformation of consumption into TB as an archetypal example of a process by which diseases are understood metaphorically until their pathology becomes clear. The philosopher Michel Foucault captures this process in postulating that modern medicine began when doctors stopped asking patients, "What is the matter with you?"—a question that invited a complex personal response— and began asking, "Where does it hurt?" instead, a question that focuses solely on biology.

Although these processes are driven by scientific discoveries, social attitudes have to shift in order for science to investigate. Moreover, people have to believe scientific findings before they act upon them. From a distance, one paradigm seems to succeed another in the blink of history's eye, but in their era they surrender slowly, and lives are lived and lost in the interim. Ideas can be slow to catch on: germ theory, for example, had been articulated but not popularized by the time of the Civil War, so soldiers blithely drank from rivers that other regiments used as toilets upstream. And there are always naysayers: bloodletting was discredited years before George Washington was bled on his deathbed by his physicians. Nitrous oxide and ether (the gases used for the first form of surgical anesthesia) had been discovered decades before anyone thought to employ them during agonizing operations.

How did the news of the discovery of tuberculosis arrive at the sanatorium? Did the residents read of it in the newspaper? Did their relatives pay a visit or send a telegram? *It's not you—it's a bacterium! Strange— you seemed so consumptive.* Did the news make them rethink the story of their sickness and realize it had nothing to do with a spiritualizing struggle? Or did they regard the news in the way one takes in scientific advances about black holes or the bones of primitive man—interesting, but personally irrelevant? After all, there was still no cure. Or perhaps the news never reached the sanatorium, and the consumptives perished on the magic mountain, imprisoned not only by disease, but by a host of lonely meanings.

Wouldn't understanding the nature of their suffering itself have been therapeutic? Even in the absence of treatment, epileptics may benefit from knowing that they are not possessed by spirits, and it may help depressed people to know that their condition is not a failure of character. Surely the consumptives would have felt relief, mixed with wonder, to finally know what their disease was—and what it was not. It was not a curse. It was not an expression of personality or a punishment. For better and for worse, it was and is a disease.

To be in physical pain is to find yourself in a different realm—a state of being unlike any other, a magic mountain as far removed from the familiar world as a dreamscape. Usually, pain subsides; one wakes from it as from a nightmare, trying to forget it as quickly as possible. But what of pain that persists? The longer it endures, the more excruciating the exile becomes. *Will you ever go home?* you begin to wonder, home to your normal body, thoughts, life?

Ordinarily, pain is protective—a finely wired system warning the body of tissue damage or disease and enforcing rest for the bone to knit or the fever to run its course. This is known as acute pain; when the tissue heals, the pain disappears. When pain persists long after it has served its function, however, it transforms into the pathology of chronic pain. Chronic pain is the fraction of pain that nature cannot heal, that does not resolve over time, but worsens. It can begin in many ways—as trivial as a minor injury or as grave as cancer or gangrene. Eventually, the tissue heals, the diseased limb is amputated, or the cancer goes into remission, and yet the pain continues and begins to assume a life of its own.

The doctor assures the patient she is fine, but the pain worsens, the body sensitizes, and other parts begin to hurt, too. She has trouble sleeping; she stumbles through her days. Her sense of her body as a source of pleasure changes to a sense of it as a source of pain. She feels haunted, persecuted by an unseen tormentor. Depression sets in. It feels wrong . . . maddening . . . delusional. She tries to describe her torment, but others respond with skepticism or contempt. She consults doctors, to no avail. Her original affliction—whatever it may have been—has been superseded by the new disease of pain.

Chronic pain is a specter in our time: a serious, widespread, misunderstood, misdiagnosed, and undertreated disease. Estimates vary widely, but a 2009 report by the Mayday Fund, a nonprofit group, found that chronic pain afflicts more than 70 million Americans and costs the economy more than $100 billion per year. Another study in the United States indicates that as much as 44 percent of the population experiences pain on a regular basis, and nearly one in five people describes himself or herself as having had pain for three months or more. Much of the degraded quality of life from diseases such as cancer, diabetes, multiple sclerosis, and arthritis stems from persistent pain. In one survey, most chronic pain patients said that their pain was "a normal part of their medical condition and something with which they must live." One-third of the patients said that their pain's severity was "sometimes so bad [they] want to die." Almost one-half said they would spend all they have on treatment if they could be assured it would banish their pain.

Yet treatment for chronic pain is often inadequate. In part, this is because it is only in recent years that chronic pain has been understood to be a condition with a distinct neuropathology—untreated pain can eventually rewrite the central nervous system, causing pathological changes to the brain and spinal cord that in turn cause greater pain—though this new understanding is not widely known. Chronic pain is sometimes defined as continuous pain that lasts longer than six months, yet chronic is not ordinary pain that endures, but a different condition, in the same way an alcoholic's drinking differs from that of a social drinker. It is not the duration of pain that characterizes chronic pain, but the inability of the body to restore normal functioning.

"The history of man is the history of pain," declares Pnin, a character in a Nabokov novel of the same name (a name that is itself just one letter removed from the word *pain*). The longing to understand physical pain and to alleviate it has threaded through all of human history, from the earliest records of thought. No single discipline seems adequate to address or represent pain, because every lens through which one tries to examine it— personal, cultural, historical, scientific, medical, religious, philosophical, artistic, literary—fractures pain into a different light.

In the Sanskrit Hindu scripture, the *Bhagavad Gita*, the god Krishna speaks of "life, which is the place of pain . . ." What is pain whose place in life is so central? To unravel its riddles, we must look at the ways in which pain has been understood and interpreted. These understandings seem to fall into three basic paradigms. First, there is what we might call the pre-modern view, in which pain is never simply a bodily experience, but reflects a spiritual realm suffused with meanings and metaphors, from the pain-causing demons of ancient Mesopotamia who spread their wings wide, to the Judeo-Christian tradition in which pain begins with the expulsion from Eden. "Thorns also and thistles shall [the ground] bring forth to thee," God condemns Adam—a curse that is transformed, in Christianity, into a means of redemption.

Pain was also seen as a force that could be used for positive spiritual transformation. Pilgrims and ascetics in many different traditions elected to draw closer to God by undergoing painful rites, and martyrs embraced painful death. Belief in pain's spiritual properties made pain the critical instrument of jurisprudence in the premodern world—not only as the appropriate punishment for crimes but also for determining guilt, both through torture and through the curious precursor to the jury trial known as "trial by ordeal," in which the suspects were subjected to painful rituals (such as holding a hot iron, walking on hot coals, or plunging a hand into boiling water). If God failed to protect them from pain, they were deemed guilty.

The premodern paradigm is not entirely obsolete; although it has been supplanted, it has not been expunged. To understand our attitudes toward pain today, we must understand the legacy we inherit from five thousand years' worth of struggle to make sense of this mortal condition. Suffering was—and still is—regarded by many as something that can, must, or ought to be endured. Although it is difficult to believe, the invention of surgical anesthesia (through the inhalation of ether gas) by an American dentist in the mid-nineteenth century was controversial at the time. Many agreed with the president of the American Dental Association, who declared, "I am against these satanic agencies which prevent men from going through what God intended them to go through." The use of anesthesia during childbirth was especially controversial, as it was believed to circumvent the divine injunction to bring forth children in pain. Even after the invention of anesthesia, many surgeons continued to perform surgery without it, including experimental surgeries on slave women who were said not to suffer the same pain as their mistresses.

The premodern understanding of pain was replaced in the mid-nineteenth century by a new biological view of pain as simple, mechanistic sensation: a function of nerve endings that send predictable pain signals to the brain, which responds passively in turn with a proportionate amount of pain. Influenced by Darwin, the biological view of pain saw all pain as protective—serving, usefully, as a warning of tissue damage. The remedy for pain seemed plain: treat the disease or injury, and the pain should take care of itself. This model prevailed for most of the twentieth century and, indeed, is still commonly held, not only by patients but also by physicians.

While this view has helped us make strides in managing *acute* pain and spurred on the development of anesthesia, it has impeded and continues to impede our ability to recognize and understand *chronic* pain. It cannot explain why some pain continues to worsen of its own accord. Even for acute pain, the model does not suffice, for it cannot explain why in a lab experiment the same heat stimulus may hurt one person more than another, or why injuries that are severe may hurt someone only mildly while mild injuries may be agonizing for others. Moreover, the model cannot explain treatments that target *only* the mind, such as the forgotten nineteenth-century technique of mesmerism (a form of hypnotism), so effective that it enabled surgery to be performed painlessly.

The biological view of pain is in conflict not only with the way man through the ages has regarded pain, but with the way in which pain is *experienced*, not as an ordinary physical function, but as an extraordinary state of being. Unlike the premodern paradigm, the biological model cannot explain the disconcerting flexibility of meaning in pain, or why the meaning of the pain changes the pain itself. Why does the pain of loss of virginity seem to differ so profoundly from the pain of rape, or the pain of sadomasochism differ from the pain of sexual abuse? How can the pilgrims I witnessed in the Hindu celebration at Thaipusam in Kuala Lumpur claim that not only are they not in pain, but they feel *joy* while fishhooks decorate their backs and skewers pierce their mouths?

In recent years, a new, third paradigm of pain has emerged, a synthesis that embodies elements of both earlier traditions. The contemporary model of pain sees it as a complex interaction among parts of the brain. While founded on the same scientific traditions that gave rise to the nineteenth-century view, it has also revealed the truth embedded in the nonscientific, premodern model by showing the way in which pain is inherently meaningful because it is not simply a matter of nerves firing, but an experience created by meaning-making parts of the brain.

Like the consumptives stranded in the half century after science had discovered the nature of their disease but had not yet yielded a cure, those who suffer from persistent pain in our era are caught in an uneasy moment. Pain is one of the most promising fields of medical research today: new tools in the form of advanced imaging techniques are taking the first pictures of the brain in pain, and techniques of gene analysis are identifying which genes are active in the presence of pain. Yet the pain clinic lags far behind the research lab. Patients languish because of lack of access to good treatment and because even the best treatment that exists today is often inadequate.

When we read about the conceptions of pain throughout history—of the ancient Babylonian tablets, for example, that situate the origin of toothache in the making of the world—we are thankful to live in the modern world with modern medicine. What would it be like to have toothache figure so prominently in consciousness that its origin merited inclusion in the story of all creation? When we read of their remedies—a word spell said over a plant poultice—we feel sorry for the Babylonians.

But when others look back on our treatments, they will feel sorry for us—both for the limitations of our knowledge and for our reluctance to use the knowledge we have. They will shiver at the thought that people lived with chronic pain—as we do now when we read the accounts of surgery without anesthesia, an idea so dreadful as to be almost unimaginable. Just as we are amazed that anesthesia could have been controversial, they will be surprised at the way some of the most powerful pain medications we have—opiate and opioid medications such as Percocet and OxyContin—are misunderstood and misused, withheld from those who would benefit from them and given to those who are harmed by them.

Pain takes sufferers' own worlds away and leaves them on a magic mountain of isolation and despair. To understand that chronic pain is a disease is the first step off the mountain of lonely meanings.

Curiously, the progression of my understanding of my own pain mirrored the larger progression of the understanding of pain in history. In 2001, I was given an assignment by *The New York Times Magazine* to write an article about chronic pain. Although I had suffered from pain myself for a number of years, it wasn't until I began researching my article that I gained any real understanding of my condition, what pain is, and what the treatment options are. I had seen a variety of doctors, both good and bad, but I had difficulty distinguishing between the two, changed doctors frequently, and complied erratically with treatment plans. Coming to understand pain as a disease changed my relationship to it, from seeing it as a personal affliction, failure, or curse to seeing it as a manageable medical problem.

For many years, I kept a record of my quest toward healing: a pain diary that documented the meanings I made of pain as it wreathed my personal and romantic life like a choking vine. The metaphors that obscured my medical situation were of my own making. Although my rheumatologist had suggested keeping the diary as a helpful tool, the diary itself became a place for embroidering my pain with pernicious meanings. When, as a journalist, I had the opportunity to read other patients' pain diaries, I was struck by how many others did the same.

While researching my article, I was able to interview the most distinguished pain specialists—researchers and physicians—throughout the country, and I spent time in seven of the best pain clinics, which served such diverse populations as coal miners in West Virginia, cancer patients in New York, and pediatric patients in Boston. I followed the director of each clinic on his or her daily rounds and appointments, studying patient charts and sitting in on difficult case conferences for periods of time ranging from a day to a month. I saw the questions they confront: How do you measure a patient's pain? What if he or she is fabricating it? How do you choose a treatment plan? How do you know which patients will abuse drugs? Are some people genetically more prone to developing chronic pain? What is the relationship between pain and depression? Why are there so many female patients? Most of all, I was struck by the *contrast* between the physician's and the patient's points of view: the difference between patients' understanding of their suffering and doctors' understanding, and the complex nature of the medical encounter.

The Victorians believed in an invisible hierarchy of feeling in which the young were more pain sensitive than the old, females were more sensitive than males, and rich, educated whites (the inventors of the theory) naturally found themselves to be infinitely more pain sensitive than the poor, the unschooled, the enslaved, and indigenous peoples. Surprisingly, modern research has found that physiological pain sensitivity *is* affected by race, gender, and age—but not at all in the way the Victorians believed.

I eventually observed several hundred patients. At times, visiting pain clinics felt like descending into Dante's *Inferno*. Some were crushed in industrial accidents or suffering from degenerative nerve and autoimmune diseases, while others had ordinary complaints such as backaches or headaches that were causing them extraordinary pain. I kept in touch with patients over the course of eight years to try to answer the question: Why did some people get better and not others? Does the answer lie in the nature of the patients or in the doctors or in the treatment methods used? How does religious faith affect pain, disability, and mortality? Does churchgoing or prayer ameliorate pain?

I met a young woman who acquired chronic back pain from a five-minute demonstration of a chiropractic maneuver which she'd been talked into by a trainer at the gym one day. Over the course of the next eight years, she supplemented her insurance with six figures of her own money, seeing every well-known doctor and trying every type of treatment she had heard of before she found one that worked. Eight years! But she got better.

Pain, like any extreme situation, brings out the best or the worst in people. Pain makes a hero of some: a woman paralyzed by a routine pain surgery for a bulging disk in her neck who coped with her new, much more terrible affliction of spinal cord injury pain. A train conductor who lost three of his limbs when he fell off a train and suffered from phantom limb pain taught his doctor about the mystery of resilience. Yet other patients were suicidal, and others (including myself) found that we were acting in ways unrecognizable to ourselves and collaborating in our pain rather than combating it.

This book is divided into five sections: "Pain as Metaphor," in which pain is seen through the lens of the meanings that have been made of it from ancient times onward; "Pain as History," which traces the discovery of anesthesia in the mid-nineteenth century and the collapse of the religious model of pain; "Pain as Disease," which discusses the state of pain treatment and pain research today; "Pain as Narrative," which follows the experience of patients undergoing pain treatment and the way in which pain changes and is changed by life as it is lived; and finally, "Pain as Perception," which unites the varying paradoxical aspects of pain through the contemporary understanding of how pain works in the brain. Woven throughout is my own story, based on the pain diary that I kept.

Every one of us will know pain in our lives, and none of us knows when it will come or how long it will stay. Although we will one day have effective treatment for the disease of chronic pain, we can never eradicate pain itself, because our bodies require it. Pain is a defining aspect of mortal life, a hallmark of what it means to be human. It often stamps both the beginning and the end of life. It threatens our deepest sense of ourselves and—portending death—reminds us of the ultimate disappearance of that self. It is the most vivid experience we can never quite describe, returning us to the wordless misery of infancy. It seems to rend a hole in ordinary reality; it is intrinsic to the human body, yet feels alien. And it is the aspect of mortality that we like least; we abhor pain more, even, than death.

Pain is like a poison from whose cup everyone has sipped; there is no one who cannot recall its taste and fear a deeper draught. *Take this cup from us*, we say, while knowing no reprieve is permanent.

This is a book about the nature of that poison—its peculiar taste, its mysterious effects—and its antidotes.

I

THE VALE OF PAIN, THE VEIL OF PAIN:

Pain as Metaphor

DOLOR DICTAT

Mortals have not yet come into ownership of their own nature. Death withdraws into the enigmatic. The mystery of pain remains veiled," the German philosopher Martin Heidegger writes. Does metaphor unveil pain to reveal its true nature, or is metaphor the veil that surrounds pain—and makes it so hard for us to see pain as it is?

Pain is necessarily veiled, David B. Morris writes in *The Culture of Pain*, because, to a physician, pain is a puzzle, but to a patient it is a mystery, in the ancient sense of the word—a truth necessarily closed off from full understanding, which refuses to yield every quantum of its darkness: "a landscape where nothing looks entirely familiar and where even the familiar takes on an uncanny strangeness."

But "illness is not a metaphor," Susan Sontag sharply asserts in *Illness as Metaphor*. "The most truthful way of regarding illness—and the healthiest way of being ill—is one most purified of, and resistant to, metaphoric thinking. Yet," she complains, "it is hardly possible to take up one's residence in the kingdom of the ill unprejudiced by the lurid metaphors with which it has been landscaped."

How true this sounds! I read it again and again to feel its full weight—how helpful and clarifying it is. Sontag's point seems to turn on what one might think of as the different resonances of the words *illness* and *disease*. While disease refers to biological pathology, illness opens the door to a world of wider meanings—the very meanings, Sontag says, that burden and confuse the patient. When the pathology of the illness is finally understood, metaphors will fade away, she asserts, in the way that consumption became TB. Cancer is not an expression of repression, it is a cluster of abnormally dividing and enduring cells; AIDS is not retribution for homosexuality, it is an immune deficiency. Pain is not a pen dipped in blood, scribbling on the body in illegible script, nor is it a mystery to be divined; it is a biological process, the product of a healthy nervous system in the case of acute pain and a diseased one in that of chronic pain.

True, true. Yet even when pain is understood this way, its metaphors endure. When pain persists, a biological disease becomes a personal illness. The illness changes the person, and the changed person reinterprets the illness in the context of her life, experience, personality, and temperament. A thousand associations spring to mind—personal, situational, cultural, and historical.

As soon as we reject certain metaphors, others immediately take their place. Foucault's modern doctor may ask, "Where does it hurt?" but the patient will ceaselessly—idly and intently, consciously and unconsciously—contemplate the old question, "What is the matter with me?" and this wrongness cannot be illuminated by the word *pain*.

More, perhaps, than any other illness, protracted pain spawns metaphor. As has often been observed, pain never simply "hurts." It insults, puzzles, disturbs, dislocates, devastates. It demands interpretation yet makes nonsense of the answers. Persistent pain has the opaque cruelty of a torturer who seems to taunt us toward imagining there is an answer that would stop the next blow. But whatever we come up with does not suffice. We are left like Job, bowing before the whirlwind.

On one hand, nothing is more purely corporeal than physical pain. It is pure sensation. Indeed, it often figures in literature as a symbol of illegibility and emptiness. As Elaine Scarry writes in *The Body in Pain*, pain is uniquely lacking in a so-called objective correlative—an object in the external world to match with and link to our internal state. We tend to "have feelings *for* somebody or something, that love is love of x, fear is fear of y...," she explains, but "physical pain—unlike any other state of consciousness—has no referential content. It is not *of* or *for* anything."

As Emily Dickinson puts it, "Pain has an element of blank." Yet it is the very blankness of pain—the lack of anything it is truly like or about—that cries out for metaphor, the way a blank chalkboard invites scribbling.

As soon as Dickinson tries to describe this great blank, she grasps for metaphor:

Pain—has an Element of Blank—
It cannot recollect
When it begun—or if there were
A day when it was not—

It has no Future—but itself—
Its Infinite contain
Its Past—enlightened to perceive
New Periods—of Pain.

You try to wake yourself out of pain—*it's not an infinite realm, it's a neurological disease*—but you can't. You are in a dreamscape that is familiar yet horribly altered, one in which you are yourself—but not. You want to return to your real self—life and body—but the dream goes on and on. You tell yourself it's only a nightmare—a product of not-yet-fully-understood brain chemistry. But to be in pain is to be unable to awaken: the veil of pain through which you cannot see, the vale of pain in which you have lost your way.

To be in pain is to be alone, to imagine that no one else can imagine the world you inhabit. Yet the world of pain is one that all humans must, at times, inhabit, and their representations of it pierce us through the ages. "Head pain has surged up upon me from the breast of hell," laments a Babylonian in a story three millennia old. The agony of the ancient sculpture of the Trojan priest Laocoön and his sons as they are strangled by sea serpents still contorts the ancient marble, as does the very different agony of Jesus' crucifixion in Matthias Grünewald's Renaissance altarpiece.

Dolor dictat, the Romans said—pain dictates, dominates, commands. Pain erases and effaces. We try to write our way out of its dominion. *How savage its practices, how dark its vales!* we exclaim, this unhappy country on whose shores we have washed up after a voyage upon which we never sought to embark.

"I would have made a fine explorer in Central Africa," the nineteenth-century French novelist Alphonse Daudet writes in his slim volume of notes about suffering from the pain of syphilis, published as *In the Land of*

Pain after his death. "I've got the sunken ribs, the eternally tightened belt, the rifts of pain, and I've lost forever the taste for food," he laments.

If only Daudet *were* in Africa, instead of in Pain, he would know that one day he could return home and leave his tribulations behind. His scribblings might then seem to be tall tales: Was he really pricked with a thousand arrow points while his feet were held in fire? But if others were skeptical, he wouldn't mind. He'd no longer need anyone to walk in that lonely place with him. Indeed, he would hardly recall it himself.

But Pain is not a place easily left behind. We inhabit Pain. Pain inhabits us.

Dolor dictat.

We write about pain, but pain rewrites us.

Pain Diary:

I Keep a Secret

ONSET: When did your pain begin? Was there any triggering event or special circumstances that surrounded it?

In the beginning, it was secret.

It began when I was visiting my best friend, Cynthia, and her friend Kurt in Nantucket. Kurt had been Cynthia's boyfriend for many years, but that had been many years before. By the time of my visit, they had been friends longer than they had ever been lovers, and everything was easy. Their relationship was the kind of thing people say never works, but it did, so that was part of the fun, too.

Kurt lay on his back in the sun, reading Foucault, while Cynthia swam the perimeter of the pond. She was wearing a cardinal-colored bathing suit, her dark curls tucked under a cap. They were both academics, a decade or so older than I. Even though I was twenty-nine, I felt a bit like a child around them—bright, but slightly ignorant. Cynthia had adopted me when she was a seventh-year English Ph.D. student and I was a first-year creative writing one, and it had been my dearest hope that she'd become my friend. Kurt never would have paid attention to me, I knew, but for Cynthia. Her gaze always put me in the best light—a prettier, cleverer light.

I lay beside Kurt, covered by a frayed magenta beach towel. It's hard to recall how I felt about my body at that time, but it involved a dim sense of unease that led me to conceal it. I remind myself of this sometimes now: I didn't enjoy my body that much even before I got pain, so pain didn't ruin as much as it should have. I wonder now, if I had known that that afternoon was, in one sense, the beginning of pain and that henceforth my opportunities to take pleasure in my body would be numbered, would I have thrown aside the towel?

I wanted to swim straight across the pond, as I had as a child. Then, my father had always followed me in a rowboat, which I was glad about because I was afraid of eels. Cynthia climbed out of the water and stretched out on the beach.

"Would you swim to the other shore with me?" I asked Kurt. My heart beat as if I had propositioned him.

Kurt looked up with a lazy, skeptical glance. He gazed at the pond and wrinkled his nose. "It's too far," he said.

"Go with her," Cynthia said.

"Now?" he said.

We swam and swam, arms curving over heads, pausing to look up as the families on the far shore came into clearer view. Closer, breath, closer. The straps of my white suit tangled, and the top slipped down. I wondered whether my breasts, pointing down pale in the dark water, looked like eels' faces to the eels waiting below. Finally we flopped on the wooden dock, clean and hot and cold and wet, alone together—a pond away from where we began.

"We really went the distance, didn't we?" Kurt said later as we climbed back to the shore and collapsed, shivering, onto the warm sand at Cynthia's feet.

I looked up at Cynthia and saw something register. In a novel, this would be a tragic turning point: the older woman realizes that her young friend wants her former lover, and even though the woman doesn't want him anymore, even though the woman might have in fact—as Cynthia had—left the man years ago, there's always a price for desire: someone has to drown. Our story is so different, though, I thought, because Cynthia is different—I felt her generosity, her easy love, as she rubbed suntan lotion into my back. "You and Kurt are such matched swimmers," she said reflectively. And then: "You should go inside, sweetie. You're starting to burn."

Sunset fell as Kurt played guitar on the deck. The light changed on the water, and the shrubs sloping toward the sea darkened and merged into the hill. We drank and listened, and as I listened, pain set in.

It began in my neck and poured through my right shoulder, down into my arm and hand. It felt as if my right side were sunburned, but inside out, reddening and beginning to pucker and blister beneath the skin.

I usually drink wine, but I poured a glass of gin. It tasted as anesthetic as it looked, clear and cooling. But the pain seemed to be drinking, too, and as it drank, it grew bold and began to mock and turn on me.

"I think I am not feeling well," I announced, puzzled, and went downstairs to bed.

My right side refused to fall asleep. It throbbed, reminding me of a horror movie I saw once, in which a transplanted limb is still possessed by the angry spirit of its original owner. I slipped into Kurt's room to look in the long mirror. I turned at different angles, but my right and left shoulders looked the same.

The pain continued, lively through the night. I heard Kurt and Cynthia whispering in the hall, and the closing of doors, and then I went up to the living room and wrapped myself in a blanket on the couch and drank more gin.

I woke from a dream of terrible pain—of reaching for something you shouldn't and arriving to find yourself stranded in a place you never wished to be.

"*Hey,*" Kurt said, puzzled, as he came up the stairs.

I sat up on the couch, cradling my arm, blinking, confused, waiting for the usual feeling of emerging from a nightmare. But the pain lingered, veiling the ordinary world.

"You look—What? Are you okay?"

"Yes—yes. I liked swimming across the pond with you," I said with unplanned passion. Why was I revealing feelings for him? Why was I concealing the pain?

He offered a mug of tea. I reached for it with my bad arm, as if to illustrate that nothing was wrong.

"Perhaps we could go again today," I said. But the cup was oddly heavy in my hand; I could barely bring it to my trembling lips.

POENA

Romantic and physical pain have nothing to do with each other, I firmly believed at that time, just as there is no likeness between a broken heart and a heart attack. A broken heart is a metaphor; a myocardial infarction is a cardiovascular event. Indeed, even as a metaphor, a broken heart seems antiquated now that we know emotion stems from the brain.

"How do you know the nature of your ailment?" my favorite grandmother—a Christian Scientist—used to inquire when I had a headache. "How do you know that it isn't a spiritual problem?"

"Because I know," I would say. "Because I'm not confused."

The feeling of Kurt and the feeling of pain had a certain similar emotional hue. And because they began at the same time, the narrative of pain and the narrative of the romance began to entwine and become a single story in my mind.

Three years later I lay in Kurt's bed for the first time, shivery and sleepless with the hope and fear that accompanies great change—and with pain, the same ghostly pain that had arisen for no reason that weekend three years before and then disappeared beneath the surface of my body.

That day, I had taken the train to Providence to visit Kurt, something I had never done without Cynthia. Cynthia—who had recently married and liked the idea of her two friends pairing—had actually arranged for the date. I had asked if we could go swimming that afternoon, in memory of the afternoon in Nantucket. We swam past scores of anxious parents bent on keeping their children from slipping under the white rope separating them from deeper waters, and then we lay on the dock on the far shore. It was so sunny, it was as if we were still swimming in the sun-air. We lay resting on the wooden slats, gauging each other's desire to lie there forever against the knowledge that the longer you wait, the harder it is to swim back. He was ready and then I was ready, but he closed his eyes again. I had just slipped into sleep when I felt his foot on my back, and I understood that we would sleep together that night.

I am not given to large romantic hopes—to imagining that a given boyfriend could be the last boyfriend—and I've never understood how that feeling seems to come so easily to most people. But that night, as I lay beside him in the dark, a sense of possibility began to dawn. The night I lost my virginity, I had stayed awake with the sense of irrevocable transformation, but since then, sex had all been erasable, like scribbling on one of those childhood magic slates that you can shake blank so the game can go on and on. Could this be different?

But I also had pain again. The old, eerie pain, familiar and strange. In the years since that day on Nantucket, I had felt a brush of this pain from time to time—a pointless ache in my neck and shoulders, which I dimly attributed to structural weakness in my body. I have a large head—poorly supported by a long neck and narrow shoulders—which I carry in a forward position, giving the impression at times that it is in danger of toppling off. I knew I should work on my posture, but it was on the list of boring beauty routines, such as working on my nails or my tan, that I had no real intention of undertaking. And the occasional achiness had become as normal as the sight of my unpolished nails and sunless skin.

Only once in that period had the pain been something odder and more urgent. I was at a roof-deck garden party on the Upper East Side of Manhattan when a forgotten friend handed me a gigantic baby—a baby I hadn't even known existed. I stood there alone momentarily, gaping at the baby, when pain sidled up and put a hand around my neck. I thrust the baby back into his mother's arms immediately, smarting, but the touch of pain tingled as dusk gathered and the air began to chill. I continued my conversations. I thought of it as a brush of mortality, a reminder that these parties could not go on forever.

Light began to fill Kurt's bedroom, and pain filled the house of my body like smoke. I thought of a deer I had seen once as a child on a hiking trip in a summer nature camp. Its leg had disappeared beneath a tangle of roots. As our troop came near, the animal began to thrash, making a huge rustling noise, twisting its neck in desperation. Our leader made us stand back as he went up to examine it. When he came back, he said the deer's leg was fractured and there was nothing to do. "It's nature's way," he said. Some of the children began to cry. How could that be nature's way? What was nature thinking? The deer would die in pain.

I finally fell asleep, but woke from a dream about the deer. I had this dream every few years, but this time my body was merging with the deer, its leg turning into my arm, disappearing into the earth, like Persephone struggling to loose herself from her captor. When I woke, the image disappeared and the dream pain remained.

"Why aren't you sleeping?" Kurt said, stirring beside me. "I can feel you not sleeping."

"No, nothing," I murmured. If he became my true love, I would look back on this night and realize that it had been the happiest night of my life because it had led to lasting happiness. But I had pain. Happiness and pain. The two nested familiarly together in my mind.

Yet—*why?* Was pain the price of happiness—or a punishment for having it? Pain, from the Latin *poena*, "punishment for an offense," and surviving in the English phrase *on pain of death*; the Greek *poine*, from the verb "to pay, atone, compensate"; and old French, *peine*, "punishment, or suffering thought to be endured by souls in hell."

But what was there to pay for? I had committed no offense. But there it was: I wanted Kurt, and I got pain. I slept with Kurt, and the pain returned. Those two facts nestled against each other, and (in the terms with which we will one day describe everything) with the miraculous neuroplasticity of the brain, began to develop neural connections. The sex mixed with the pain: the weight of his hands, pressing, imprinting, hurting my body, irrevocable as love.

It wasn't love, though, that turned out to be irrevocable. I never didn't have pain again.

Of course, I know now that the pain was related not to Kurt, but to swimming! Although I had occasionally splashed around hotel pools, the only times I swam long distances were with Kurt. That day, I had strained my neck and shoulder, beginning a cascade of symptoms stemming from an underlying condition of which I had been unaware. But what did I know of *cervical spondylosis, spinal stenosis, occipital neuralgia, impingement syndrome, rotator cuff disease*?

I was years away, at that point, not only from having that information but from seeking or valuing or, one might even say, believing in it—at least with any of the same depth with which I felt the truth of other, unacknowledged meanings. As soon as I got pain, the thin veneer of science schooling began to crack, revealing conceptions of pain formed over millennia by art and literature, philosophy and religion.

THE DESCENT OF PAIN

I t's a small space, a crevice over which tangled roots cross like hands. The deer takes an idle leap; her hoof falls through the lattice. She tries to leap again, but pain holds fast and her body quivers and falls. She pants, panicked, but the desire to flee is checked against pain. She tries to stand once again, but pain tightens its grip.

In the deer's leg, sensory receptors known as *nociceptors* are activated in the basic process of tissue protection common to many multicelled creatures, from horses to earthworms. This process is known as *nociception*, from the Latin *nocere*, "to hurt or injure," and the root *-cept*, which can mean "begin." These receptors are, indeed, "the beginning of hurt," responsible for sending nerve signals warning of a bodily threat.

Nociceptors register mechanical (crushing), chemical (poisons), thermal (burns), or other stimuli that have the potential to damage cells. The threshold for activating normal pain-detecting nociceptors is similar among all members of a species: in humans, for example, the pain threshold for heat is about 108° F. At a lower temperature, the water feels pleasantly warm, but right around 108° F the pain-detecting neurons activate and send an alarm.

Nociceptors are attached to two different types of nerve fibers, A-delta fibers and C fibers, which transmit information from the periphery of the body to specialized receptors in the spinal cord. A-delta fibers are nature's warning alarm; they produce a fast, sharp, distinctly localized pain. Indeed, the information conveyed by the A-delta fibers doesn't even need to reach the brain to have an effect; when the signals reach the nociceptors that sit in the spinal cord, they trigger an immediate muscular action that causes the creature's body to move away from the harm. C fibers, on the other hand, are activated after the alarm has sounded and damage has already occurred. They produce a slow, persistent, diffuse pain that indicates continuing injury and forces the creature to tend to its wound after the danger has passed.

The other deer continue to trot, disappearing into the woods. Yet vast respiratory and cardiovascular changes take place in the injured animal as the brain stem reacts to news of the injury by activating the autonomic nervous system (the part of the nervous system that regulates heart rate, breathing, and so forth) and triggering a massive release of adrenaline and other hormones. The vital purpose of the hormones is to pump up the immune system and help the liver and muscles produce and absorb more sugar, which will generate more energy to flee or fight. Rising heart rate and blood pressure prepare the deer to escape.

While danger causes the body to generate energy initially, the wounds—along with the subsiding of endorphins, adrenaline, and the other hormones—later create a sense of sluggishness to force rest. Pain activates the immune system as the injured tissue causes an inflammatory reaction that sensitizes nerves, which causes greater pain. White blood cells release substances that promote fever and sleepiness, helping healing by increasing blood flow to the area, consuming dead cells, and delivering nutrients to the site. The entire area becomes sensitized so that even a light touch there will hurt. This sensitivity is adaptive because it ensures that the site of the injury is protected and rested.

Pain also affects the hypothalamus, the part of the brain that controls hormone release, sleepiness, waking, hunger, thirst, and sexual drive. In the hierarchy of drives, pain is the highest—the most important to survival—so all other drives are stilled. As the feeling of agitation and alertness ebbs, the deer begins to feel heavy, warm, drowsy.

Each of these reactions—together composing the body's response to grave wounds—is a product of a neurobiology millions of years in the making. The basic sequence of responses to pain is common across many species: vigorous activity to escape danger, combined with unresponsiveness to all other external stimuli, followed by guarding of the wound and lethargy during recovery.

There are also characteristic behavioral responses, such as repetitive motions (e.g., rocking to and fro), vocalization, grimacing, crying, or whimpering, which serve to warn others in the group of danger and to impress upon them the severity of the threat. Although human pain behavior seems designed to evoke care from others, when most animals are wounded, others of their species will instinctively keep their distance to let the injured member of the group heal. Moreover, the animal isolates itself from its own herd or family for fear its injury will be jostled. When a human comes near, it will try ever more frantically to escape. If the human tried to examine the leg, the deer would desperately thrash her head and kick with her other legs. If the deer were a fox or a wolf, she would bite.

If the deer were a worm who had just lost the tail of its body, it would slither away without a second thought—or, indeed, a first one. Nature endows even invertebrates, like sponges and leeches, with the damage-sensing nociceptors of mammals and the reflexes to withdraw from danger, but with one key difference: this stimulus-response is not thought to cause the invertebrate pain.

Since nature didn't give invertebrates the thinking parts of the brain that would enable them to recall dangers and avoid them in the future, she also didn't curse them with the apparatus of a central nervous system to make them suffer from their blunders. Instead, she gave the worm, like plants, spare or replaceable parts to cover mishaps. Anyway, nature (it feels unnatural to write about nature without personification) is not concerned with the worm's death, because the worm has dozens—perhaps hundreds—of offspring.

The deer, on the other hand, is dear. Nature has a limited supply: deer produce few offspring, and they take a long time to mature. Mammals have no spare body parts and cannot grow new ones; a broken leg is the deer's demise. So nature endows the deer with a cortex to generate pain to ensure that she will protect her leg.

Even fish have an efficient nociceptive sensory apparatus involving nerves, a spinal cord, and a primitive cortex to process nociceptive signals. Moreover, they respond with behaviors characteristic of animals with more complex cortices (like mammals) in pain, and these behaviors can be reduced by opiate pain medication. Still, pain involves not only detecting harmful stimuli but also having a negative psychological experience, and some researchers argue that the brain of a fish lacks the complexity that is necessary for consciousness. Pain requires—indeed, is *a function of*—consciousness: the greater the level of cortical development, the greater the capacity to feel pain. Fish have small, primitive cortices. Mammals' cortices are much more complex than those of other animals, and primates' are the most so. Moreover, only primates possess an *interoceptive cortex*—a part of the brain believed to be critical in pain perception. The human interoceptive cortex is greatly enlarged.

We, mammals with few natural defenses (lacking claws, camouflage, and saber teeth) and limited reproductive capability (having few offspring, who take many years to reach maturity), are the most closely guarded by a hypervigilant nervous system and a brain with special capacities for generating pain and turning it into a world of unhappy associations and emotions—of dread, loss, anguish, anxiety, regret, and suffering.

THEIR EYES WERE OPEN TO SUFFERING

A woman whose leg is caught in a crevice would feel pain commensurate with the threat the injury poses to her survival, just as a deer would. But as evening descends, another feeling would begin to set in. Although her brain would release the same neuropeptides that allow the deer to sleep off the pain, the woman would lie awake, contemplating this pain and its implications. What if no one comes to help her? She pictures the life that she had, and already it appears both near and impossibly far, like a garden from which she has been suddenly exiled. Along with fever, the sense of *'etsev* (עֶצֶב—a Hebrew word with the various meanings of "hurt, pain, worrisome toil, pang, sorrow, hardship, forsakenness, grief, and affliction"), to which Eve was condemned, sets in. Her eyes are open to suffering.

The multiplicity of meanings of *'etsev* reveals what is human about human pain: the way pain is always steeped in sorrow and other negative emotions (a result of a development, unique to humans, of certain kinds of neural bridges connecting the emotional, cognitive, and sensory parts of the brain).

Why? the woman protests. Of course, she comprehends her situation in the same basic way the deer may (she fell; she was injured; she can't get up). But we cannot picture a human for whom this explanation would fully suffice, because from ancient times onward, humans have also asked a question of a different sort—one that cannot be answered with reference to the material world, but rather that conjures a hidden world of meaning. The question is "why?" in the peculiar sense of "why *me?*"

This human *why—why is this my story and what story is this?*—does not seem to serve any evolutionary function. Yet the question is so universal, appearing across diverse cultures over thousands of years, as to seem genetically coded into the experience of prolonged pain, like inflammation and drowsiness.

Why must I suffer? we ask haplessly, fearing the answer and fearing the absence of an answer. And the longer the pain persists, the more the question presses.

The deer's stumble hurts her, but only the human falls into *'etsev.*

EVIL, HURTFUL THINGS OF DARKNESS

The same questions would pain a woman who fell in the forest today as a woman four millennia ago. The earliest records of history—the cuneiform tablets of ancient Mesopotamia—reflect the urgency to understand bodily pain: how to parse its spiritual significance and alleviate its physical consequences. If the injured woman were an ancient Babylonian stranded somewhere on the Mesopotamian plain, she would understand her pain and injury in a particular way, and indeed, the frame would not be that different if she were Sumerian, Akkadian, Assyrian, ancient Egyptian, Roman, Greek, or Indian.

If I were that woman, I would know that pain, illness, and death arise from a vast, invisible cosmological contest between the opposing malevolent and beneficent demons and deities that control the natural world and compete for domination over mortals. Hosts of demons could enter the body through the unguarded openings of the eyes, mouth, nostrils, and ears, where they would suck the marrow out of bones, drink blood, and devour organs until—save for the intervention of a benevolent deity—the victim perished. Protection could come only from the gods, who, though unreliable and inattentive, must be petitioned for aid. If I were a Babylonian, I would have a personal god whom I cultivated with prayers and offerings and invocations. "One who has no god, as he walks along the street, Headache envelops him like a garment," warns a Babylonian fragment.

For the ancient Egyptians, the body was divided into thirty-six parts, each one the province of a particular god or goddess. In some traditions, demons shared their names with the specific maladies they inflicted. The ancient Indians were tormented by Grahi ("she who seizes")—a she-demon who caused convulsions. For the Akkadians the Dï'û demon caused headaches. Indeed, Dï'û *was* headache—to have a headache was to be possessed by the demon, so there is no other Akkadian word for "headache." In Babylonian texts, the words for "sin," "sickness," and "demon possession" are closely related and often used interchangeably.

How might I rid myself of these demons? In the ancient world, ritual magic could be used to dispossess demons, or pain could be transferred from one person to another. In Babylonia there was a special class of priest, called *gala-tur*, who could absorb an ailment from a living person and carry it into the netherworld and dispense it there. A suckling pig or kid could be sacrificed, and the demon could be transferred to the animal's body. In some cases, expelling demons from the body called for graver measures, such as trepanation—drilling holes through the skulls of the sick to release the demons causing migraines as well as seizures and other ills.

While demons, ghosts, and other evil spirits were more common than gods, in most cultures the powers of the gods were superior. So although the gods could not eliminate the demons—who were also immortals—they could control them. I might turn to the Ebers Papyrus, a compendium of ancient Egyptian prescriptions, spells, and enchantments from 1552 B.C.E. that is one of the oldest medical documents in existence, to find an invocation to the gods, imploring them to "free me from all possible evil, hurtful things of darkness."

I would know, though, that unfortunately, pain and disease could arise directly from the gods themselves. Some gods were consistently adversarial, but most were mercurial and might be swayed by entreaties for assistance and dissuasion from harm. Arrows thrown by Rudra, the ancient Indian Vedic storm god, brought humans sudden pricks of sharp pain. But his hands also contained "a thousand remedies," and his urine, the sacred element of rain, was an anodyne. The Greek god Apollo shot invisible arrows and spears at men, causing illness and death—sufferers were "Apollo-" or "sun-struck"—while his twin sister, Artemis, afflicted "Artemis-" or "moon-struck" women with female maladies. Yet Apollo was also known as a healer: sacred hymns that pleased him might lull him into ending plagues, while Artemis was also known as a goddess-physician, specializing in obstetrics and gynecology.

If I were a Babylonian, I would implore my personal god to lobby for me in the pantheon of gods, as in this invocation in which Marduk, the patron deity of the city of Babylon, consulted his father, the god Ea, about an innocent human victim: "Oh Father, Headache has set out from the Underworld . . . whatever this man has done, he doesn't know it; however will he be relieved?"

Comfortingly, the gods themselves were vulnerable to pain and disease and used spells and curses to rid themselves of pain, which mortals could imitate for their own cures. For example, the Egyptian god Horus was tormented by catfish demons that caused him migraines so severe he sometimes resorted to living in the dark. The great sun god Ra (who suffered from eye diseases, which manifested as eclipses) helped Horus by threatening to cut off the catfish demons' heads with his *tmmt*-loop, his sacred scepter. If I were suffering from a migraine and I incanted this story while my head was rubbed with a *tmmt*-loop made of snake, the demons might flee from me as well. Alternatively, the demon could be dispossessed by rubbing my skull with the ashes of the bones of catfish boiled in oil for four consecutive days.

I could read stories of cures of both gods and men on the walls of temples dedicated to the healing gods in ancient Mesopotamia, Egypt, Greece, and Rome. I might even sleep in the temple, undergoing purification rituals of fasting and bathing, and make an offering to the god or his animal representative. During the night, the gods might reciprocate by transmitting cryptic clues for cures in the form of opaque dreams, which would be interpreted by priests in the morning. If I were too ill to travel to the temple, my family or friends might make the pilgrimage on my behalf, as when Alexander the Great lay dying in Babylon and his generals slept in the temple of Marduk on his behalf. Evening rites often involved the use of opium, which would lull pain and induce vivid dreams for the priests to interpret. If a cure did not arise, I could continue to stay in the temple and further entreat the god. (Dying patients, however, having been scorned by the gods, would be cast out by the priests lest they pollute the temple.)

If I were Greek, I might sleep in the temple of Asclepius, the god of medicine, whose followers—priest-physicians, such as Hippocrates, who claimed to be his descendants—took an oath to heal, to cause no harm, and to keep secret their sacred medical knowledge, a pledge that may be a template for the modern Hippocratic oath. Statues of Asclepius often feature him with his symbol, a serpent-entwined staff that expressed the ancients' belief in the twinning of divine help and harm—the intimate relationship between poisons and remedies, healers and destroyers. Even today, a version of the serpent-entwined staff survives as a symbol on ambulances and hospitals: an indirect tribute to the god—or plea, perhaps, for his protection—who, in the words of the fifth-century B.C.E. poet Pindar, "first taught pain the writhing wretch to spare."

Words themselves could become medicine, as in the Egyptian practice of writing down an incantation or spell with edible ink, dissolving the letters in liquid, and then drinking it. But spells and incantations were often paired with natural remedies such as herbs, roots, or the testicles of an exotic animal, with which they worked synergistically. Babylonian tablets dating back to the third millennium B.C.E. detail how each ailment corresponded to a particular deity or demon and required an individual remedy. If I were a Babylonian with a toothache, I would know that it was caused by the sucking of a primal demon-worm. When the worm was first created, a god offered her some nice food to eat, but the worm rejected the food, saying, "What are a ripe fig and an apple to me? / Set me to dwell between teeth and jaw, / That I may suck the blood of the jaw / That I may chew on the bits [of food] stuck in the jaw." The worm's request was granted, but she was cursed for her bloodthirstiness. Invoking the curse by reciting the story of the worm's creation three times over a poultice of beer, oil, and a (now-unidentifiable) plant and applying it to the tooth would cause the toothache to resolve.

As the Egyptian Ebers Papyrus explains, "Magic is effective together with medicine. Medicine is effective together with magic." Although it would take millennia to understand why, magic *is* effective together with medicine and medicine *is* effective together with magic: words (when given the power of belief) do affect pain—and words in combination with physical treatment can alleviate pain in ways better than either treatment alone.

NO GOD CAME TO THE RESCUE,
NO GODDESS TOOK PITY ON ME

B
ut sometimes all remedies failed. As civilizations developed, anthropologists have observed, the gods tended to grow in power while the demons' status diminished. Over the course of the ancient Mesopotamian empire, for example, as the Sumerians gave way to the Babylonians and Assyrians, it was increasingly believed that demons could only act as permitted by the gods—or as enabled by their absence or indifference. Thus pain and illness raised the haunting question of why the gods were failing to intervene. A Babylonian monologue from the fourteenth century B.C.E. known as the Poem of the Righteous Sufferer concerns the plight of a nobleman who is inexplicably cursed with misfortune, pain, and illness.

> *My own god threw me over and disappeared,*
> *My goddess broke rank and vanished.*
> *The benevolent angel who [walked] beside me split off*
> *My protecting spirit retreated, to seek out someone else . . .*
> *I called to my god, he did not show his face*
> *I prayed to my goddess, she did not raise her head.*

The nobleman details his faithful efforts to conciliate the gods. Despite his piousness:

> *Debilitating disease is let loose upon me . . .*
> *Head pain has surged up upon me from the breast of hell,*

A malignant specter has come forth from its hidden depth . . .
A demon has clothed himself in my body for a garment . . .
My flesh was a shackle, my arms being useless . . .
A crop lacerated me, cruel with thorns
No god came to the rescue, nor lent me a hand
No goddess took pity on me, nor went at my side
My grave was open, my funeral goods ready . . .

At the poem's conclusion, the sufferer has a dream in which the god Marduk belatedly heals him:

My illness was quickly over, [my fetters] were broken . . .
He bore off [the head pain] to the breast of hell,
[He sent] down the malignant specter to its hidden depth,
The relentless ghost he returned [to] its dwelling.

Yet it is the anguish of the abandonment that lingers. Why do the gods desert us?

Pain Diary:

I Avoid Diagnosis

Confronted with the mystery of physical pain, "willingly or unwillingly, we enter a realm that is somehow set apart," David B. Morris writes in *The Culture of Pain*. "We might even say it is the most earnest wish of almost every patient, ancient or modern, to be released not just from pain, but from the requirement of dwelling within its mysteries."

I did not wish to dwell in a mystery. I wanted to live in my old life and my old body, just as I always had.

PAIN HISTORY: Describe your symptoms and their progression. How did you treat it? What aggravated your pain; what ameliorated it?

The morning after Kurt and I first spent the night together, I took the train back to New York City, and Pain came with me. This came as a great surprise, though I realized unhappily that there should be nothing to be surprised about. Pain was there on the train, and there in the taxi from the train, and there as I told the doorman I had a good trip and opened the door to my apartment world.

Everything was just as I liked and had left it: my smoky blue Siamese perched on the velvet sofa I had matched to her coat, my Depression-era teapot collection lined up in optimistic pastels on the window ledge overlooking the courtyard. I settled into an armchair to read my mail, but the chair no longer fit my body. It was impossible to get comfortable with Pain sitting there, too. I rose, and Pain rose with me.

A terrible thought occurred. What if Pain were planning to stay? What if I were never again free to read, because I'd always be reading with Pain? What if I never slept, because I was sleeping with Pain?

I decided to go out to buy Tylenol. The ordinariness of the errand—going to the corner drugstore as if I simply had cramps—was soothing, though the pills made no difference.

"Throughout life I have seldom known respite from pain, having had at least two hundred days of suffering each year," Nietzsche writes. In his final stage of syphilis, consumed by burning nerve pain, he declares, "I have given a name to my pain and call it 'dog.' It is just as faithful, just as obtrusive and shameless, just as entertaining, just as clever as any other dog—and I can scold it and vent my bad mood on it, as others do with dogs, servants and wives."

I had always liked this saying. I had copied it down in a notebook upon first reading it. Yet the image struck me as fatuous now—I didn't believe even Nietzsche truly felt that way. Was he trying to cheer himself up by pretending he was master? Was he not in pain when he wrote it? *Was he kidding?*

Pain began to establish dominion in my world. Pain was not like a violent intruder who batters his way in, wreaks havoc, and departs. It was more like a sour domestic partner—intimate and ugly; a threatening, dirtying, distracting presence, yet one who refused to move out. I did not like waking up to feel its grubby hands on me; I did not like it hanging about in the kitchen, making me drop heavy dishes; I did not like it interrupting my phone calls, especially when a friend was confiding a sorrow I cared to hear. I cared, but not the way I used to care, because part of me now cared only about Pain.

My neck hurts, I checked myself from interjecting, plaintively, while my friends discussed their marriages and miscarriages. *My arm hurts, too.* It sounded like a little kid's complaint: *I have sand in my shoe.*

Pain: it seemed like such a trivial kind of problem to have, categorically different from the deep, meaningful problems with which I liked to think I was preoccupied. It offered nothing to think about, no psychological or spiritual tangle you might unravel in a long, satisfying conversation with a friend while walking around the reservoir in Central Park or drinking tea in a favorite café.

"Pain, while always new to you, quickly becomes repetitive and banal to your intimates," Daudet observes. But I was not only afraid of boring others, I was bored with pain myself—bored to tears. I had never had a problem so utterly consuming and so intellectually empty.

How did I get pain? I didn't seem to have an injury. Several times a day I found myself peering into a mirror, but there was never anything to see. I had endless variants of dreams where I was being hurt—stabbed or twisted or burned—from which I would wake to realize that I had moved the wrong way in my sleep and my sleeping brain was trying to understand the pain, to give it a narrative.

I'd wake, shaking off the foggy images, reminding myself of all that I was not. I was not sleeping in a temple to Asclepius, waking to find the clues to my cure contained in a dream. I was not a Babylonian fettered by pain and no god came to the rescue and no goddess took pity on me; nor was I a Ghanaian man I had read about in a newspaper who was hung by an arm for days and even now, years later in a torture treatment program in Michigan, still weeps to recall it. I was a woman in real silk pajamas lying on a king-size Tempur-Pedic mattress under a white Shabby Chic comforter in a room with a really decent view. In *Manhattan*.

And yet . . . *what*?

I knew, of course, that I should see a doctor. I didn't like the idea that I was *not* seeing a doctor, since that would be weird: a normal urban American with health insurance always sees a doctor when she has a medical problem. And there were many bodily complaints for which I had done exactly that—and benefited. But those were cases, I realized now, in which I already knew what was wrong. I was prone to coughs; I loved watching my primary care physician write prescriptions, knowing that in forty-eight hours I'd feel better. *Always*. It offered a kind of ritual satisfaction. As he recited the instructions with which I was so familiar, I'd take the first easy breath. In an important sense, it seemed to me, the cough actually ended when he handed me the prescription, as if the prescription were a telegram announcing that the enemy was retreating; the fighting might drag on for a few days, but the war was effectively over.

Beneath this satisfying exchange, however, there was always the threat of another possibility. Perhaps one day there'd be no prescription to give. The doctor wouldn't know what was wrong—or he would, and I wouldn't want to know, because there would be no remedy.

It wasn't that I thought the diagnosis created the illness. My father's parents had been Christian Scientists who thought disease was an illusion—that you are only as sick as you think you are—but I had never been persuaded. Perhaps, nevertheless, there was some way in which you weren't fully sick—*sick* sick—without the pronouncement that you were. After all, observation changes its object. Perhaps an undiagnosed illness might be a tree falling in the forest without making a sound, a matter of at least debatable ontological status. If I wasn't listening to my pain, how real could it be? If I went to the doctor, I'd be not only listening but soliciting a witness—a professional witness—to listen, too.

Of course, I didn't really believe any of this. It was inconsistent with the basic way I understood the world. But who knows? Reality can surprise. As long as I didn't make an appointment, it was possible—or rather it was not *impossible*—that a devastating diagnosis was being adeptly avoided.

On the subway one day, I sat in a free handicapped seat. Holding the pulley hurt my arm now, like trying to hold on to the leash of an angry animal. At the next stop, however, a pregnant woman lumbered toward me. I looked at my lap for a minute before standing up, tears of resentment springing to my eyes. *She's not handicapped—she's healthy. She's so healthy, she's conjuring new life. I am*—what?

A doctor would fix the problem, I told myself. She would fix it or reassure me that it was nothing, and then it would actually be nothing.

I asked a friend who was a doctor whom I should see, and he suggested that I consult a neurologist. I thought the specialty had an ominous ring, but I began to feel better in the neurologist's waiting room. Flipping through a women's magazine, I discovered an article about the body's miraculous healing powers: "90% of pain resolves itself in six to twelve weeks, regardless of the method of treatment used," the article stated. Though the primordial jungles had been a dangerous place—roots to trip on, thorns to pierce—our ancestors healed themselves without any help from neurologists. I began to feel I had simply been impatient; surely my body would reveal its healing powers.

"No injury?" the neurologist asked. She moved my limbs as if they belonged to an antique doll whose face looked young but whose parts no longer moved well. She smiled at me, a frank "at your service" smile.

"I'd call it cervical strain," she declared. On her desk, a picture of a little girl with straight brown bangs stared out, seriously. I averted my eyes.

"Cervical?"

"The cervical spine is the neck. As opposed to the lumbar spine."

"Ah." I returned the girl's stare. "So you think it'll get better?"

"Sure."

"Why does my arm hurt, too?

"You know that children's song: 'the neck bone's connected to the shoulder bone; the shoulder bone's connected to the . . .'" Her voice turned into a lullaby.

"So, it'll get better, right?"

Could I have asked any more anxiously? I reproached myself. What if the doctor was of the mind-set that where there is smoke, there is fire?

In fact, my anxiety had the opposite effect, and she became reassuring. "I wouldn't worry about it," she said.

I beamed at her.

"Sometimes we carry tension in our neck and shoulders. How are things going, personally, for you?" she asked. "Are you under stress? As you know, there's a connection between the body and the psyche."

"Oh, absolutely. I am under stress."

On my way out of the room I pinched the magazine with the healing article. I thought of this article frequently as the six to twelve weeks I gave my pain to improve turned into six to twelve months without improvement. In fact, though I told myself it couldn't be, I suspected at times that the pain was growing.

ACUTE AND CHRONIC PAIN

The article I read was correct, but it neglected to explain that its description of natural healing applies only to acute pain, not to chronic pain—a distinction with which I was not familiar at that time.

Acute pain is a healthy reaction to tissue damage, steering us away from threats, alerting us to injury, and resolving when the injury does, often without any treatment at all. Acute pain is often referred to as protective pain because its messages are helpful and should be heeded. It's the body's warning that you are beginning to bend your knee in the wrong direction, or a louder distress message telling you that you have done so. The protection of pain is one of the most important survival tools, its value eerily illustrated by patients who suffer from some form of the rare genetic disease called *congenital insensitivity to pain* (or *congenital analgesia*)—an indifference to physical pain of any kind. People suffering from this condition—suffering, one might say, from a lack of physical suffering—often die young, having destroyed their bodies by inadvertently walking on broken ankles, scratching their eyes, and chewing their tongues.

An oft-used metaphor for chronic and acute pain is that of a fire alarm. Acute pain is like a well-functioning alarm signaling danger; it ends when the fire does. Chronic pain is not protective; its intensity bears no relation to the amount of tissue damage and may, in fact, arise without any apparent damage at all. It is like a broken alarm that rings continuously, signaling only its own brokenness. There may be no fire; the original injury may be long healed. Or there may not have been an injury in the first place; the problem lies in the alarm system itself. It is as if a wire has been cut and the whole system begins to malfunction.

Imagine a home-security alarm that is first triggered by a cat, then a breeze, and then, for no reason, begins to ring randomly or continuously. As it continues to ring, it triggers other noises in the house: the radio and television start to blare; the oven timer dings; the doorbell buzzes repeatedly; and the phone rings maniacally even though no one has placed a call. It's as if a demon has entered the house. This is *neuropathic pain*—a pathology of the central nervous system and the basis of much chronic pain.

My own conception of pain was primarily as something to overcome. It was a challenge to which I fancied myself fully equal—which my life provided ample opportunities to demonstrate. The phrase *accident-prone* has a passive ring; my style had involved a more vigorous courting of disaster. Mine was a willful blitheness, a loose-limbed, gangly clumsiness married to an adolescent impetuousness I had never chosen to outgrow. I consistently overestimated my physical abilities. The black diamond ski trail looked good to me, though the green circle matched my skill. There was no time to walk down the stairs when I was late, though leaping sometimes landed me in a pile at the bottom. If you're not afraid of ladders, why bother with the safety latch—the function of which I recalled only when, standing at the top, I felt the ladder folding up beneath me.

But I was not traumatized. These incidents did not keep me, for example, from buying a wild horse and assuring its previous owners that I was *an expert rider*, though my last lessons had occurred during fifth-grade sleepover camp, and when I got home from camp, my mother—who has a fear of horses—discontinued them. In my twenties, I broke a bone each year for three years in a row and sported a variety of bruises, sprains, and burns. But I recovered splendidly from everything. How had I lost the knack?

"Perhaps you could be a little more careful," Cynthia had suggested sweetly as she carted me around in my casts. But I didn't want to be. Carelessness felt like carefreeness; carefulness, like an acknowledgment of aging, fragility, and mortality. And breaks hurt less than one might imagine. At first, I found, you can stave off the pain by concentrating on how you're going to get help, when, for example, the horse has ditched you an unknown number of miles in the woods and is trotting back solo for its dinner. By the time the pain catches up with you again, you're safe in a cozy cast, coddling the fractured limb like a baby bird in its shell.

My greatest triumph over pain occurred on a warm March day. I was in graduate school, living in a country cottage ten miles outside Ithaca, New York. For no good reason I began to leap down the thawing driveway. My foot landed on a patch of ice. I tumbled forward, flinging out my right arm to break the fall, and felt a jarring pain.

I drove myself into town, steering with my left arm and whimpering. I had a psychoanalysis session, and since my analyst's office was near the student health services center, I decided to stop and explain the situation.

"Do you want to sit down?" my analyst asked, and the sound of her calm voice seemed so restful. I realized that I was tired from the effort of getting there. I lay down on the couch for a minute, explaining that I wouldn't be able to stay long because of the pain. Yet, as I began to talk, I was amazed to find that when I concentrated on the session, the pain became less urgent. It was as if Pain and I had been alone, and then when another person entered, Pain tactfully disappeared into a back room in my mind. I knew Pain was still in the house, but my analyst and I had been left to ourselves to have a private conversation.

As soon as I went back out to the street, Pain met me again. Still, I thought I'd stop off for a milk shake, as I was in the habit of doing after therapy. But as I stared at the menu on the wall, I realized there was no time.

At the student health center, the doctor noticed that the tissue of my arm had swollen and asked what time the accident had occurred. Although I nodded, chastened, as he lectured me on the importance of seeking immediate medical attention lest an infection such as gangrene set in, I felt triumphant inside. *So,* I thought, *emotional pain is greater than physical pain; psychotherapy trumps orthopedics; the mind transcends the body.*

This template for understanding pain stayed with me for many years and seemed borne out by other mishaps in the years that followed. Then, toward the end of my twenties, I got tired of accidents. My New Year's resolution the year I was twenty-eight was to have a break-, sprain-, and burn-free year. So it seemed unfair to me that, having more or less kept the resolution, I had now acquired a different affliction—an illogical, unhealing harm.

There is a certain pleasure in ordinary, acute pain: the pleasure of seeing the body work. You think your body is like china—as if you have dropped your favorite teacup and it's ruined forever. But it's not. The bones knit, the cast is cut open, and you feel the forgiveness of healing, the erasure of mistakes, again and again.

The experience of chronic pain, on the other hand, is one of defeat. The memory of transcending prior pains reproached me, as did stories of football players finishing a play despite broken legs and soldiers soldiering on despite grievous injuries. Whatever was wrong with my neck and arm now, I kept telling myself, they weren't as bad off as if they had been broken. So why couldn't I anesthetize them?

What I (like most people) didn't know is that there is a simple physiological answer to this question. It has nothing to do with the triumph of the will, but with a quirky aspect of acute pain. Although the intensity of acute pain generally reflects the degree of injury, there's a neat trick by which grave injuries can temporarily not hurt at all. After an injury, the brain can sometimes stave off pain by temporarily switching on powerful pain-inhibiting mechanisms and releasing its own painkillers, such as endorphins, into the spinal cord, in a process known as *descending analgesia*. This phenomenon conferred a survival advantage upon our ancestors and thus became an evolutionarily selected trait, allowing them to leap away after being bitten by a saber-toothed tiger on a pain-free high of adrenaline and endorphins instead of bursting into tears.

Such *stress-induced descending analgesia* was necessarily temporary, however, or its pain-blocking powers would have turned into a survival disadvantage by keeping us from tending to our wounds back in the cave (or allowing us to go out for a milk shake with a broken arm instead of seeking medical attention). And sometimes stress-induced descending analgesia proves harmful: even temporary ignorance of an injury may lead to further damage (as in a sport, in which the player finishes the match unaware of a broken limb and ends his or her career).

What is all this blood? shark attack victims wonder as they paddle toward shore. *Is my leg still there?* Unintentionally expressing nature's rationale, teenage surfer Bethany Hamilton, whose arm was bitten off by a shark, recalled, "I didn't feel any pain—I'm really lucky, because if I felt pain, things might not have gone as well." Undistracted by pain, she was able to focus on paddling to shore. A flood of nervous impulses from the damaged tissue would have interfered with her brain's ability to formulate and execute a plan for survival.

Some stress-induced descending analgesia can be activated by simple aerobic exercise. A 1981 study of Boston runners showed that beta-endorphins (the brain's internal opiate-like neurotransmitters) are released along with adrenaline, creating the "runner's high" that allows them not to feel blisters and muscle aches until they cross the finish line.

Acute pain—as Dr. Patrick David Wall, a preeminent British pain researcher, theorized—is not a general perception by the brain: it is a perception *about an action that needs to be taken.* The brain can process the sensory information necessary for only one decision at a time. When you are swimming from a shark, fighting a battle, running a race, or even preoccupied with an important psychotherapy session, your brain is preoccupied with that goal; thus it fails to heed sensory inputs from injuries and generate an experience of pain. Indeed, many of those impulses never even reach the brain: the "gate-control" theory that Wall and his colleague Ronald Melzack developed in 1965 states that there are a series of neurochemical "gates" in the spinal cord that close off unwanted information.

During the Yom Kippur War of 1973, Wall's research team interviewed Israeli soldiers who had lost limbs. The team found that the soldiers' initial wounds had not hurt most of them. But the descending analgesia proved limited to the area of injury: the same soldiers who didn't feel pain from their wounds also teared up when pierced by an IV needle. A day later all of the men were in pain. A majority of them went on to develop *phantom limb pain*—pain that is experienced as coming from the missing limb (which afflicts between half and two-thirds of amputees). Fifteen years later, those cramping and burning sensations had not eased with time. The descending analgesia that had erased their pain on that first day never reappeared. Rather, their pain had become chronic, and chronic pain is, by definition, pain that the brain fails to modulate.

DESTROYER OF GRIEF

I wanted a holiday from pain—an hour or two, smooth and round as my old hours. I did not want aspirin, Motrin, or Aleve. I wanted the ancient medicinal herbs that date back, the Rig Veda explains, three ages before the gods were born, or the wine potion that Helen of Troy gave grieving visitors—what was it called?—that lulled pain and brought forgetfulness of every sorrow.

Those ancient medicinal herbs . . . Cannabis, the vapors of which, writes Herodotus, caused "the wounded Scythians to howl with relief and joy" in healing huts where the seeds were thrown on hot red stones. Black henbane, the "killer of hens," whose yellow-veined flowers crowned the dead in Hades and which was used in witches' brews to induce visions and convulsions and to confuse memory of pain. Mandrake, whose twisted human-shaped root was said to grow under scaffolds from the ejaculation of hanged men's final death spasms. When uprooted, it shrieked in pain, killing those that heard its cry, yet it could be made into a potion that eased the pain of the living. According to a medieval heresy, it was mandrake mixed into vinegar that caused Jesus to fall into sleep for three days, after which he awakened in the tomb, as if resurrected.

But the "key to paradise" has always been opium, the ancient Sumerians' *hul gil* ("plant of joy") that "induces deep slumber and steeps the vanquished suffering eyes in Lethean night," as Ovid wrote. Opium was said to console the goddess Demeter herself when she wandered the earth to search for Persephone, for when she suckled its milk, she momentarily forgot her grief and fell into the twilight sleep that is halfway to Hades. How did mortals figure out the secret of how to extract the drug from the white opium-rich *Papaver somniferum* ("the poppy that brings sleep")? Only in the brief interval in which the petals begin to drop can the fat, round capsules containing the unripe seeds be tapped, through an incision out of which the "Milk of Paradise," the cloudy fluid also known as "poppy tears," seeps. But it is not until it dries and oxidizes that it turns into a sticky, black opium-containing gum.

"I possess a secret remedy which I call laudanum ['to be praised'] and which is superior to all others' heroic remedies," the sixteenth-century alchemist and physician Paracelsus proclaimed. Laudanum—and other potions of opium dissolved in alcohol—soon became a staple of a well-supplied cupboard. There are a number of versions of Paracelsus' recipe, calling for opium mixed with such ingredients as henbane, an Arabic drug called mummy, oils, amber, musk, crushed pearls, coral, stag heart, and unicorn.

In my medicine cabinet I had a few tablets of Darvocet—a narcotic pain medication that Cynthia's husband, Jim, a physician, gave her for cramps, which she had generously saved to share with me. One morning I stood in the bathroom holding a fat magenta pill in my palm, as anxious and excited as a teen taking drugs. Milk of Paradise, Hand of God, Destroyer of Grief. "How divine this repose is," Coleridge wrote of opium, "what a spot of enchantment, a green spot of fountain and flowers and trees, in the very heart of a waste of sands."

I took half a pill and then went out to do errands. I felt a dizzy nausea and had to find a bench to sit down. But as the pill dissolved in my stomach, I had the sensation that a genie emerged, looked around at my insides, and said, *I know what you want.*

It wasn't the key to paradise, but it did seem to offer a modicum of blurry magic. After a few hours, though, the genie wearied of my wish and left me with the pain again. I tried taking a whole pill but became so dizzy I had to lie down on the couch. But I was not in pain. *I must appreciate not being in pain*, I thought. But I felt too vague to do anything but flip through an old magazine and wait for the drug to wear off.

I thought of how medieval love potions were made with poppies, as the flower was sometimes said to spring first from the tears of the goddess Aphrodite as she mourned her lost lover Adonis. On Saint Andrew's Day, in one tradition, a maiden could write a secret question about love on a piece of paper, tuck it into an empty poppy pod under her pillow, and have it answered in a dream. Sleepless with pain one night, I took the last magenta pill and fell into a brief, restless sleep. I woke before dawn from a dream in which I had told Kurt that my arm was hurting and he suggested that I cut it off. I did, but then I needed to use it, so I tried to reglue it with Krazy Glue, but I couldn't make the nerves align, so it didn't stick, and when I tried to use it, it toppled off. Then I remembered reading about phantom limb pain—terrible, intractable pain. I realized with particular dream-horror that I had made an irreversible mistake.

"I didn't say you *should* cut it off," Kurt clarified coolly in the dream. "I said it was an option."

The only question in my heart—the one I wanted to tuck into the empty Darvocet bottle—was, *Why am I in pain?*

The pain I had felt lying awake that first night with Kurt had seemed then like *poena*—the price for what I imagined would be the happiness of the relationship. But, as the happiness had failed to materialize, the pain had metamorphosed in my mind into a symbol of unhappiness: a mysterious unhappiness, mysteriously conjoined to mysterious pain.

THE PLAN

The months turned into a year and continued to accumulate. When I think back on the time that elapsed between the day the pain first settled in and the day I finally got a diagnosis, I think of the joke about the drunk looking for his keys under the streetlamp— even though he has lost them farther down the block—because "that's where the light is." For me, the light shines most appealingly on the self. I wanted to imagine it was a problem, just like my other problems, best solved by me.

All the things on my to-do list, big and small, got checked off. I moved to LA for a job teaching fiction writing; I moved back to New York; I moved to a cheaper apartment in New York. I published several long, difficult magazine articles on murder. I located a Depression-era jadeite reamer, which also served as a measuring cup, to replace a favorite I had chipped. But pain—which topped my thoughts continuously—was somehow never on that list. Rather, it was on a different list, an invisible list that went something like this:

Plan A: Ignore it.
Plan B: Try alternative medicine. Since I didn't really believe in alternative medicine, if it didn't work, I didn't need to feel I had exhausted all the good options. I could still move on to:
Plan C: Find a doctor and get treatment.

Plan A had failed. Plan B would fail. As long as I didn't try Plan C, I could believe that I could still get truly serious about getting well, click my heels like Dorothy and say, *I want to go home*—home, home, home to my normal body—and wake from the dreamy delusion of pain. I didn't want to try Plan C and find that medicine would not offer me ruby slippers.

Like most people, I had never heard of a pain specialist or a pain clinic. So by the time I resolved to see a doctor, I had no idea what kind of doctor to see. I didn't know that one's choice of doctor partly determines one's diagnosis. I went to see an orthopedist who specialized in athletic injuries, which is what he found me to have.

The other patients seemed unsurprised by the two-hour wait to see him, as if they knew that to have a medical problem is to be cast out of the realm of busy people (like the doctor). The sick have no schedule, their time is of no value. "Illness is as much a failure as poverty," wrote the Parisian syphilitic Xavier Aubryet in 1870. The patients waiting with me had the resigned shabbiness of the unemployed waiting to see their caseworkers.

The orthopedist had the hearty self-assurance, square jaw, and heavy build of a former athlete. But he wore an incongruous gold necklace and a large decorative ring—a tiny, opaque bit of self-expression that I fastened on as a positive sign.

"Rotator cuff injury," he announced after examining my shoulder. He scribbled a diagram with a ballpoint pen on the white paper covering the examining table. I had no idea what the diagram said, but I sensed that he felt he had exerted himself to explain this. He had drawn an illustration for a patient—the kind of thing one of those mandatory touchy-feely continuing education courses suggests: *Patients need to see it.*

I didn't see it, though; it was just a mess of lines.

"Could I tear this out?" I asked timidly, thinking that perhaps if I studied it at home, it would reveal its meaning, the way a difficult poem sometimes opens up late at night.

He waved away the idea, as if I had asked something absurd. Then he wrote me a prescription for eight weeks of physical therapy.

"That should—" My voice cracked as, half naked in the paper gown, I revealed my deepest desire. "That will make it better?"

"Yes."

Years later, after I figured out that patients should always request copies of the notes doctors make after a consultation, and as I was gathering my old records, I called the orthopedist's secretary to request my notes. Although I had seen him numerous times, she said she could locate only two of them, an initial impression and a follow-up. The history was brief:

HISTORY:
Patient, for approximately a year, has had pain in and about the shoulder secondary to a bicycle/pedestrian accident.
PHYSICAL EXAM:
Physical exam demonstrates the patient to have lack of range of motion of 20 degrees in all planes, with crepitation in the subacromial space. There is pain on palpation of the greater tuberosity and bicipital groove.
IMPRESSION:
Adhesive capsulitis
RECOMMENDATION:
Patient is advised as to her condition . . . She is referred for physical therapy.

Had he hesitated, feeling a slight annoyance as he tried to recall my story, or had his mind automatically invented a narrative as he dictated the notes, in the same way my mind invented narratives for my pain? Had he confused me with another patient he had seen before or after me? By the time I read his notes, it had been years since I had seen him. I wasn't going to go back to complain, so there was no one to blame but myself for not insisting that I be understood. Still, I found myself mentally protesting: *A bicycle accident is the one kind of accident I have never had.*

If the orthopedist's office had looked like an unemployment office, the physical therapy office to which he referred me looked like a place where the unemployed received pro forma job training—the kind that didn't seem like it was going to help them find jobs any more than basket weaving helps the mentally ill. Just as these attempts at help only underscored the recipient's helplessness, lifting small weights that were now too heavy for my hand seemed to be turning me into a cripple.

I shrank away from the other patients, afraid to be grouped with the tired, old, sick, disabled, and sad. Although there was a stray college athlete with a chipped bone, en route to health, most of the patients looked like inhabitants of a village of the damned.

I disliked my physical therapist, a married, middle-aged German woman. I could see in her eyes that she thought I was one of those pathetic thirty-something waifs—a New York City breed, a decade too old to be a waif, but still lost.

"You live alone?" she asked the first day.

She nodded knowingly at my answer. "There is no one to take care of you," she announced.

I could have said I had a boyfriend. I had Kurt, after all. But I told myself that this wasn't any of her business. And something in me also knew it wasn't true. The true answer was that I was alone.

"What have you eaten today?" she often asked when I came in. I would stammer, realizing it was something weird, like a piece of shrink-wrapped deli pound cake, because that was the only thing that had appealed. I had lost a lot of weight, which I attributed to pain curdling my appetite, but I now realize the nausea was more likely to have come from the Tylenol, Advil, Motrin, aspirin, and Aleve, which I believed worked best in combination, with a dash of Maker's Mark at night. I can't recall if I noticed the warnings on the drug labels not to combine these medications, not to take any of them regularly for more than two weeks, and not to consume them with alcohol. I didn't believe anything sold over the counter could be all that dangerous, and anyway, what was fine print compared with the urgency of my pain?

"Do you think you're fat?" my physical therapist would ask patronizingly, her smug, well-fed face assuming the faux concern and veiled contempt of a high school gym teacher for an anorexic girl sitting on the sidelines at a soccer match.

"No," I would say. "My shoulder hurts."

I did not *not* do the exercises. I said I was doing them, and I sort of did, for a while. At home, I occasionally picked up my Thera-Band—a piece of rubbery material that was supposed to provide resistance for stretching—and I certainly looked at those heavy weights that I had placed on the mantelpiece. But my arm no longer seemed suited for lifting five, or four, or even three pounds, and whenever I tried, the pain sparked like kindling set on embers. Since I didn't understand the logic behind physical therapy, I had no framework of belief that would have encouraged me to do something that not only didn't seem to be making me better, but felt like it was making me worse.

Since pain is an alarm bell—or, as Patrick Wall put it, a perception about an action that needs to be taken—the body responds to pain by going into its emergency mode. Muscles contract and joints stiffen in order to immobilize the area of injury. When the injury heals, the pain goes away and the muscles return to their normal state. But when pain persists, these changes begin to be a source of pain themselves. Contracted muscles clamp down on nerves and cause pain. The rigid muscles cause postural changes that strain other muscles. Using the affected area hurts, so one guards it, which deprives it of exercise, which makes the muscles atrophy, which in turn makes it harder to use that area and causes more pain. Physical therapy aims both to strengthen muscles and to relax them, through heat packs or massage.

In my unhappiness, I discontinued even the daily walking I had done. Walking would not have hurt me; in fact, aerobic exercise has been shown to stimulate beta-endorphins, which anesthetize one against pain (as well as stimulating serotonin, which elevates mood and also mitigates pain). But since I didn't know this, and the idea of exercising a body part that was in pain felt completely counterintuitive, I'd show up late for physical therapy. Since I hadn't been practicing, I wasn't getting stronger. Yet the therapist continued to graduate me to heavier weights and more resistant Thera-Bands, so that the exercises hurt more and more. Under her disapproving gaze I'd have a slight feeling of paranoia, as if the exercises were designed to hurt me and to keep her—in collaboration with the orthopedist—supplied with weak pain patients.

I didn't want to be a weak pain patient; I wanted to walk out of there. And when I did, I successfully put the experience out of my mind. I came late and left early, and in between appointments I tried not to think about physical therapy.

THE PLACEBO DILEMMA

A friend of my mother's told me he had a Q-Ray bracelet that warded off his knee pain with magnetic rays. Previously hobbled by pain, he could now run for miles. He had researched the bracelet and was dismayed to discover a study showing it to be a placebo, which he didn't believe. Once, he took the bracelet off and realized he had forgotten to put it back only when the pain caught him by surprise.

"Perhaps your subconscious knew," I suggested.

My mother gave me a look.

A woman in my building showed me the copper bracelet that had cured her arthritic elbow. She wore the homely piece of metal every day along with her art deco cocktail rings and diamond tennis bracelet. *What do you think the connection between copper and arthritis exactly is?* I started to say, but thought better of it. Why spoil it for her? Was I jealous of her relief?

One night, I stared at a candle and had the impulse to burn myself and remind my body what normal pain was—the kind that could be bandaged. I tried to understand pain through psychoanalysis. (Why my *right* side? Is it connected to *writing*, since I'm right-handed?) Was I looking for a sub-conscious excuse to avoid work—to feel literally pained when I did it? That was how the Victorian affliction of hysteria worked.

I tried positive visual imagery, using a workbook on illness and posi-tive thinking, but the blue, celestial light with which I tried to imagine my pain turned to an evil, ashy gray. I tried acupuncture, massage, and herbal remedies.

"I'll take all of them," I told the surprised salesman in the health food store after listening to all his recommendations for pain relief remedies.

I had always been skeptical about natural remedies because, in addition to not having been tested for efficacy or safety, they aren't natural. Although they *derive* from plants they are actually formulations of compounds isolated from plants and presented in hundreds or thousands of times the concentration in which they are found in nature.

But if I took these remedies with a dose of skepticism, would they definitely fail? I didn't understand how placebo works at a physiological level, but I had heard many times that if you believe you are being relieved of pain, you will experience (deluded?) pain relief. Yet I always got stuck on what I thought of as the Placebo Dilemma: Knowing that the relief was a result of placebo, how could I believe in it? In order to work, didn't placebo require precisely *the belief that the treatment was something other than placebo*? Yet, if the effectiveness of the placebo testifies to the transformative reality of belief, shouldn't that make it easier for me to believe? I felt like doubting Thomas asking Jesus to remove his unbelief. *In order for God to save me, all I have to do is believe He exists.*

There is a story about a famous physicist who put a horseshoe on his office wall. "I thought you didn't believe in that kind of thing," remarked a puzzled graduate student.

"They say you don't have to believe in it for it to work," he replied.

If I wore a copper bracelet, was I revealing my desperation, my willingness to forsake the person I used to be, who knew that copper doesn't penetrate skin (luckily, as it is poisonous), or was I demonstrating to the universe that I was open to being healed in any way, including ways I didn't believe in?

I kept flashing back to a conversation I once had on a reporting trip in Addis Ababa, on a day when I was wandering around stricken by inexplicable pain. On a street corner I had seen a leper whose arm was dissolving. His right hand was dripping off like a melting candle; in his left, he held a mango. He seemed to understand my question, as he laughed shyly and said he was "okay."

"No pain?" I repeated, staring at him amazed, and then went back to the hotel, ashamed, and got a massage. As the therapist put her warm hands on my shoulders, I closed my eyes and remembered how the leper ate the mango and laughed at me.

REPRESSED NEGATIVE EMOTIONS

I arrived to visit friends at their beach house for the weekend in a daze of pain. Although I didn't want to explain, I had a neck wrap in my suitcase that I was longing to use.

"I have this—uhh—stupid pain," I said. "I have this wrap that is heated in the microwave—"

"Chuck used to have back pain!" Erin said. Her husband's back pain, she told me, had melted—*melted*—away when he enrolled in the treatment program of Dr. John Sarno, a New York physician whose bestselling book, *Healing Back Pain*, they still had in the house. He had told our mutual friend Daniel about the book, too; Daniel went to the bookstore to check it out, hunched over with pain, but by the time he walked to the cash register— having read only a few chapters in the aisle—he was standing straight.

Sarno explains that the major cause of most back, neck, shoulder, and limb pain is a syndrome that he terms *tension myositis syndrome* (TMS), which is a controversial notion. By assigning their pain a medical-sounding term (which means—more or less—tense, painful muscle syndrome) people can feel validated with a medical diagnosis. However, people with TMS pain are also reassured that (unlike for most medical conditions) the cure lies entirely within their control.

Sarno asserts that repressed negative emotions such as stress, anger, and anxiety are the major causes of TMS, decreasing blood flow to muscles, nerves, or tendons, resulting in mild oxygen deprivation, which is experienced as pain and muscle tension. He has subsequently revised some aspects of his theory, but the fundamental tenets remain the same: when the negative emotions are addressed, the tension and pain disappear. His treatment works on the same principles as Freud's treatment of hysteria: acknowledging the underlying emotional problems causes their physical manifestations to disappear. Although Dr. Sarno concedes that sometimes testing may be necessary to ensure that the pain is not from, for example, a tumor or a fracture, once these are ruled out, he believes that other pain is psychosomatic and that its function is to distract the conscious mind from its true sources of stress. Even when the pain syndrome begins after an injury, Dr. Sarno asserts, "despite the perception of an injury, patients are not injured. The physical occurrence has given the brain an opportunity to begin an attack of TMS."

In Dr. Sarno's work, patients are told that they must discontinue all physical treatments, such as physical therapy, medication, injections, chiropractic adjustments, acupuncture, or any other conventional form of treatment because these harmfully reinforce the mistaken notion that there is a structural causation for patients' chronic pain when, he argues, "their physical condition is actually benign and . . . any disability they have is a function of pain-related fear and deconditioning." Instead, they should resume all previous activities and the normal physical activity that pain had interrupted, while attending support meetings, writing about their emotional issues, and keeping a daily journal. Failing to acknowledge the psychological nature of pain is "to doom oneself to perpetual pain and disability."

"You must renounce all treatments," Chuck said, "and believe that your pain is all in your mind."

"I know. But what if—" I said timidly.

"It would show up in an MRI. But you don't need an MRI. Don't baby your neck, don't take Tylenol, ditch the microwave wrap! Just chill out and have a good weekend. Let's hit the beach."

In the months that followed, I faithfully scrutinized my life for *repressed negative emotions*: "abuse or lack of love," "personality traits such as a strong need to be liked by everyone," and "current life pressures."

Unfortunately, all that self-scrutiny about stress was itself extremely stressful. Was it my relationship with Kurt, or was it a problem within myself? My neck and shoulders looked the same as always, but perhaps inside, something had crumbled. I've always had a sense of a certain inner crippledness, of my character as less than fully sturdy. There were mistakes in construction, internal beams that are weak. I reinforce them as best I can, but most of them are inaccessible—too much of my personality is built upon them. I had been depressed before. I always thought of depression like misty rain, the way the gray blankets consciousness, making it difficult to see. Pain felt more like a thunderstorm. There was an edge of violence amidst the rain—as the familiar terrain of the body becomes eerily illuminated—and then the futile scramble for shelter.

"Pain upsets and destroys the nature of the person who feels it," Aristotle observed. The McGill Pain Questionnaire (the standard pain-assessment technique) asks sufferers about their pain using clusters of words that describe the sensory or affective dimensions of pain. Is the pain *Flickering, Pulsing, Quivering, Throbbing, Beating, Pounding*? Or is it *Sickening, Suffocating, Fearful, Frightful, Terrifying, Punishing, Grueling, Cruel, Vicious, Killing, Wretched, Binding, Nagging, Nauseating, Agonizing, Dreadful, Torturing*?

I had been given the questionnaire once years before, when consulting a neurologist about migraines, and at the time the questions had seemed laughable. My headaches throbbed, but they were not cruel. But now I understood. This new pain *was* cruel—Cruel, Vicious, and Killing.

Time felt different. Pain, I realized, is not just every day, but *every hour of every day. Every minute of every hour.* When too many pain minutes pass, the hourglass balance between bearable and unbearable changes and the shape of self collapses. The more desperate I felt, the more I wondered if—as Dr. Sarno says—desperation itself was the problem. I remembered how I had stayed up late that night at my friends' beach house reading Sarno's book. But eventually, sleepless with pain, I crept back into the kitchen to heat my microwave wrap. The machine made a deep whirring noise; I pictured Chuck and Erin waking to hear me and thinking that I wasn't ready to be well.

THISTLES TO THEE

W estern medicine is one way to think about illness," my grand-mother Bea was fond of saying, *"but it's not the only way."* When I was a child, she gave me the central Christian Science text, *Science and Health with Key to the Scriptures*, a book I treasured, believing it contained the secret recipe to reality, a truth from which my secular parents were excluded (my father is an atheist and my mother a secular Jew). But although I love religion and sacred texts, the passion I once had for it—the sense that it held truths that might illuminate my life—had waned over the years, so that by the time I got pain in my early thirties, my interest in the subject was almost entirely academic.

For some reason, my neck and right arm were hurting. When I woke exiled by pain from sleep, I reminded myself that the reasons for this were not clear, but surely it was not a test or a punishment, or a payment for sin or a bid for immortality, or a curse, or a spell or an ordeal, or an opportunity for self-transcendence, or anything of the like. Not at all, actually. Those ideas come from the world of religion, in which I did not personally believe.

Whenever the thought of *poena* would suggest itself or I'd notice that the pain was surrounded by some other vague, dark cluster of thoughts, I would dismiss them. Again and again I dismissed them. And the thoughts were always there to dismiss.

Why me? Why must I suffer?

There is a curious teleological evolution of the meaning of pain in religions; indeed, the task of accounting for the presence of physical pain and suffering is so critical and so difficult that religions are defined by their various answers to that question. If I were a Hindu, a Buddhist, or a Jew, my faith would invest pain with a different meaning from the religions of ancient Egypt, Greece, Rome, and Mesopotamia. And if I were a Christian, a distinct conception of pain's meaning would reside at the very center of my faith.

In the most ancient religions, pain and suffering pose no theological problem, because the gods, like the universe, are cruel. The karmic religions of Hinduism and Buddhism, by contrast, posit the framework of a just universe. The doctrine of reincarnation neatly removes pain and suffering from the unreliable hands of the ancient Indian gods and satisfyingly reinterprets it as *poena*—karmic retribution for transgressions committed in previous incarnations. In the monotheistic traditions, God is loving, attentive, and just. But what about pain and suffering? The problem is explored through three central characters—Adam, Job, and Jesus—who grapple with different conceptions of pain.

Physical pain comes into the biblical world with the Fall. Only after Adam and Eve steal godly knowledge and become self-conscious are they cursed, like animals, with pain and the struggle for existence. Both Adam's and Eve's pain are described with related Hebrew words derived from the same root. Adam uses the word '*itstsabown* (עצבון—"labor, toil, pain, sorrow, worrisomeness"), but Eve's pain is described using the word '*etsev* as well. The pain and sorrow to which Adam is condemned concerns the struggle for survival, while Eve's involves reproduction.

The passage in which Adam is cursed in his struggle to draw subsistence from the ground employs not only images of toil but also of physical pain and the threat of wounds ("thorns also and thistles shall [the ground] bring forth to thee"). In Eve's case, the sorrowful pain of childbirth stands as a metaphor for all pain, christening our very entrance into the world, as if setting the stage for a lifetime of suffering. The curse involves an exile from what one might conceive of as a natural state. One might imagine that the most basic functions that allow for the species to propagate— eating and reproducing—should not cause pain and suffering. And pain *feels* unnatural; while we can't imagine human life without hunger or thirst, it is easy to fantasize about a life without pain and to picture that life as one to which we could or should return.

While embodying this fantasy, Genesis also seems to resolve it. Eating the fruit of the tree of knowledge created self-consciousness ("the eyes of them both were opened, and they knew that they were naked"). In biological terms, pain is indeed a function of consciousness, as the ability to suffer the former increases proportionally with the latter—with, that is, the complexity of the cortical development of a species. Do we really wish not to have tasted that fruit? Wouldn't that be like wishing that we were still apes—or that we were a kind of creature who feels no pain at all, such as the centipede? Pain's origin is thus justified in Genesis as the price of the consciousness that makes us fully human.

Why must I suffer?

Even if generally viewed as the price of consciousness, pain still seems unfairly distributed. Like the Righteous Sufferer in the Babylonian Poem, Job questions Genesis's account of pain, asking not why does pain exist, but why does *he*, in particular, suffer from it?

Job's trial begins when Satan suggests to God that Job's piety has no value, since he is constantly rewarded for it; perhaps, after all, it is the reward Job loves, not the Lord. The trial of Job is progressive. First his livestock is taken, then his servants and children. Yet these hardships prove insufficient; he accepts them as the will of the Lord, prostrating himself and declaring, "The Lord gave, and the Lord hath taken away; Blessed be the name of the Lord." God then gives Satan permission to subject Job to the ultimate test: physical pain. Job's pain is nothing if not visceral. He feels as if he is being crushed, shriveled, about to burst open, torn; his kidneys feel pierced, his intestines boiled, and his skin grows black and peels.

As Job's suffering continues, three of his friends insist that if he is suffering, he must deserve it and he should repent of his sins. The text refers to them as the three "miserable comforters." Belief that suffering is deserved can be comforting, since a deserved sickness is just and curable by repentance. When people are casting about for explanations of sickness, they often point to sin because, after all, everyone has sinned. But Job *hasn't* sinned; his case gives lie to the doctrine that pain is always *poena* and suffering is always divine retribution. Job's wife believes that he has not sinned, but she shares the comforters' theology. Unable to reconceive God, she becomes disillusioned and tells Job to curse God and die.

Eventually, Job breaks down and reproaches God. Late in the story, a prophetic figure enters who, in contrast to the comforters, declares that Job's sin is imagining that he can judge God and reproach him for making him suffer. It is this point of view that the story endorses. When God finally speaks, it is not to answer Job, but to tell him that he cannot understand pain any more than he understands other mysteries of nature. ("Where were you when I laid the earth's foundation?" God asks.)

The book of Job is not what one might expect from a theodicy. Although God explicitly condemns the theology of the comforters, He does not offer an alternate explanation for Job's pain (or for why He is wagering with Satan). Job must bow before the whirlwind and accept that—although pain cannot be understood—its meaning somehow must not be incompatible with religious faith. The book of Job thus defines faith as *that which is upheld in the face of inexplicable pain and suffering.*

The book of Job ends the same way the Poem of the Righteous Sufferer does, with the restoration of health. Job prostrates himself and repents of his arrogance in questioning God, and God restores Job to health and gives him riches, long life, and even replacement children. Seen from one perspective, Job's passing the test reveals the test to have been unnecessary, indicating that his suffering was pointless and that God should not have permitted it to happen. Yet seen from another perspective, Job's pain tests his faith, not only by causing him to demonstrate it, but also by *creating* it, in the way fire and hammering forge a sword. According to this model, pain is not extrinsic to faith, but rather is the ground from which faith grows and into which it sinks and extends deep roots—an idea that becomes the dominant conception of the New Testament.

Why must I suffer?

The Gospels reframe pain not as a problem for faith to overcome, but as faith's central mechanism. The curse of mortality becomes *the solution to mortality*—the very means to eternal life. The God of the Gospels answers the problem of pain not by removing it from human life, but by sharing it, becoming human in the form of Jesus and paying his own *poena*. In so doing, he forever inverts pain's significance. Just as God became man when Jesus shouldered Adam's curse, man can become godly by accepting pain as Jesus did. By so doing, man transforms *poena* into passion, as Christ willingly submitted to crucifixion and its pain. In an era when people of many faiths wore amulets to ward off pain and disease, Christians began cradling an image of torture close to their hearts.

JESUS' PAIN

The conception of pain and suffering in Jewish and Christian scripture had implications for medicine that were profoundly different from those in the theology of magic-based religions. In the latter, the right magical formula could eradicate a fever-causing demon as surely as the right plant leaves could ease a fever. The spell targeted an underlying supernatural cause, whereas the potion treated its manifestation in the natural world, but both had the same result. *Magic is effective together with medicine. Medicine is effective together with magic.* Replacing magical practices with religious ones, however, called for a more complicated internal response of repentance and prayer. This followed from the biblical premise that God cannot be manipulated through incantations or herbs to serve human desires (although God can play an opaque role in healing: paradoxically, once Job humbles himself, God restores his health).

The New Testament departs radically from Judaism here. Christianity promises the faithful not physical health, but spiritual salvation—goals that are aligned in Judaism but actually *opposed* in Jesus' story. Egyptian and Greek medical remedies imitated the gods' remedies for the successful assuaging of their pains. The Christian ideal of imitating Christ, *imitatio Christi*, stands in contrast. Unlike Horus, who is rescued from the headache-causing catfish demon, Christ is not freed from the pain of crucifixion. Rather, he suffers unto death, showing Christians not how to evade pain, but how to welcome its redemptive possibilities.

The canonical Gospels don't describe Jesus' pain during the crucifixion, although the Gospel of Saint Peter, one of the Gnostic Gospels, contrasts Jesus with the thieves being crucified by his side, saying he "was silent as one who experiences no pain." But mainstream Christian theology asserts that Jesus did suffer pain; that to be fully human he had to do so; and that in doing so, he paid the price for humanity's redemption. (After all, how much of a sacrifice is it for an immortal merely to painlessly shed the human body he temporarily inhabited and reassume his place in heaven?)

Jesus suffered in what can be described as a peculiarly human way: torture by crucifixion is designed to take advantage of pain-sensing capacities specific to human anatomy. The universal eloquence of wounds to the hands and feet—the instinctive horror an image of them evokes—derives from the evolutionary importance of those parts and their consequential ability to feel pain.

Since the human palm is not substantial enough to support the weight of a human's body on a cross without the nails tearing out, some historians argue that nails were driven either through Jesus' wrists, where they would have been held in place by carpal bones, or between the radius and ulna bones in his forearm, as is consistent with the one extant skeleton of a man crucified in that period. Regardless, nails through either the wrists or the hands would damage the median nerves that supply the hands, causing excruciating pain (from the Latin *cruciare*, "to torment, crucify"). The pain of carpal tunnel syndrome can come as a result of the median nerves merely being compressed by surrounding tissue.

Body parts are protected by nerves in proportion to their importance for survival. A cut to the lips, hands, or testicles—or the nerve branches that supply them—hurts more than a cut to the back or arm, where a wound is less likely to threaten a vital function. Wrapping around the top of the human brain is an area known as the sensory cortex, which functions as a map of the body and its sensations. Information coming from the sensory nerves is registered by the corresponding parts of this map: input from the hands is mapped to the hand regions of the sensory cortex. This cortical map is sometimes referred to as the *sensory homunculus* (Latin for "little man"). It can be thought of as "the body in the brain." Thus, although we may experience pain as coming from our hands, what actually hurts are the hands of the homunculus.

Since the parts of this body represent the actual body in proportion to the nerves it contains, rather than to its actual size, the homunculus has a giant head with swollen lips and tongue, large genitals, massive hands with big fingers and a giant thumb, and feet with ballooning toes. Human hands are so dense with nerves that a homunculus's hands are bigger than the entire trunk of its body! Artistic depictions of the crucifixion in which Jesus' hands, feet, and face are exaggerated can be thought of as renderings of a homunculus, rather than of a body, and are therefore truer to our experience of our bodies.

THE MARTYR'S PARADOX

The idea of pain as spiritual transformation offends me. It seems, in a word, perverse. Pain is useless to the pained, the Greek physician Galen said (*dolor dolentibus inutilis est*), and almost everyone today decidedly agrees. If we try to describe the particular terror of pain, it seems to lie in the way that it kidnaps consciousness, annihilating the ordinary self. Yet many religious traditions insist that this terrible annihilation opens the possibility of self-transcendence, since the self is, in many religions, what separates us from the divine. Pain is an "alchemy of the soul"—melting, purifying, and reshaping sin. Pain is a means of devotion central to ascetic traditions. Its devotees range from self-flagellating Christians and Shi'ites to Muslims who wage internal jihad against the raging ego of the sinful self. Certain painful meditation methods of Yogis (involving icy water or holding uncomfortable positions for long periods of time) are said to strengthen the spirit as well as the body. The training of shamans typically involves painful rites.

Religions find so many uses for pain! It can be a payment for sin, preempting the even-worse pain of the afterlife. The medieval Christian theologian Thomas à Kempis advised that it is better "to suffer little things now that you may not have to suffer greater ones in eternity. If you can suffer only a little now, how will you be able to endure eternal torment?" In some religions, pain can be a penalty not only for one's own sins but also for the sins of others. Self-inflicted pain in the Taoist tradition can not only atone for others, it can even rescue dead sinners who are already writhing in hell. In the Hindu and Buddhist karmic systems, pain can be a payment for transgressions from previous incarnations.

To embrace pain requires overcoming the most primal instincts. It requires privileging cultural beliefs (that pain may be desirable) over biological instincts (that it is always negative) and choosing a spiritual meaning that is normally overwhelmed by a corporeal one. Saints and martyrs are celebrated because they have achieved this unhuman or superhuman relationship to their own pain. Ironically, the bodies of saints are consecrated—and treasured in the form of relics—precisely because saints treat their bodies as something to discard.

In many traditions, martyrdom is the ultimate test of religious conviction, the most important opportunity for distinguishing the faithful from the apostates. In Hebrew, a term for martyrdom, *Kiddush Hashem*, means "sanctification of God's name." Martyrdom is the greatest act of *Kiddush Hashem*. For Christians, undergoing pain is the ultimate act of *imitatio Christi*. "Allow me to be eaten by the beasts, which are my way of reaching to God. I am God's wheat, and I am to be ground by the teeth of wild beasts, so that I may become the pure bread of Christ," wrote Saint Ignatius of Antioch in his second-century "Letter to the Romans." His prayer was granted: the Romans fed him to the lions. (While praying for martyrdom was acceptable, seeking it out was not. Some would-be martyrs became frustrated by the Romans' "don't ask, don't tell" policy toward Christians and turned themselves in for prosecution. But theological opinion determined that they were not virtuously withstanding martyrdom, but sinfully committing suicide.)

Yet how painful is willing pain? Do those who embrace suffering really suffer? Oddly, the ability to appear unaffected by torments seems central to the mythology of martyrs and saints—a mark of their special nature. While representations of sinners in hell show them writhing in torment, saints are usually pictured looking upward, their gaze sad and abstracted, such as Saint Sebastian, for whom being shot full of arrows seems only to have induced a deep reverie. "We pray you torment us further for we suffer not," the brother physicians Cosmas and Damian legendarily implored their Roman torturers, who stoned them, drew them on a rack, and finally resorted to beheading them.

John Foxe's beloved 1563 *Book of Martyrs* relates with adulation how, when Bishop John Hooper was condemned to be burned alive, he praised God for the opportunity to demonstrate faith to his former flock. And demonstrate it he did—praying aloud to Jesus Christ as the flames consumed his body—in gruesome detail. He continued to pray "when he was black in the mouth, and his tongue so swollen that he could not speak, yet his lips went until they were shrunk to the gums."

Yet, Foxe noted, he prayed "as one without pain." Therein lies the paradox of martyrdom: its virtue lies in embracing pain, but that embrace seems to inure the martyr against the very pain that defines a martyr!

TRIAL BY ORDEAL

Personally, it was hard for me to take much inspiration from stories of the martyrs welcoming their pain, when my pain felt so unwelcome—forced upon me, I sometimes fancied, like the ancient practice of trial by ordeal that had fascinated me as a child.

In trial by ordeal, which flourished for thousands of years in cultures from ancient Mesopotamia, Greece, and India to Europe, the accused underwent a ritual in which—through magic or divine aid—guilt or innocence was established. In one type of ordeal, judges forced the accused to walk through flames or over hot plowshares for a certain distance, or to plunge his hands in boiling water or—worse—lead or oil. Astonishingly, betraying pain or injury constituted proof of guilt. In short, in order to prove their innocence, the accused had to show that they were protected from pain as martyr mythology insisted.

Sometimes signs of tissue damage itself were considered damning; in other instances, victims were permitted to suffer tissue damage as long as they maintained the equanimity of a martyr. In a form of trial by fire, the burns were inspected after three days, and if the wound persisted, the accused's guilt was sealed. In short, the belief in pain as *poena* was so deeply rooted that suffering pain in and of itself *proved the sufferer deserving of* poena.

Hindu law has specifically endorsed the fire ordeal. In the *Manusmriti* it is said, "When the blazing fire does not burn a man . . . he should be judged innocent." In the Ordeal of the Bitter Water in the Jewish Torah, a woman suspected of adultery was forced to drink a concoction known as "bitter water" (which most scholars now believe was poisonous). If the drink caused her belly to swell—or, if, indeed, she perished—her guilt was established. In Europe, fire ordeals tended to be reserved for the upper class and water ordeals for commoners and witches. A famous eleventh-century English adultery case is typical. Queen Emma of Normandy was accused of committing adultery with the bishop of Winchester. When she walked absentmindedly over red-hot plowshares and asked when her trial would begin, she necessitated a finding in her favor.

In the early tenth century, King Athelstan of England codified the laws governing ordeals, decreeing that for one of the ordeals, the accused must pluck a stone from boiling water, submerging his or her hand up to the wrist or the elbow (depending on the severity of the accusation). The hands of the accused would then be bound and examined three days later. If the wounds were healing, the accused was deemed innocent, as God had healed them, but if the wounds were "foul," the accused was condemned. Other types of ordeals involved games of chance such as jousting matches or drawing lots, with the idea that God would rig the games so that the innocent would win. A particularly nasty variety was the Babylonian river ordeal, in which guilt would be fatally assessed by the river deity after the accused was tossed into the rushing Euphrates.

In the thirteenth century, ordeals finally gave way to trial by jury (indeed, the jury system is thought to have been invented partly in response to the pressure of growing skepticism about the ordeal). Torture-provoked confession remained routine long after the demise of the ordeal, and some scholars argue that it was practiced in good faith, so to speak. From a modern perspective (recent events in American history notwithstanding), torture seems obviously flawed as a means of discerning guilt; indeed, the very fact of coercion seems to discredit the information it elicits. Yet according to a worldview that sanctified pain, torture was believed to enlighten not only the torturer but his victim as well. "The witch is executed in an exceptionally painful manner because her death is conceived, obscenely to be sure, as spiritual passage, initiatory rite, or saving violence, not merely a removal from society," Ariel Glucklich writes in his extraordinary book *Sacred Pain*. Mercy for the witch would have been misdirected because it was the witchcraft, not the woman, that was being burned out or boiled away, in a terrible baptism of sorts. The woman was being redeemed as pain performed its fearful alchemy.

Pain Diary:

I Decide to Get a Diagnosis

"What are you doing at the moment?"
"I'm in pain."

—Daudet

"Pain strengthens the religious person's bond with God and other persons," Ariel Glucklich writes in *Sacred Pain*. "Of course, since not all pain is voluntary or self-inflicted," he adds helpfully, "one mystery of the religious life is how unwanted suffering can become transformed into sacred pain."

A mystery, to be sure. The ancient religious traditions of self-inflicted pain still linger in some corners of the contemporary world. They flourish in the Philippine celebrations of Easter, where each year volunteers are nailed to crosses before enthusiastic crowds, and in the Hindu festival of Thaipusam in India and Malaysia, when pilgrims regularly mortify their flesh—hanging weighted fishhooks from their chests or threading skewers through their cheeks and tongues—and say they feel no pain. I had seen gruesome photographs of the mutilated flesh and serene faces. But what did any of it have to do with me?

Crossing the street against the light one day in Providence, where I was visiting Kurt, I found myself caught on the traffic island. The day was unusually hot. It struck me how different that heat on my neck—just the other side of pleasant—was from the sensation *in* my neck, which burned in a different way, like the scald of dry ice. How odd it was that the world

outside my body no longer seemed to come inside it! The day did not melt
the dry ice and ease my pain into the ordinary crankiness of August on
the East Coast.

With cars crisscrossing in both directions, the city shimmered as if it
were not a familiar, but an allegorical landscape in a story, a movie, or a
dream. What if I was not in pain, but in Pain: a large, busy city filled with
other unfortunates, next door to Samara. If I were in Pain, what should
I do?

Take up your cross.

I was surprised to find the phrase surface in my mind, because I've
never really understood it. The idea made my brain feel fuzzy.

Take up your cross and follow Me.

Uhh . . . What cross was that? Most of the time I feared I was insuffi-
ciently committed to being happy. Was embracing crosses really a healthy
goal? How could you distinguish a sacred cross from a penchant for masochism or simple misfortune? What if you picked the wrong cross?

Take up your cross and follow Me.

What if I tried to value my pain and see it as an opportunity for *imitatio Christi*? Could Pain—this pain that, for no reason, had come upon
me—be my cross? Should I try picking it up?

Why? I felt diminished—degraded, even, by pain—not only physically
but spiritually as well. I thought of a favorite Kafka short story, "In the
Penal Colony," that parodies the religious belief that physical pain can
inscribe our bodies in sacred script.

In the story, a traveler visits a penal colony where an old Officer demonstrates his prized instrument of torture: a machine, called a Harrow,
that literally uses needles to carve on the body of a prisoner a description
of his crime, with pressure that increases over the course of twelve hours.
The Officer explains that the nature of the prisoner's crime is not told to
him, but that six hours on the Harrow takes him to the point of enlightenment where he "deciphers it with his wounds" and there is a "transfigured
expression from the tortured face"—a "glow of that justice, attained at
long last and already fading!"

But the machine is rarely used anymore, the Officer laments: faith in
its powers has been replaced by faith in modern jurisprudence. The spec-
tacle of torture no longer draws happy crowds. Instead, the Officer per-
forms his duty alone, executing the occasional prisoner. The torturer's
belief in the beneficent effect of torture on his victims proves wholly,

shockingly sincere. The story at first appears to be a simple critique of torture, yet it turns out to be a critique of the broader idea of pain as passion, when, sparing the prisoner, the Officer unexpectedly throws himself on the machine.

"When pain transgresses the limits, it becomes medicine," commends the nineteenth-century Sufi mystic Ghalib. Yet the Officer's sacrifice only destroys the machine; its gears break, its needles pierce rather than inscribe his flesh, and their message is lost in blood. The Traveler "could discover no sign of the promised transfiguration" in the mutilated corpse, no moment in which the Officer had tasted, as Saint Teresa of Avila puts it, "the sweetness of this greatest pain." Yet the blank stupidity of the Officer's conviction appears unshaken: "His lips were pressed firmly together, his eyes were open and looked as they had when he was alive, his gaze was calm and convinced. The tip of a large iron needle had gone through his forehead."

Pain inscribes the body in Kafka's world, but the words turn out to be gibberish.

Take up your cross . . .

I didn't want to be in Pain; I didn't want to want it. Pain is not a cross; it's a Harrow. There is nothing to decipher; the language of pain dissolves in suffering.

I scrapped the idea.

THE BODY IN PAIN

The longer I didn't tell Kurt, the harder it was to begin.

I am afflicted by terrible pain, I would say.

Weird, he would reply. *For how long?*

A year and a half.

What? Why didn't you say something?

I don't know.

When did it start?

The day we were first together. Really. Precisely then.

What?

I would seem like I was hostile, hypochondriacal, or crazy.

Oddly, he himself suffered from neck pain, which should have made it easier, but it actually made it more difficult. He was a decade older. I was supposed to be the young, healthy one. He found sickly women distasteful; his mother had been sickly. I had a white lace nightgown he called "your took-sick nightgown" with the "consumptive look." I argued that it was beautiful and expensive, but in the end, I threw it away and bought pajamas.

He would twist my neck at times to kiss me, or crush my shoulder in a hug, and although I'd tear up, I'd never explain. I'd lie awake at night reading his copy of Elaine Scarry's *The Body in Pain*, thinking how true is its thesis. Philosophers are always looking for ways to define the essential difference between what we can know about ourselves and what we can know about others—and pain, Scarry explains, is a paradigmatic example of that difference: "To have great pain is to have certainty; to hear that another person has pain is to have doubt."

I am in pain, I would think, looking over at Kurt. *My body is in pain.*

When one speaks about "one's own physical pain" and "another person's physical pain," one might almost appear to be speaking about two wholly distinct orders of events. For the person whose pain it is, it is "effortlessly" grasped (that is, even with the most heroic effort it cannot *not* be grasped); while for the person outside the sufferer's body, what is "effortless" is *not* grasping it . . . And, finally, if with the best effort of successful attention one successfully apprehends it, the aversiveness of the "it" one apprehends will only be a shadowy fraction of the actual "it."

Ask me.

When one hears about another person's physical pain, the events happening within the interior of that person's body may seem to have the remote character of some deep subterranean fact, belonging to an invisible geography that, however portentous, has no reality because it has not yet manifested itself on the visible surface of the earth . . . the pains occurring in other people's bodies flicker before the mind, then disappear.

Don't ask me.

Always, I felt a little lonely in the relationship with Kurt, haunted by the sense that he didn't truly know me. Yet when I tried to think of what he didn't know about me, the only thing I could think of was pain. The pain reflected the distance, but the pain *was* the distance, too. Pain was the reason I couldn't sleep entwined in his arms the way he wanted me to. Pain was the reason I wasn't really sleeping with him at all—or watching a Bette Davis movie with him, or making dinner with him. I was doing all those things with Pain. Did I not want him to know me?

I don't recall the occasion on which I finally told Kurt about the pain, or what he said, but I know he didn't respond badly.

I was wrong to have been so anxious, I told myself—to have imagined that he might see maggots of pain crawling down my neck into my rotten arm and not want to be with a rotting person. The fear that had kept me silent for so long, I realized—the fear that my pain would mean too much to him—had actually concealed another, more realistic, fear: the fear that it would mean too little.

PIONEER GIRL

I'm not seeing you on a canoe trip," Kurt said when Cynthia and her husband invited us on a trip to West Virginia.

"I love canoeing," I retorted, although I never had before. The idea conjured a dim, unpleasant memory of a junior high school trip. But even as I said it, I could feel the tug of the pain in my right side and a self-doubt, the feeling that perhaps I had actually become the person Kurt thought I was—a person who was unable to canoe.

There was my present self, which I pictured with a gigantic head puffed up with pain, drooping from a pale, attenuated body, like a nineteenth-century neurasthenic patient. But I still had a vision of myself—of a plucky, resourceful, woodsy self, like an illustration from a Laura Ingalls Wilder book. The old self—who didn't canoe, but did climb mountains, ride horses, and ski—was my best, most attractive self. This was the self that had enticed Kurt into swimming across the pond the day I first seduced him. But it was also the self that was lost that same day—the day I acquired pain.

"You really want to?" he said. "To canoe?"

I remembered how he had looked across the pond to the far shore, wrinkling his nose with disdain at the dark distance. But he had swum with me, and so everything began.

"Okay, Pioneer Girl." He sighed.

We had been dating for several years, but it still felt as if we were nowhere. The relationship sometimes seemed as attenuated as Kurt complained my body was now, his concern laced with irritation. I dimly associated the feeling of nowhereness with the fact that we never *did* anything together—or nothing that seemed "real." We went to movies and watched simulations of people's lives. We went out to dinner and ate food other people had cooked. We talked, endlessly, about our hypothetical future: about whether to spend our lives together. But it never felt as if we were *already* together, as if the building of a life had begun. Whenever I left his house in Providence and took the train back to New York, I felt as if I was finally home. We had a thousand and one dates, but we never cooperated on a task or an errand or even went grocery shopping together. Now, perhaps, we could make a tent-home in the wilderness.

"If you say so," he said.

The night before we left, I reminded him of the problem with my arm. "I told you about my arm," I said carefully. "So I might not be able to paddle that much."

"Why does this not surprise me?"

"Or at all."

"Don't worry," he said curtly. "I'll handle it."

I sat in the front of the boat on the river, sunshine pouring around my big straw hat with a bow on the brim, while he maneuvered the boat. I beamed at him. I felt a happiness that was as light and dappled as the trembling green lace of the trees. The boat with Cynthia and her husband was just ahead. I could hear them laughing.

"You look pretty in your floppy hat," Kurt said. "Like a heroine in a Venetian gondola in a Merchant-Ivory movie." But he hated Merchant-Ivory movies—he refused to go to them with me. The boat drifted sideways as he paused. He struggled to right it against the current. Although he had let go for only a moment, it took several minutes to correct.

"It's funny how hard it is to get on track once you lose your course," he said. "Doesn't that seem resonant?"

"Of my whole life," I said. *Until I met you*, I wanted to add because I knew it would be a sweet thing to say. But I was silenced by the thought that perhaps being with him was the ultimate wrong turn and that, weakened as I was now, I might never be strong enough to set myself back on course. Anyone would want to be with him. His beautiful face and mind, his brilliance, his wit, his blue-gray eyes. The thought of his desirability confused me, as it had confused me for the length of the relationship. The longing I felt for him still ran as quick as it always had. Yet somehow, the force of the relationship pulled me away—away from health and strength and capableness and honesty. Here I was, now: almost crippled, a person who couldn't paddle or even open a jar of jam some mornings—and then who pretended not to want jam. I was always anxious about presenting myself poorly—seeming pathetic or pitiful—and burdening or irritating him. So many things irritated him.

"You'll set up a good, snug tent for us tonight, Pioneer Girl," he said. He leaned on the paddle, his face flushed. The first drops of rain began to fall. "Promise me you'll take care of it."

"I'll take care of it."

It was raining steadily as I set up our tent in the last light. It had been difficult to carry the equipment up the bank to the highest ground. Kurt looked for firewood as I threaded the silvery rods through the pale green nylon. The tent puffed up, soft and fluffy as a mushroom. I was about to secure the tent when I dropped the stakes into the muddy grass. I unzipped the tent and sat inside to keep it from blowing away while I leaned out and searched. But without stakes to hold them taut, the metal rods bumped and twisted against one another, and then the cloth deflated and slowly, suffocatingly billowed down around me.

I lay on my back and laughed helplessly.

"*Goddamn* it," Kurt said. "Our tent is wet." He pushed the folds off my face. I squinted against the rain.

"So I'm a bad pioneer," I said.

"That's not good *enough*," he snapped. "What if you were a pioneer? What are you going to contribute to society?"

"I'm a writer."

"There are no writers. Everyone is struggling to survive." He leaned in close. "What is your function? You can't paddle, and you can't build us a home to keep us dry. Everyone contributes to the community's survival—or they die."

He pinned my wrists on the fallen floor.

"You're hurting me." The weight of his body pressed into my shoulder, which felt as unstable as the tent poles.

"You're starving. What is your function?"

"I don't know."

"What is your function?"

"I'm a prostitute." Tears mixed with rain on my face.

He let my wrists go and knelt in the grass, looking for the missing stakes.

Sitting around the campfire later, I told the group the story of the leper I had seen in Addis Ababa.

"He was *laughing*," I said. As I pictured him, he laughed at me again.

"Perhaps he wasn't in pain," suggested Cynthia's husband, Jim, a physician.

"His hand was falling off."

"Well, leprosy creates peripheral neuropathies. The bacteria eat away at the peripheral nerves, so the person becomes insensate. Without the protection of pain, limbs get damaged."

The leper stopped laughing. To the extent that I thought of leprosy at all, it dimly stood in my mind as a biblical curse or an inexplicable horror. I had never thought to consider it as a disease and wonder about its mechanisms rather than its metaphors. The leper hadn't transcended pain; he wasn't in pain. *I* was in pain. When we returned to civilization, I decided, I would get an MRI and find out why.

II

THE SPELL OF SURGICAL SLEEP:

Pain as History

CONQUERING PAIN

At a particular juncture in the mid-nineteenth century, pain was transformed from the spiritual signifier it had always been to a merely biological phenomenon, in light of a single medical discovery. This particular discovery changed not only thinking about pain, but separated medicine itself from its ancient embrace of religion and situated it in the realm of science.

"WE HAVE CONQUERED PAIN," announced *The People's Journal* of London in 1847, with capital-lettered jubilance at the discovery that surgical anesthesia could be achieved through the inhalation of ether gas. "Oh, what delight for every feeling heart to find the new year ushered in with the announcement of this noble discovery of the power to still the sense of pain, and veil the eye and memory from all the horrors of an operation," it waxed. In that giddy hour, it seemed that not merely surgical pain, but all pain would soon bow to human ingenuity.

The development of anesthesia, scholars have suggested, resulted from cultural changes in the late eighteenth and early nineteenth centuries that demanded pain's abolition. The German romantic poet Heinrich Heine's ironic comment about his experience of dental work seems to embody this change of attitude: "Psychic pain is easier to endure than physical, and if *I* had to choose between an evil conscience and an aching tooth, I would prefer the former," he grumbled. "Ah! there is nothing so horrible as toothache."

From ancient times, cultures had always entwined the spiritual and material realms, as in the myth of the Babylonian tooth worm. While primitive, Greco-Roman, karmically based, and Judeo-Christian views of pain differed in their interpretations, they all had in common the belief that pain required interpretation because physical pain was never simply physical, but was suffused with metaphysical meaning. For them to decouple the two, as Heine did—flippantly privileging a bad tooth over an evil conscience—would have made no sense, since toothache was believed to *reflect* moral decay. On this theory, solutions for the former would necessarily have to address the latter.

The astonishing efficacy of anesthesia, however, seemed to belie this. Science's new ability to dispel the pain of saints and sinners alike disenchanted pain of its ancient meanings. Stolen from the province of the gods, pain was no longer *poena*, passion, or ordeal, but simply a biological function that could be controlled by men. Anesthesia, followed by Darwin's theory of evolution, resituated man in the cosmos. Although religion itself did not die out, of course, secular scientific modes of thought became the culturally dominant ways of regarding the body.

Interest in synthetic chemistry and atmospheric gases in the late eighteenth century led to experimentation with ether, nitrous oxide, and chloroform. Coincidentally, it was observed that the inhalation of these gases induced giddiness and excitation, which were quickly followed by a brief yet extraordinarily deep sleep—a sleep from which the patient could not be roused.

Ordinarily, the sleep-arousal mechanism in the brain is highly responsive and can be activated by as little as a caress—not to mention the serious assault on bodily integrity of a surgeon's knife. Only in the case of grave neurological injury does the brain shut down enough to disable this mechanism and leave the body vulnerable to assault. Inhalation anesthesia (the precursor to modern anesthesia) used ether, nitrous oxide, or chloroform to allow for the creation of a coma-at-will: a predictable faux coma, as it were, with none of coma's ill effects.

It was an effect physicians had been trying to achieve for centuries, with desperate attempts such as "concussion anesthesia," which involved knocking the patient out through a blow to the jaw or by placing his head in a leather helmet and hitting it with a wooden hammer! Occasionally, concussion anesthesia worked. But most of the time, patients only incurred a head injury without losing consciousness, or they lost consciousness and woke in the middle of the surgery—or never again. Interestingly, ether and nitrous oxide were well known and had been used recreationally (sometimes even in the treatment of disease) since the early nineteenth century—almost a half century before they were used in surgery. During that time, changes in cultural conditions that had begun in the eighteenth century accelerated in ways that rendered the horror of surgical pain increasingly intolerable.

Pain—whether inflicted by nature or man—has always been an ordinary part of life. Indeed, beholding the pain of others, in the form of surgeries or executions, was once rabble-rousing entertainment. "Out to Charing Cross to see Major-general Harrison, hanged, drawn and quartered," the great literary raconteur Samuel Pepys recorded in his seventeenth-century diary of London life, adding wittily that the major general himself (who had the misfortune to side with Parliament in the English civil war) was "looking as cheerful as any man could do in that condition." Afterward Pepys took friends "to the Sun Tavern, and did give them some oysters." The prisoner himself was forced to be a spectator to his own dismemberment by being only partially asphyxiated during the hanging, so as to be conscious while being drawn and quartered (the details of which I will spare the reader).

Brutality began to recede from daily life during the late eighteenth and nineteenth centuries. The practice of capital punishment declined in England. Torturing convicts to death became less acceptable. In 1814, it was decreed that a prisoner should be hanged until dead before being drawn and quartered, but by 1870, even mutilating a corpse came to be seen as indecent, and the entire practice of drawing and quartering was prohibited. Women who murdered their husbands were no longer burned at the stake. Slavery was abolished in America and in the British colonies. Other humanitarian reforms addressed labor and the welfare of women and children.

The American and French revolutions ushered in a new preoccupation with individual rights. Along with the rights of man, there arrived a radical concept: the right to happiness. The novelty of this idea—a cornerstone of the modern ethos—is lost to us. Certainly, nowhere in the Bible does God enjoin man to pursue happiness; to the contrary, Adam and Eve are cursed to a life of thorns. Most other religions agree with the Buddha's

First Noble Truth that life is *dukkha*—suffering, grief, and pain (and not just any pain, but burning pain, from the Sanskrit root *du*, "to be burned or consumed by fire"). Acceptance of suffering is a central task of the faithful (a principle of great utility to governments!).

In the modern self created by the Romantic movement, however, identity ceased to derive from connection to God and community, but from individualism, according to which happiness was valued over self-sacrifice and self-transcendence. And happiness seemed increasingly possible as the Industrial Revolution spread prosperity, creating a large middle class for the first time in England and America. People began to expect alleviation from pain.

The Christian conception of the necessity of pain was undercut by the Darwinian (and later the Freudian) template of human nature as driven to seek pleasure and avoid pain. Far from divinely ordained, pain and suffering in Darwin's theory were simply part of the process of evolution, contingent on environment and physiology. And Christianity itself was influenced by the intellectual currents of the day. Reflecting the humanistic tradition that saw man as essentially good, Victorian Christianity posited a more benevolent God than that of earlier ages, a loving father figure who would not inflict *poena* upon His children—at least not the obedient ones. Although good characters die in Victorian novels, they die painlessly—especially children (Charlotte Brontë's Helen Burns, Harriet Beecher Stowe's Eva St. Clare). Dickens extolled Little Nell's corpse as "so free from trace of pain, so fair to look upon. She seemed . . . not one who had lived and suffered death," as if death were an ordeal her virtue allowed her to painlessly pass.

Pharmacies helped relieve pain by providing a huge, cheap supply of unregulated opiate-alcohol concoctions, such as Mrs. Winslow's Soothing Syrup, with which many Victorians kept themselves and their children continually dosed. Even so, opiates were insufficient (except in dangerous doses) to banish the agony of surgery.

With the vast migration to the cities, medicine began to industrialize. Physicians had been trusted community leaders with long, intimate knowledge of their patients and many means of healing, few of which were physiological. The new breed of doctor in the hospital or city clinic could only ask, "Where does it hurt?" and hope that a description of tissue damage would point to a deeper cause. It frequently failed to do so, of course. But developing an understanding of *why*—and of all the pain phenomena that defy such a model, such as the twin Victorian fads of mesmerism (pain relief through no apparent physiological mechanism) and hysteria (pain with no apparent physiological cause)—would take another century. Although the mechanisms of anesthesia were not understood (and curiously remain poorly understood even today), the simplicity of its effect made pain itself seem simple and—momentarily, thrillingly—conquerable.

THE CRAFT AND ITS TERRORS

Our craft has, once for all, been robbed of its terrors," announced Dr. Henry Bigelow on October 16, 1846, as he rose, agape, from the audience at the first successful demonstration of surgical anesthesia using ether gas.

How terrible surgery had been, "ensanguined like a slaughter-yard, the air rent with the shrieks of the unhappy victims quivering under the knife," as another surgeon later recalled. Surgeries were public spectacles, like executions, at which crowds gathered in operating theaters to watch a surgeon who—as the Scottish anatomist John Hunter described—resembled "an armed savage who attempts to get that by force which a civilized man would get by stratagem."

No stratagems were possible as long as the body's integrity was so well guarded by pain. The field of surgery had reached an impasse. Before anesthesia, the body's surface remained opaque, with the glimpses afforded by the carving knife brief and blurry. Anesthesia allowed surgeons to carefully study the inside of a living body and meticulously fix its problems. Surgeons knew how to perform delicate operations, such as removing stomachs or lungs, on the corpses of humans and animals. But the difference—as a surgeon at the time put it—between "moving, bleeding flesh and a passive carcass" meant that they could not perform such operations while patients screamed and thrashed about. Although patients were frequently blindfolded and gagged—and although some medical textbooks typically included recommendations for the number of able-bodied assistants required to restrain patients (four, in most cases)—it was impossible to fully immobilize a conscious person.

Speed was the crucial factor in a surgeon's skill; the Napoleonic surgeon Langeback bragged that he could "amputate a shoulder in the time it took to take a pinch of snuff." Tellingly, surgeons originally belonged to the guild of barbers (in England, the Company of Barber-Surgeons), as if snipping locks and limbs entailed a single skill. Botched operations were the rule: in 1834 a surgeon generated controversy when he was quoted saying candidly that before a man could successfully perform cataract surgeries, he must first "spoil a hatful of eyes." But it was true. About a third of patients died from such surgeries.

The invention of anesthesia (along with, at about the same time, the adoption of antiseptic techniques, such as sterilizing instruments, to prevent infection) had a startling effect on patient mortality. As part of a crusade to win social acceptance for the practice, the Scottish obstetrician Sir James Young Simpson compiled statistics to show that anesthesia had reduced mortality owing to amputation at the thigh—a particularly perilous operation—from one in two to one in three.

"How often have I dreaded that some unfortunate struggle of the patient would deviate the knife a little from its proper course," the prominent Columbia University surgeon Valentine Mott wrote of his practice before the use of anesthesia, "and that I, who fain would be the deliverer, should involuntarily become the executioner, seeing my patient perish in my hands by the most appalling form of death!" Not infrequently an artery would be accidentally severed, causing the patient to bleed to death on the table.

Prior to the nineteenth century, surgeons were typically of the lower class; an occupation that entailed torture seemed hardly fit for a gentleman—and, indeed, repulsed the compassionate of every class. In fact, it was the violence of surgery that helped dissuade Charles Darwin from choosing a medical career. While in medical school in 1820s Edinburgh, Darwin witnessed two operations in an amphitheater—one on a child—and rushed from the room in horror. The memory, he wrote later, "fairly haunted me for many a long year."

A tolerance for inflicting pain was required of surgeons. A surgeon had to have a mind "resolute and merciless," Ambroise Paré declared in the sixteenth century, so that "he be not moved to make more haste than the thing requires, or to cut less than is needful, but does all things as if he were not affected by their cries." Yet, Paré—royal surgeon to four French kings—recognized the importance of the physician's relationship with his patient. He wrote persuasively that the "indications of the patient's state of mind, determination and strength must take precedence over everything else. If he is weak or in terror, it is necessary to forsake all other things in order to be helpful to him. If the patient lacks the necessary strength of mind, operations should be postponed—if possible. Nothing can be gained from surgery if the patient is unwilling to face his ordeal."

How? How did anyone have the strength of mind to face such an ordeal when, for example, the surgeon arrived the day before to draw on the patient's body a diagram of the incisions to come, leaving him to contemplate the map of his own dismemberment?

Surgeons' records lament the great number of patients who preferred to die, succumbing to infections such as gangrene, rather than suffer an amputation knowing that many of those who submitted to the agony of an operation perished anyway. Fear of pain often trumped fear of death. Of the many experiences of premodern life inaccessible to us now in the developed world, few seem more so than preanesthetic surgery (although, shockingly, in China and Africa and during wartime, such surgeries still sometimes take place). In the West, remarkably few pathographies (patient accounts) of the experience of premodern surgery exist. Studies of nineteenth-century surgeons' records rarely include the mention of a patient's pain; the few allusions that exist limit themselves to comments such as, concerning an 1832 amputation, "during the operation the patient did not seem to suffer greatly"! How little suffering could sawing through the two bones of the forearm to amputate an arm above the elbow joint have involved?

Surgeons liked to make a point of recounting stories of patients who refrained from burdening them with their pain, such as one who cajoled a seven-year-old boy, "I suppose, my little fellow, that you would not mind having this knee removed, which pained you so much and made you so very ill." The boy replied, "Oh no, for mammy has told me that I ought."

One might imagine that such patients endured agony by "blanking out" via shock or some other mechanism that rendered them oblivious to their plight. In fact, however, intense pain creates extraordinarily clear awareness of surroundings; as people sense mortal danger, they become hyperalert, fixing details in memory. Time seems to slow (a sensation familiar to people who've been in car accidents). And, as ascetics attest, intense pain can also create a sense of disassociation, in which one is merely observing one's own agony. For example, far from being distracted by the pain of his testicle's amputation, a patient of Dr. Robert Keate's attended with keen awareness to the attitude of the surgeon's assistants, watching as one of them paused during the operation to dab at a spot of blood on his own white pants! Although the patient had intended to tip the assistant twenty guineas, he told Dr. Keate afterward that, as the fellow "regarded the purity of his trousers as more important than my sufferings, I will not give him a farthing."

While the details of the environment surrounding the person in pain remain seared in memory, the actual sensation of the pain is hard not only to describe, but even to recollect, since the rupture it creates *in* the self cannot be integrated into memory *of* the self. George Wilson's description of the amputation of his foot in 1842 (just four years prior to the invention of anesthesia) illuminates the relationship between pain, memory, and language—how, as Wilson said, "at the extremities of human experience, we can observe only a kind of silence." But whereas the sensory quality of pain disappears from memory, the emotions surrounding it do not.

Wilson was then a twenty-four-year-old medical student in Edinburgh, and his ankle had become infected. "During the operation, in spite of the pain it occasioned, my senses were preternaturally acute," he wrote in a letter to Sir James Young Simpson. "I watched all that the surgeons did with a fascinated intensity. Of the agony it occasioned, I will say nothing. Suffering so great as I underwent cannot be expressed in words, and thus fortunately cannot be recalled. The particular pangs are now forgotten; but the black whirlwind of emotion, the horror of great darkness, and the sense of desertion by God and man, bordering close upon despair, which swept through my mind and overwhelmed my heart, I can never forget, however gladly I would do so."

A TERROR THAT SURPASSES
ALL DESCRIPTION

One of the very few attempts to recall and express "particular pangs" is to be found in an 1812 letter by the English novelist and memoirist Fanny Burney to her sister, describing the mastectomy she had undergone in Paris the year before. Fanny Burney's letter is considered one of the most vivid pieces of writing on physical pain of any era.

A painful abscess had developed in Fanny's right breast almost twenty years earlier. She had fasted, drunk asses' milk, and rested, and it had gone away. In 1810 the pain returned. Her "doom" was pronounced by three doctors: she was "formally condemned to an operation." She was "as much astonished as disappointed," for "the poor breast was no where discoloured, & not much larger than its healthy neighbor." Fanny herself may have been the only one in possession of this knowledge, for the mores of the time meant that the doctors most likely did not actually *examine* her breast. Indeed, the first time they touched it was probably with their scalpels. Fanny was spared, however, the opinion of subsequent historians that she did not, in fact, have a malignant tumor (else she would not have survived with it for two decades before and three afterward), but rather an inflammatory condition that did not require a mastectomy.

As the wife of a French nobleman, Fanny was operated on by Napoleon's chief surgeon, Baron Dominique-Jean Larrey, who (fortunately—or not) happened temporarily to be between wars. This respite offered the baron the leisure to operate meticulously. At the Battle of Borodino in Russia, in contrast, he recorded in his memoir, he performed some two hundred amputations in one twenty-four-hour period! Fanny wrote about the operation as a medieval morality play in which the pain is an evil that the doctors must exorcise; indeed, she "felt the evil to be deep, so deep, that I often thought if it could not be dissolved, it could only with life be extirpated." Fanny's letter testifies to the importance of a strong surgeon-patient relationship prior to anesthesia, one in which the patient can balance the sensory experience of the torture of surgery against belief in the physician's benevolence. Viewing the pain as an evil required turning Dr. Larrey into a savior. Yet the extreme nature of the experience makes help and harm both merge and split, as images of the physician as savior, saint, healer, and torturer, butcher, executioner, compete and become confused and conflated. She wrote that "the good Dr. Larrey . . . had now tears in his eyes," yet her descriptions of the operation suggest an assault, a rape, and an execution.

Dr. Larrey refused to tell Fanny what day they would operate and to let her make preparations for it, promising only four hours' warning (a strategy surgeons employed to prevent patients from committing suicide on the eve of an operation). "After sentence thus passed, I was in hourly expectation of a summons to execution," she wrote. "Judge, then, my surprise to be suffered to go on [a] full 3 weeks in the same state!"

Then one morning, a letter from Dr. Larrey was delivered to her bedside, informing her that he would arrive shortly. She arranged for a pretext to cause her husband to leave the house, in order to spare him "the unavailing wretchedness of witnessing what I must go through." She was alone when the team of doctors and assistants—"7 Men in black"—arrived. The doctors told her "to mount the Bedstead. I stood, suspended, for a moment, whether I should abruptly escape—I looked at the door, the windows—I felt desperate."

The maid and one of the nurses ran off in terror. The doctor began to issue commands, using military language. Fanny was compelled to take off her long dressing gown, which she had somehow imagined she might retain. No attempt at analgesia was made: in an era when nursing mothers would smear opium concoctions on their nipples to quiet their babies, Fanny's breast was lopped off after giving her only a wine cordial to sip.

She threw herself into her fate. Finally, she "mounted, unbidden, the Bed," and the doctor spread a cambric handkerchief upon her face. "Bright through the cambric" she glimpsed "the glitter of polished Steel." She watched as—without touching her—the doctor made the sign of a cross and a circle with his finger over her breast "intimating that the Whole was to be taken off."

She threw off the handkerchief and protested that the breast hurt in only one place. The doctors veiled her face again. She saw one doctor make the gesture a second time, and she "closed once more [her] Eyes, relinquishing all watching, all resistance, all interference & sadly resolute to be wholly resigned."

An 1837 medical textbook instructed that in the case of mastectomies, "no half-measures will answer . . . the duration of the proceeding must not for once be considered. Many operations can be done quickly and well . . . this is not one of them."

Fanny's operation was anything but quick. She felt:

> a terror that surpasses all description & the most torturing pain . . . when the dreadful steel was plunged into the breast—cutting through veins—arteries, flesh, nerves . . . I began a scream that lasted unintermittingly during the whole time of the incision, and I almost marvel that it rings not in my Ears still! So excruciating was the agony . . . When the wound was made and the instrument withdrawn, the pain seemed undiminished, for the air that suddenly rushed into those delicate parts felt like a mass of minute but sharp poniards that were tearing the edges of the wound—but when again I felt the instrument, describing a curve, cutting against the grain . . . while the flesh resisted in a manner so forcible as to oppose and tire the hand . . . then, indeed, I thought I must have expired.

She lost consciousness twice during the operation. Even when no one was touching her, the finger of the doctor "literally *felt* elevated over the wound . . . so indescribably sensitive was the spot." The operation lasted a full twenty minutes. She tried to bear it as courageously as she could, she writes, and "never moved, nor stopt them, nor resisted nor remonstrated, nor spoke," except to piteously thank the doctors for their attention. When she opened her eyes, she saw that the "good Dr. Larrey himself was pale nearly as myself, his face streaked with blood, and its expression depicting grief, apprehension, & almost horrour."

Afterward, "not for days, not for Weeks, but for Months I could not speak of this terrible business without nearly again going through it! . . . I have a headache from going on with this account! & this miserable account, which I began 3 Months ago, at least, I dare not revise, nor read, the recollection is still so painful."

DROWSY POTIONS

By the time of Fanny Burney's operation, many techniques for mitigating pain during surgery had been experimented with throughout the ages, but all were dangerous, insufficient, or both. In his 1812 memoir, Dominique-Jean Larrey—Fanny Burney's surgeon—related the anecdote of operating on a colonel during a battle by punching him on the chin. Dr. Larrey also wrote of employing "refrigeration anesthesia" (snow or ice), noting that the frozen conditions of the Russian battlefields eased the pain of operations. But while cold interferes with nerve conduction, freezing flesh makes it difficult to cut and puts a patient at risk of frostbite, leading to infection. The ideal was a "drowsy syrup" that would cause the patient to sleep through the surgery, but what elixir would allow (as the thirteenth-century Catalan alchemist and physician Arnold of Villanova bragged of his own potion) a patient to be "cut and [he] will feel nothing, as though he were dead" without *being* dead?

Like Villanova, many healers claimed such powers, of course, but they were all wise enough to keep their recipes secret. The most powerful secret ingredient was doubtless placebo. It's interesting to imagine what the history of medicine would be like without the placebo effect: in a sense, there might not have *been* a history of medicine before modern times without the placebo effect, because it would have been obvious that most treatments made no difference. Disease might have been relegated, like earthquakes and volcanoes, to the province of religion, seen as something that could not reliably be manipulated (even if the gods might be implored to ameliorate it). While the tendency of a disease toward resolution might sometimes have been mistaken for the effectiveness of a medical intervention, only the placebo effect granted healers uncanny power.

Pain relief is the task for which placebo is most effective. Unlike modern physicians, who focus on curing disease, ancient healers were primarily renowned for their anodynes. And when healers achieved relief, they enhanced their reputations, which might yield a stronger placebo effect for the next patient, which could in turn further enhance the physicians' reputations, maintaining a positive feedback loop.

What were the medicinal substances of the ancient world? Of all the plant anodynes, only a few were true analgesics: opium from poppies, alcohol, cocaine from the coca plant, henbane, mandrake (mandragora), deadly nightshade (belladonna), cannabis (marijuana), and salicylic acid (similar to aspirin) found in willow bark or dried myrtle leaves.

Willow bark was commended by Hippocrates to reduce the pain of childbirth and fever. The ancient remedy was rediscovered by the Reverend Edmund Stone one evening in 1758 when he was strolling in a meadow in Chipping Norton, England. Stone was a believer in the "general maxim that many natural maladies carry their cures along with them, or that their remedies lie not far from their causes," as he later wrote to the Royal Society. As the willow grew in wet soil, which was widely believed to give rise to disease, Stone surmised that the willow might provide an antidote. Breaking off a bit of bark, he found that its bitter taste reminded him of a costly imported medicine made from the bark of the South American cinchona, dubbed the fever bark tree, which contained quinine and had been discovered to have an extraordinary effect on a particular ague— malaria.

This daft chain of thought led to a real discovery. Stone gathered and dried willow bark and ground it into a powder that he tested on fifty of his parishioners. It was effective, he discovered, not only against fevers but as a general anodyne against pains of all sorts. Thereafter, willow bark medicine—crushed, powdered, and mixed into alcohol—led to such a craze in England that the willow population declined until stripping its bark was outlawed. (At the end of the Victorian era, a synthesized form of salicylic acid became the first popular synthesized drug, in the form of aspirin, beginning the modern pharmaceutical industry.)

Still, although aspirin could mitigate the inflammation that followed surgery, it could not ease the pain of surgery itself. Many plants' components are mildly soporific, but only henbane, mandrake, and opium could create a drowsy potion sufficient for surgery. Henbane and mandrake were too dangerous: both are intimately related to poisons. Although deadly night-shade was also poisonous, combined with opium it produced a twilight sleep that blurred the memory of pain. (These may have been the ingredients in nepenthe—Helen of Troy's wine potion that brought forgetfulness of pain and sorrow.)

Opium is the oldest and most important medicinal substance, the discovery of which is believed to predate even that of alcohol. Because opium has various effects (like alcohol, it initially has a stimulating effect that eventually turns to drowsiness), it could be used to kindle bravery in battle, as well as for celebrations, sacred rites, divinations, and to induce prophetic dreams. In some societies, opium's use was restricted to shamans and priests. In the Victorian age, Infants' Quietness and other "soothing syrups" of opium dissolved in alcohol—each of which possessed its own signature twist, from frog sperm to witch hazel—were prescribed for pains of all sorts, ranging from teething to neurasthenia, the fashionable ailment of Victorian women. Because, like alcohol, opiates depress respiration, they were useful in stilling the agonizing cough of tuberculosis. They could also stop life-threatening diarrhea by stilling contractions of the intestines, and they could alleviate the chronic pain of malnutrition by depressing appetite.

By inducing feelings of well-being, the syrups could soothe the cares of both the upper and lower classes. They also functioned as babysitters; although they jaundiced children's skin, they also kept them docile. Elizabeth Gaskell's novel *Mary Barton*, about the poor of Manchester, England, praised opium as "mother's mercy" for its ability to soothe the pangs of starving children: "Many a penny that would have gone little way enough in oatmeal or potatoes, bought opium to still the hungry little ones, and make them forget their uneasiness in heavy troubled sleep." Eventually, however, concerns about (among other things) the number of infants who were lulled to death after being dosed with such effective "baby-calmers" led to the first regulations on opiates in England in the late nineteenth century and America in the early twentieth.

The most potent analgesic in opium had been isolated early in the nineteenth century by a German chemist who named it *morphine* after the Greek word for *shapes*. (It is often erroneously thought to allude to

Morpheus, the god of dreams; in fact, the chemist originally called it "the shape of dreams," shortened to "shapes," or morphine). Yet the mystery of how it worked lingered. In the fourth century B.C.E., Diocles of Carystos, a Greek physician, mused about the "wondrous flower" that refused to "give up its secrets." Why did it "soothe some, but cast others into melancholy"? Why was its effect on some immediate and on others delayed? Why did it have a curious effect such that "even when it does not abolish pain, the pain no longer preys on the person's mind"?

It was not until the discovery of the opiate receptor in 1972 that the pod began to yield its secrets. The belief that opium was "God's own medicine" turned out to capture a biological truth: opiates work by mimicking the chemicals in the body's own pain-modulating system. The chemical structure of opiates is sufficiently similar that they can bind to the same receptor on nerve cells in the brain and spinal cord, where they change the way those neurons function, interfering with the transmission of pain signals in the spinal cord.

The effect of opiates is different from that of anesthetic agents, such as ether, that render people completely unconscious. A person on opiates seems to have all his senses about him—he can still run a marathon and will still cry out in pain if he falls and hurts himself—yet his relationship to pain is strangely altered. In addition to blocking the transmission of pain signals, opiates—as Diocles of Carystos observed—change one's relation to pain, so that the pain no longer preys on one's mind. This more complicated effect may be due to the way in which opiates boost the level of dopamine in the brain, creating a sense of pleasantness or even euphoria.

Yet despite its wondrous properties, opium was a perilous analgesic for surgery. Because opiate receptors are distributed in many parts of our bodies, opiates affect multiple systems throughout the body in addition to pain modulation, including those governing respiration, heartbeat, blood vessels, and the cough reflex. Opium increases bleeding by dilating blood vessels, which counteracts the body's way of adaptively responding to injury by constricting blood vessels and directing blood toward the vital organs. Opium shares the same perils as alcohol. They both induce nausea, putting the patient at risk of vomiting stomach acid onto the delicate lining of her lungs and fatally asphyxiating. Most perilously, by depressing respiration, as a sixteenth-century medical text cautioned, opium "causeth deepe deadly sleapes."

Of all the ancient remedies, only cocaine was suitable for surgery. In addition to the psychotropic effects with which we associate it today, cocaine is a topical anesthetic that acts on peripheral nerves (inhibiting the transmission of nociceptive impulses between cells) to cause localized numbness. The ancient Incans used the leaves of the sacred coca plant to perform operations such as trepanations. As they bored holes into their patients' skulls to allow the illness-causing demons to escape, the shamans chewed the leaves so that the cocaine dissolved in their saliva, and then they spit into wounds—a perfect double treatment, as the cocaine both inspired and focused the shamans and numbed their victims' peripheral nerves. While European trepanations in the eighteenth and early nineteenth centuries usually resulted in the patients' deaths, archaeological evidence reveals a surprisingly higher survival rate after ancient Peruvian trepanations (an examination found that the majority of trepanned skulls showed signs of healing). The success of the prehistoric trepanations is thought to stem from the sterilizing effect of cocaine.

The conquistadores figured out that cocaine was a useful addiction for their slaves: it acted as both a stimulant and an appetite depressant, energizing the starving natives and spurring on hard labor in the gold mines, for which the conquistadores would compensate their slaves with more cocaine. For unclear reasons, however, the plant was not exported and arrived in Europe only in the late nineteenth century, after the discovery of general anesthetics made it largely medically irrelevant (although it was and still is sometimes used as a local anesthetic in eye and throat surgery).

MESMERIZED

The most effective treatment for pain relief prior to anesthesia lay in the mind itself. It was long known that religious belief could assuage pain. Muhammad tells the faithful, "When anyone suffers from toothache, let him lay a finger upon the sore spot and recite the sixth sura." Thomas Aquinas writes how "the blessed delight which comes from the contemplation of divine things suffices to reduce bodily pain." Hindu Yogis cultivate indifference to pain as well as to pleasure. A typical tale from a book of Yogic philosophy involves a master who refuses anesthetic before an operation and then proceeds to calmly expound upon his philosophy to all present throughout the procedure. Afterward, when the dumbstruck surgeon asks if he felt any pain, he replies, "How could I? I was absent from that part of the Universe where you were working. I was present in this part where I discussed philosophy."

Contemplation of philosophy itself (philosophers claim) may equally suffice. In "On the Power of the Mind to Master Morbid Feelings by Sheer Resolution," Immanuel Kant writes of how, one night, kept awake by the pain of gout in his swollen toes, "I soon had recourse to my Stoic remedy of fixing my thought forcibly on some neutral object that I chose at random (for example, the name Cicero, which contains many associated ideas), and so diverting my attention from that sensation. The result was that the sensation was dulled, even quickly so, and outweighed by drowsiness; and I can repeat this procedure with equally good results every time that attacks of this kind recur."

How does an ordinary person achieve such control? At the time of Fanny Burney's surgery, a form of hypnotism known as *mesmerism* or animal magnetism (whose legacy is the verb *mesmerize*) had already been shown to induce analgesia, as well as to heal patients of other ills. Of all the techniques (opium, alcohol, freezing, inducing concussion, and so forth) that might have been used in Burney's parlor, mesmerism would have been the best—and indeed, in 1829 it was successfully used during another mastectomy in France. Following the undisputed success of that operation, performed by the surgeon Jules Cloquet in front of a dozen witnesses, mesmerism went on to be successfully used in several hundred surgeries. Unfortunately, however, it never achieved acceptance in mainstream medicine, and most surgeries continued to be performed without it—or any other analgesia—until the discovery of ether anesthesia.

Like a shaman, Franz Mesmer, a German physician trained in Vienna, used various impressive-looking props to induce a trance in his subjects, after which he would declare them healed. Instead of religious belief, however, his methods were wrapped in a dressing of Enlightenment science. Chief among them was the idea of a vital spirit or life force animating all beings (as well as planets and the earth), a biological correlate of the soul that (as with the Eastern idea of *chi*) was believed to be blocked in sickness. Following their mid-eighteenth-century commercialization, magnets and their invisible force were objects of particular scientific interest. Mesmer believed that just as a magnet could compel a piece of metal to move through space, channeling magnetic *fluidum* could restore the flow of vitality in a body and dissipate disease.

In 1774 Mesmer had a patient swallow a mixture that contained iron, and then he attached magnets to various parts of her body. The patient reported that she felt "streams of fluid" running through her body, which relieved her of pain for several hours. Soon, however, Mesmer discovered that he was able to achieve the same effects simply by touching patients, and he posited that the healing resulted from the transfer of his own magnetism to the patient. Notably, he recorded two conditions of success as necessary for hypnosis, which are true (and relevant to placebo in general): first, that the patient have a desire to be healed, and second, that the healer have a personal relationship with the patient.

Overwhelmed with individual patients, Mesmer took to treating people in groups. Clad like a magician in a violet-colored silk robe, he

presided over wooden tubs he called "banquets" that were filled with water and iron rods, in which the sick could be magnetized. The patients
would fall into a trance, sometimes even hallucinating or convulsing,
which Mesmer referred to as a "crisis." Afterward, he would declare the
patients cured and play music on a glass harmonica. He was even summoned by Queen Marie Antoinette to magnetize her poodle, Marionette.

The greater mesmerism's popular success, the more hostility it faced
from the medical establishment. In her book *Mesmerized: Powers of Mind
in Victorian Britain*, Alison Winter argues that the competition from mesmerists was actually the catalyst for the development of inhalation anesthesia. The extent to which the two were in competition is evident in the
British surgeon Robert Liston's famous (if perhaps apocryphal) quip upon
first using the new ether anesthesia from America during an amputation:
"This Yankee dodge beats mesmerism hollow . . . Hurray! Rejoice! Mesmerism and its professors have met with a heavy blow."

To the dismay of physicians who saw the technique as competition,
mesmerism swept through Europe, eventually spreading to Britain and
America. Mesmer moved his practice from Vienna to Paris, where he set
about trying to obtain the endorsement of the French scientific community. Mesmer's opportunity for validation came in 1784, when King Louis
XVI appointed an investigative committee composed of prominent members of the Faculty of Medicine and the Royal Academy of Sciences. The
committee considered not the *effects* of Mesmer's technique on patients,
but only the *theory* by which he explained it, which they swiftly debunked.
After all, the eighteenth century had seen great advances in the study of
anatomy, yet none of it had turned up magnetic forces or vital fluid. Mesmer left Paris just before the French Revolution, and mesmerism died with
him in exile. It enjoyed a revival in the 1830s and '40s. Public demonstrations by traveling mesmerists became popular in England and America;
they would put a subject (usually a comely young woman) in a trance, then
show that she would remain unresponsive to smelling salts, pinpricks, or
even acid poured on her skin!

More startling were reports of almost three hundred painless surgeries
performed under mesmerism. In 1842 a Nottinghamshire surgeon amputated the leg of a farm laborer. A skeptical lawyer named William Topham
witnessed the operation. Topham watched as the surgeon plunged the
knife into the laborer's thigh, all the way down to the bone, while the

laborer continued to sleep, moaning softly at times. Topham was stunned: "I saw" and "was convinced . . . There can be few, even of the most bigoted objectors, who will deny its powers," he wrote.

Yet they did. After debate, the Royal Medical and Chirurgical Society declared Topham's account "humbug" and censured him. A medical professor at the University College Hospital defended his interest in mesmerism, writing, "These phenomena I know to be real . . . independent of imagination . . . of the most interesting, most extraordinary & important character." He was ridiculed as a "tom-fool" and forced to resign.

The Enlightenment yielded a binary opposition between the subjective experiences of magic and faith healing on one hand and, on the other, the ideal of objective medical treatment having the same effect on every patient, regardless of whether they believed in it. There was no understanding that belief and other subjective mental states—and the role a healer could have in conjuring them—could *themselves* be objective phenomena, real yet also dependent on imagination.

Trance states were also seen as morally degrading. An 1851 article in *Blackwood's Edinburgh Magazine* denounced mesmerism as requiring "a ready abandonment of the will" along with "every endowment which makes man *human*" and concluded that it was "a disgusting condition which is characteristic only of the most abject specimens of our species." Some surgeons attempted mesmerism, but the patients failed to fall into a trance, or the trance did not last and they woke up screaming partway through the surgery. For a patient to achieve a trance, practice is usually required (and not everyone is able to learn it). Moreover, the crowded amphitheaters in which surgeries were typically performed in Europe were not conducive to achieving such a state. Horribly surprised, doctor and patient alike joined the backlash when mesmerism failed.

With the development of anesthesia, mesmerism was permanently abandoned. However, in the mid-nineteenth century, the Scottish physician James Braid (although he criticized the "immoral tendency" of "the irresistible power of . . . the mesmerizers") revived the practice of employing the trance to treat disease, naming it hypnotism. Self-hypnotism has been shown to be of use during medical procedures and to reduce the amount of anesthesia required.

Although ether was accompanied by more risks and side effects than mesmerism was, it was clearly a superior mechanism for controlling pain, because it did not require a particular mental state on the part of the surgeon or the patient. Yet the puzzle lingered for those who had witnessed operations or public demonstrations under mesmerism. How did mesmerism actually work? How had the knife been plunged painlessly to the bone or acid poured on the somnolent demonstrator's skin?

The puzzle would have to wait for the invention of brain imaging to see how the hypnotized brain can block (or create) pain, and why some people are susceptible to hypnotism while others are not. Mesmer's magnetic *fluidum* might not exist, but the phenomena he observed are indeed real.

A CHIMERA NOT PERMITTED

The puzzle of the history of anesthesia—one on which every medical history speculates to incomplete effect—is why it wasn't practiced earlier. By the time of Fanny Burney's operation in 1812, the anesthetic effects of inhaling the gases ether and nitrous oxide had long been known by British chemists. Yet decades of gruesome surgeries would transpire before an American dentist finally brought the gases into the operating room.

In his book *Romance, Poetry, and Surgical Sleep*, the distinguished anesthesiologist E. M. Papper theorizes that anesthesia could only have been invented in America because its development depended on a democratic society in which the pain and suffering of the masses mattered. But many Americans lived in misery, and regardless, the suffering of certain Englishmen certainly counted in the British mind. So why didn't the elite demand anesthesia?

Part of the answer seems to involve opposition from surgeons. Throughout British medical history, pain and surgery had been linked, and thus, attempts at uncoupling them struck many as impossible, unnatural, or dangerous. The profession required people who were willing to inflict severe pain on others, and who—having done so—were invested in seeing that pain as appropriate. Pain is "necessary to our existence," argued the Scottish surgeon Sir Charles Bell in 1806. "To imagine the absence of pain is not only to imagine a new state of being, but a change in the earth and all upon it."

The idea of such a change was viewed with alarm. "To escape pain in surgical operations is a chimera which it is idle to follow up today," declared the great French surgeon Alfred Velpeau in 1839. "Knife and pain in surgery are two words which are always inseparable in the minds of patients, and this necessary association must be conceded."

It is worth contemplating what Velpeau means by *chimera*. Is painless surgery a chimera in the sense of a mythical creature that does not exist, even if we wish it did, or a chimera in the sense of a monstrous creature that *should* not exist—a goat with a lion's head—whose very existence is a subversion of the natural order? After the Fall, aren't we *supposed* to suffer pain?

Every surgeon was familiar with the moment at which a patient became eerily quiet. Because unconsciousness usually prefigures death (both imitating and presaging it), crying was considered a sign of health, a manifestation of the vital spirit. Moreover, consciousness was considered an emanation of the soul; to extinguish consciousness was to play God and temporarily kill the patient.

Long after the means of anesthesia had become available, many scientists either didn't understand its potential application or were unsuccessful in convincing others of it, so the story of anesthesia's development is often told as an allegory of the difficulty of progress, the tenacity of suffering, and the conflict between science and religion. Sir Humphry Davy discovered the anesthetic properties of nitrous oxide (which he termed "laughing gas") at the turn of the nineteenth century while working at the Pneumatic Institute—a clinic that attempted to treat diseases such as TB and asthma with nitrous oxide and ether gases. One day when Davy was suffering from a terrible toothache, he experimented on himself with the gas. Suddenly, to his surprise, his pain seemed quite amusing. In his book *Nitrous Oxide*, he wrote that as the gas "appears capable of destroying physical pain, it may probably be used with advantage during surgical operations in which no great effusion of blood takes place." His apprentice, Michael Faraday, reached similar conclusions regarding ether. But when pneumatic medicine was discredited and the clinic closed, Davy lost interest in nitrous oxide and went on to be knighted for other discoveries.

The gases became popular among Romantic poets such as Samuel Taylor Coleridge and Robert Southey, who wrote of nitrous oxide as "the air in heaven this wonder working gas of delight." Ether frolics became the rage; traveling shows would demonstrate the gas's effects and invite the audience to partake. As in the case of alcohol, the effects of the gases occur in two stages: Initially it creates arousal and exhilaration, which is followed by deep sleep. The first stage seemed inappropriate for surgery: What place could a party trick have in the operating room? The doses administered at shows were usually sufficient to cause giddiness, but not to take subjects into the sleep phase befitting surgery.

BY WHOM PAIN IN SURGERY
WAS AVERTED AND ANNULLED

I n science the credit goes to the man who convinces the world, not to the man to whom the idea first occurs," observed the botanist Francis Darwin, son of Charles Darwin. William T. G. Morton's tombstone reads, "Inventor and Revealer of Anesthetic Inhalation. Before Whom, in All Time, Surgery was Agony. By Whom Pain in Surgery was Averted and Annulled. Since Whom Science has Control of Pain." Dr. Morton did not discover any new agents, but by persuading the medical establishment of ether's utility during an operation at Massachusetts General Hospital on October 16, 1846, he bifurcated medical history forever.

During the 1840s at least three Americans were experimenting with ether and nitrous oxide: among them, two New England dentists and a southern country doctor. That one of the two dentists ultimately prevailed has sometimes been attributed to the economics of dentistry; unlike most surgeries, dentistry was usually elective, and the fear of pain kept patients away from it. (But, like the idea that anesthesia could only have been invented in America, this theory seems puzzling. After all, even if the surgical profession as a whole maintained a cultural bias against anesthesia, it would have taken only one surgeon to play Morton's role.)

The earliest of the three is generally believed to be a doctor from Georgia who, after attending ether parties as a medical student, experimented with using ether during surgery on a patient in 1842. But, concerned that the technique would strike other physicians as improper, to his eternal regret, he did not publish his findings until after Dr. Morton had already claimed credit for ether's discovery.

At a popular science demonstration three years later, a Connecticut dentist named Horace Wells noticed that one of the volunteers seemed unaware of having accidentally cut his leg while leaping around the room under the influence of laughing gas. The next day, Dr. Wells had a fellow dentist pull out one of his molars while he inhaled nitrous oxide, and he found it didn't hurt at all. Dr. Wells successfully experimented on other patients (he tried ether on some as well, but decided nitrous oxide was safer, as ether can cause vomiting and is also easily flammable). Finally, Dr. Wells persuaded the eminent surgeon Dr. John Collins Warren, founder of what became *The New England Journal of Medicine* and Massachusetts General Hospital, to permit a demonstration during one of Warren's surgeries in the hospital's glass-domed amphitheater (today known as the ether dome).

The demonstration was a failure: the patient hollered at the first cut, and the crowd of surgeons and medical students jeered, "Humbug!" (Dr. Wells might have given the patient insufficient quantities of nitrous oxide, and later the patient said he had felt only a little pain but had been alarmed by the procedure.)

A year later, Dr. Wells's former colleague Dr. Morton persuaded Dr. Warren to let him demonstrate gas anesthesia, using ether instead of nitrous oxide, on a young man submitting to the removal of a tumor from his jaw. Accounts of the incident are all so vivid: the audience waiting, the tremulous young man strapped down on an operating chair on the stage of the amphitheater, the surgeon impatiently declaring, "As Dr. Morton has not arrived, I presume he is otherwise engaged," and Dr. Morton finally bursting in, explaining that he had been delayed because the custom-made device for delivering vapors of an ether-soaked sponge had not been ready. The patient inhaled the vapors from the sponge, lost consciousness, and did not awaken until after Dr. Warren had finished washing the blood off his wounds. When questioned about the pain, the patient answered that he had felt only a peculiar scratching at his cheek, like a hoe raking a field.

"Gentlemen, this is no humbug," Dr. Warren announced to the hushed crowd. Later he wrote, "The student who . . . in distant ages may visit this spot will view it with increased interest, as he remembers that here was first demonstrated one of the most glorious truths of science." Around the

world, word swiftly spread that, as a German surgeon put it, "the wonderful dream that pain has been taken away from us has become reality.
Pain . . . must now bow before the power of the human mind, before the
power of the ether vapor."

Anguished with jealousy over Dr. Morton's success, Dr. Wells suffered
a nervous breakdown after trying in vain to petition various boards for
recognition of his role in the discovery. In searching for an agent superior
to nitrous oxide, he developed an addiction to chloroform. He attacked
two prostitutes while under the influence and committed suicide shortly
before the arrival of a letter from the Paris Medical Society declaring that
he was "due all the honor" for the discovery.

In fact, he needn't have been too jealous of his old friend. Although
Dr. Morton would receive credit for the discovery of the "greatest gift ever
made to suffering humanity," the alleviation of mankind's pain came at a
personal price. Dr. Morton wasted the rest of his life in a futile attempt to
patent ether in order to profit from it (he was unable to patent it, because
he hadn't invented it). He had hoped to disguise ether's well-known reek
by mixing it with orange-scented oils and other fragrances and calling it
Letheon, after the Greek river of forgetfulness, but the ingredient was evident. He died bitter and impoverished.

THE SLAVERY OF ETHERIZATION

In a corner of the Public Garden in Boston stands an unusual monument, one that is neither to a hero nor a battle, but rather to a medical achievement: "The discovery that the inhaling of ether causes insensibility to pain. First proved to the World at the Mass General Hospital in Boston." The 1868 forty-foot rose-speckled marble and granite obelisk is the only such statue in the world. The invention of other revolutionary medications, such as the discovery of antibiotics, does not seem to call for the visual tribute of a monument—they are celebrated, one might say, by every life they save.

The commissioning of the ether memorial was controversial in its time, and its intricate surfaces make clear its real purpose: not merely to mark an achievement but also to address the source of the controversy that surrounded it by attempting to reconcile science's and religion's competing perspectives on anesthesia. The monument did so by interpreting the discovery not as a triumph of the former over the latter, but rather as a *fulfillment* of the prophecy from the book of Revelation inscribed on its east relief: "Neither Shall There Be Any More Pain." Above those words an angel of mercy descends upon a sufferer, while the south and north faces of the monument depict operations performed with anesthesia. On the west side of the monument, a female allegorical embodiment of Science perches on a throne of lab equipment, and an inscription from Isaiah insists, "This also commeth forth / from the Lord of hosts . . ."

Yet, critics of anesthesia pointed out that Revelation prophesizes that *God*—not science—"shall wipe away all tears from their eyes." And they considered anesthesia "of the devil," a deliberate flouting of Adam's curse. The benefit of anesthesia is so absurdly obvious now that it's hard for us to believe it was ever controversial, yet at the time some physicians saw only "evil" in anesthesia. It was "a questionable attempt to abrogate one of the general conditions of man," one causing "the destruction of consciousness." (Advocates countered that ordinary sleep is a nightly destruction of consciousness.)

Ether, in the view of many, was a party drug that was now being brought into the most serious of arenas, inducing a state that, in its exhilaration stage, suspiciously resembled drunkenness. "Even were the reports of persons who felt no pain during an operation credible, this would not be worth the consideration of a serious-minded doctor," a prominent surgeon declared. A full seventeen years after the discovery, New York surgeon Valentine Mott wrote a passionate defense of anesthesia, arguing that "*the insensibility* of the patient is a *great convenience to the surgeon*" (Mott's emphasis).

But some surgeons saw only inconvenience in having to share their operating rooms with a new medical specialist—an anesthesiologist—who might make them "a mere operator, a subordinate instead of a chief, who under all circumstances retains the supreme command," as one Edinburgh surgeon grumbled. Anesthesia went so far as to represent "the degradation of surgery against which all surgeons should guard with all their might."

Moreover, many surgeons considered ether "a remedy of doubtful safety," a poison that caused unnecessary bleeding, suffocation, TB, depression, insanity, or sometimes death. The experience of pain was thought to be somehow conducive to healing. "Pain during operations is, in the majority of cases, even desirable; its prevention or annihilation is, for the most part, hazardous to the patient," wrote a British physician. Unsurprisingly, military surgeons were among the most reluctant. "The shock of the knife is a powerful stimulant," a military surgeon wrote; "it is better to hear a man bawl lustily" from pain than "sink silently into the grave."

By anesthetizing patients, the physician was seen as temporarily "killing" them and imposing a "slavery of etherization." Perhaps he might even commit a crime such as rape against them. Like drunkenness, anesthesia was thought to induce lascivious dreams in female subjects. After hailing its discovery, the Boston surgeon Henry Bigelow himself soberly warned in his address to the Boston Society for Medical Improvement on November 9, 1846, "It is capable of abuse, and can readily be applied to nefarious ends." Alarmed by the depiction of such dangers, even patients themselves sometimes refused anesthesia.

Ether required patience—surgeons had to wait for it to take effect. It did not work on all patients, and even when it did, in lighter doses it created a state of semiconsciousness where patients, alarmingly, talked or sang. It could cause vomiting, and—most perilously—it was highly flammable. How to dose the drug to avoid exhilaration and induce sleep was poorly understood. Different kinds of inhalers produced different results. As an 1847 article in *The Lancet* noted, "In some cases there is perfect insensibility to pain," but "there are cases in which ether does not act at all or appears to act as a violent stimulus."

That same year, Sir James Young Simpson pioneered the use of chloroform, which caused unconsciousness without exhilaration. It swiftly replaced ether; indeed, its use became so universal that opponents of anesthesia in general were dubbed the Anti-Chloroformers. Hospital records of the era show us that many surgeons worked without any anesthesia, while others used chloroform for their initial cuts, but did without it during the rest of an operation, or limited their use of it to major operations. James Syme—the Scottish surgeon who had amputated poor George Wilson's foot—said he would use anesthesia only "if the patient has a very great dread of pain"! Factors such as sex, age, and ethnicity were considered in decisions regarding who merited anesthesia and when.

Many Christian churches strongly opposed using anesthesia during childbirth, on the grounds that it contradicted God's direct commandment to Eve. The entire city of Zurich banned anesthetics on these grounds. "Pain is the mother's safety, its absence her destruction," wrote an obstetrician. "Yet are there those bold enough to administer the vapour of ether even at this critical juncture, forgetting it has been ordered that 'in sorrow shall she bring forth.'"

Sir James Young Simpson argued that the Genesis commandment was actually to bring forth children not in "pain" but in "toil" (the Hebrew words for Eve's pain actually carry both meanings). And, Dr. Simpson argued, labor under anesthesia certainly involved toil. In 1853, chloroform received the ultimate imprimatur when Queen Victoria chose to use it to ease the birth of her eighth child, causing masses of women to demand "anesthesia *à la Reine*."

By the close of the nineteenth century—almost one hundred years after Michael Faraday suggested that nitrous oxide could ease pain in surgery—the acceptance of anesthesia was virtually universal, and with its acceptance, the meaning of pain in Western culture was forever altered. For if anesthesia had robbed the craft of surgery of its terrors, as Henry Bigelow put it, it also stole from pain some of its store of ancient meanings.

Tensions between secular and sacred conceptions of medicine had long existed, but efforts had always been made to reconcile the two. Ambroise Paré, for example, famously ended his case histories with the sentence, "I dressed him, God healed him." Since ancient times, sufferers had slept in the temples of the gods of healing *and* taken opium and willow bark, and for the most part, such actions were not considered inconsistent. In the nineteenth century, as Darwin's theory provided a biological framework for understanding pain and the discovery of anesthesia allowed for its control, the medical alliance between scientific and religious perspectives finally splintered.

In 1887, H. Cameron Gillies wrote a series of articles in *The Lancet* claiming that "Pain never comes where it can serve no good purpose," because pain is God's way of protecting the body. In reply, W. J. Collins argued that not all pain is protective: "Is this the grim comfort he [Gillies] would bring to a suffering woman, tortured slowly to death by a sloughing scirrhus of the breast, or to a man, made almost inhuman and killed by inches by the slow yet sure ravages of a rodent ulcer?"

The medical establishment dismissed Gillies. By the end of the Victorian era, the underlying debate was conclusively settled: there was no meaning to pain. Pain was not a metaphor; it was a biological by-product of disease. The body had been claimed as the province of science, the patient dispossessed. Pain was not passion, alchemy, ordeal; in the cosmological contest between demons and deities, it was man who had won. Thousands of years of thinking about pain were swept aside as the biological paradigm of pain displaced the religious one. The telegram went out: just as the consumptives came down the mountain, acute surgical pain could be controlled by anesthesia. Medical science could now turn to chronic pain, and surely it, too, would soon be mastered.

Surely.

Pain Diary:

I Get a Diagnosis

"I'm ordering scans of both your cervical spine and your right shoulder," my internist said. "It's good to get to the bottom of problems before they become chronic."

"How long does it take to become chronic?" I said.

"How long have you had it?" he said.

ONE'S WHOLE LIFE AND ONE'S FATE

I hope you get a good result," Kurt had told me with a measure of anxiety the night before my MRI—anxious for me, but not only for me. I could sense his desire not to have a girlfriend with a health problem. *A good result*—I should concentrate on hoping for a good result. But what would that be? Ordinarily, it would be no result at all, proving the test to have been superfluous.

In the basement of the hospital, I shed my earrings and rings and blouse and bra and lay still, as if in a sarcophagus, as the MRI machine illuminated not merely the vertebrae but also the tendons, cartilage, and disks of my spine. The spine: the stem of the body, the vine from which everything flowers. I could feel the pain even then, like a white electrical current in my neck that flowed quickly through my right shoulder and sizzled in my hand—a pain I had come to know so well.

I tried to calm myself with the Christian Scientist tenet my grandmother taught me: "There is no life, truth, intelligence, nor substance in matter. All is infinite Mind and its infinite manifestation, for God is All-in-all." The greatest fear of pain patients, doctors sometimes say, is that it's "all in their head." Infinitely scarier, I realized as I lay there, is the idea that it isn't. I knew the machine was seeing my body in a different way and that its record would be irrefutable. My pain would no longer be a tree falling in the forest with no one (but me) to hear it. Through feeling and thought, pretense and denial, hope and despair, the machine knew: the tree crashing, the tent bones breaking, the leper laughing—the truth.

"There are situations in life in which our body is our entire self and our entire fate. I was my body and nothing else," wrote the French philosopher Jean Améry of his time in Auschwitz. When I read his account in college, years away from pain, I thought, *Let that time never come. Let my body never be my fate.*

The next week, when I was to meet with my internist, I would know my fate; I would know, that is, whether my body was to be my fate.

"Ah yes, the films and the radiologist's report," my internist said. He tacked the films up on a lighted screen set into the wall beside a life-size yellow plastic model of a skeleton. He traced his finger over the films, referring periodically to the structures on the skeleton as he began to explain. The more he talked, the more animated he grew. He liked to explain things, I could tell; he knew the material, he felt confident.

I pictured my body as a skeleton in a medical school class.

This is an example of cervical spondylosis, the doctor was explaining to a sea of eager students. *Cervical spondylosis is a type of osteoarthritis. If you look closely at these vertebrae, you can see osteophyte formations on their surfaces. As the disks degenerated, the unprotected vertebrae rubbed against each other and developed calcium deposits, which are also known as bone spurs. The bone spurs impinge on the nerve roots, causing pain and weakness. Note that the opening of the spinal canal is abnormally narrow as well, the congenital problem of stenosis, which, in this case, aggravated the spondylosis.*

This skeleton belonged to a woman, age thirty-three. She reported right-sided pain and weakness. Looking at the skeleton as well as the MRIs, we can see that the degeneration was, in fact, more significant on the right side.

Additionally, we can see a problem with the right shoulder here. In some people the space between the undersurface of the acromion—the bone at the top of the shoulder—and the top of the humeral head is narrow. This narrow passageway squeezes the rotator cuff—the tendons that connect the shoulder to the arm and allow it to rotate—causing what is known as impingement syndrome, *with which this patient was diagnosed.*

The only unusual thing about this skeleton is the patient's age. Symptoms of cervical spondylosis typically first appear between the ages of forty and sixty, *although cases have been found in people as young as thirty. Normally, osteoarthritis is associated with aging, but in cases of premature wear such as this, the origin is presumably genetic, possibly aggravated by trauma.*

It is not known if any specific trauma brought this on, but the patient's history notes that she described herself as accident-prone and had broken this arm, as well as having incurred other injuries that may have contributed to the development of the condition.

What is the treatment?

Primarily symptomatic: physical therapy, pain management. The disease is most devastating when it begins early, as in this case. Over time, as the stenosis continues to narrow the vertebral passage, it may begin to impinge on the spinal cord itself—an emergency requiring immediate surgery to open up the vertebral spaces and try to preserve the cord. Patients must be monitored for signs of cord impingement such as loss of motor skills.

Married or single?

Single.

The relationship with Kurt—the long, false relationship—was over, I realized. Of course, of course, of course. I had deluded myself about the relationship, just as I had deluded myself about the pain. The two had seemed so confusing—confusing and confused—but now they were clear. My pain was not a manifestation of a personal, spiritual, or romantic problem and could not be alleviated by thinking of it that way; it was a biological condition, plain for a stranger to see.

"Questions?" the doctor said affably, and sat down at his desk. "Come now. What about what I said don't you understand?"

"Will it get better over time?"

"It's degenerative."

"Can it be fixed?"

"No, it's structural. Do you see?" He paused. "You'd need a new spine." He smiled.

I almost asked whether as it degenerated, I would have more pain, but I was too afraid of the answer.

I broke up with Kurt that night.

III

TERRIBLE ALCHEMY:

Pain as Disease

A PARTICULAR CHAMBER IN HELL

In an antique illustration of hell I saw once, each of the damned had his or her own chamber, equipped with particular instruments of torture designed to fit—or rather, not fit, as the case was—the inhabitants, from the long rack for the short woman to the Procrustean bed for the giant fellow. It was a clever painting, a vertical cross section, like the bisected rooms of a dollhouse. Thick, damp walls separated each grotto so that if the damned could hear the screams of others, they would sound faint and faraway, and anyway, who can listen with ears filled with one's own screams? No one came, and no one left. Even the devils seemed to have abandoned the place, leaving pain to do its perpetual work. Or perhaps the devils were pain itself: the invisible agent of agony writ on each inhabitant's face.

Pain is eerily common. A consensus estimate, widely used in the field, is that as many as one in five Americans suffers from chronic pain. Pain costs society as a whole billions of dollars in disability and lost productivity. Demographics have changed as baby boomers age, so that a growing portion of the population is at risk for the diseases that lead to chronic pain. Life expectancy continues to increase, but who wants a life lasting 120 years if the final third of it is spent in daily pain?

Although pain is one of the primary complaints for which people seek medical care in America, there are only 2,500 board-certified pain specialists in the United States—roughly one doctor for every 25,000 patients with chronic pain. According to a 2006 survey, just 5 percent of chronic pain patients ever see a pain specialist. Consequentially, the treatment of pain remains primarily in the hands of ordinary physicians, most of whom know little about pain and don't want or seek to know more. Medical schools and textbooks give the subject scant attention. Pain medicine as a specialty did not even exist until after World War II, when Dr. John J. Bonica—an anesthesiologist who had treated wounded soldiers—wrote the first comprehensive textbook on pain management in 1953 and was instrumental in the creation of the International Association for the Study of Pain, the first medical organization devoted to pain.

In the sixteenth century, Ambroise Paré defined the task of medicine as "cure occasionally, relieve often, console always." How could pain have strayed from such a compelling imperative?

The reason that pain per se has not, until recently, been a focus of research is that pain was understood as a symptom of an underlying disease. On this theory, the remedy was plain: treat the disease, and the pain should take care of itself. Specializing in pain medicine seemed as absurd as specializing in fever—a form of making the cart lead the horse. Yet the actual experience of patients frequently belied the assumption that pain was merely a symptom, for chronic pain often outlives its original causes, worsens over time, and takes on a puzzling life of its own.

The idea that pain leads a life of its own turns out to be not a metaphor, but a biological reality. There is increasing evidence that over time, untreated pain eventually rewrites the central nervous system, causing pathological changes to the brain and spinal cord, and that these in turn cause greater pain. Even more disturbingly, recent evidence suggests that prolonged pain actually damages parts of the brain, including those involved in cognition.

One way of explaining this shift is to say that pain itself can now be a diagnosis. "Ninety-eight percent of doctors still say pain is a symptom, not a disease," Scott Fishman explained to me. Dr. Fishman is chief of the Division of Pain Medicine at the University of California, Davis; head of the American Pain Foundation, an important patient advocacy group; and the author of *The War on Pain*, a genuinely helpful self-help book (that I wish I had read when I first got pain!). "Yes, pain is usually a secondary disease stemming from an underlying problem, just as blindness can be caused by diabetes. But that doesn't mean it isn't real and doesn't need to be treated. And over time, it often becomes the primary disease."

At first glance, the distinction between diagnosis and symptom might seem merely semantic. But in the medical context, semantics have proved to be of great importance. Getting depression recognized as a disease was half the battle in finding treatments and making them accessible to patients. The real question, then, is practical: What is the value of regarding pain as a disease? What are the results of doing so or not doing so?

Categorizing pain as a disease underlines the gravity of the threat it poses. "Pain can kill" is a motto of the new field of pain medicine—a motto that is not hyperbole. Far from being merely an unpleasant experience that people should endure with a stiff upper lip, prolonged pain turns out to actually harm the body by unleashing a cascade of neurochemical and hormonal changes that can adversely affect healing, immunity, and kidney function.

Evidence suggests that patients treated with adequate doses of opiates heal more quickly from surgery. Pain keeps people in bed after an operation, increasing the risks of problems such as blood clots. Chest and pulmonary injuries are associated with a high rate of death in part because the pain they cause makes patients breathe more shallowly. The air in their lungs stagnates and permits ordinarily harmless germs to settle in and cause diseases like pneumonia, necessitating the use of a respirator—which, in turn, introduces further risk of infection.

Adequate pain treatment may be important for general health and recovery from disease. Many of the hormones that regulate the processing of pain in the brain are also critical in regulating immune function. Stress hormones like cortisol increase with pain and impair immunity. Pain and immunity are both regulated by endorphins and local mediators of inflammation.

How could treating pain be controversial? one might ask. Why wouldn't it be treated? Who are the *opponents* of relief? Very few physicians would declare that they don't believe chronic pain exists, and although some might profess ignorance, few would say they are unwilling to treat chronic pain. Likewise, few members of the public would advocate suffering (especially if it's their own). Yet conceptions about pain, like those about pleasure, are deeply entrenched—culturally, socially, and psychologically. Chronic pain is a disease that resists measurement, and patients' self-reports are easy to dismiss or disbelieve. The cultural evolution of the understanding of depression may serve as a model for that of pain. Depression was once treated with denial (as not a real, medical problem), dismissal (as irrational emotion), and stigmatization (as something shameful that could and should be overcome). Eventually these attitudes gave way to the recognition of depression as an organically based, potentially fatal disease with both subjective psychological and objective physiological components.

If arriving at a new medical understanding of pain has been a difficult and protracted process, disseminating the knowledge will be more so. Although there is a scientific consensus about the reality of the disease, it has not gained widespread acceptance outside the small circle of pain specialists.

"My patients have seen an average of five doctors about their condition before they get to me—and some have seen a dozen, and gotten complicated and contradictory diagnoses—yet for the most part, their pain has not been treated in *the most obvious ways*," Dr. Fishman said. California and other states have mandated continuing education in pain management as a requirement for renewing a medical license, following court verdicts such as a $1.5 million judgment awarded in 2001 against a San Francisco–area internist for having undertreated a terminally ill patient's pain. In that case, the internist's defense team argued that he had never received any specific training in pain management and that he had treated his patient as best he knew how—which is probably true.

Jim Mickle, a family doctor in rural Pennsylvania (and my friend Cynthia's husband), described the leeriness ordinary physicians feel about treating pain: "Is it objective or subjective? How do you know you're not being tricked or taken advantage of to get narcotics? Chronic pain patients are, generally, well—a pain. Most doctors' reaction to a patient with chronic pain is to try to pass them off to someone who's sympathetic. Or just to try to pass them off."

What makes a doctor sympathetic to pain? Jim thought about it. "Someone who has pain himself," he said. "Or has an intellectual interest—who isn't interested in immediate results, doesn't want to make money, has a lot of degrees. We've had a few in this area, but then they get all the pain patients sent to them, and eventually they burn out and quit."

THE SHAPE-SHIFTER

Every pain patient is a testament to the dangers of the conservative wait-it-out approach to pain, as some weeks spent observing treatment at a pain clinic demonstrated. Inside the cement tower of the pain clinic in downtown Boston, all sights and sounds of the neighborhood—the swans in the Public Garden, the lanterns of Chinatown—disappeared, collapsing into a small examining room in which there was only this triad: the doctor, the patient, and pain. Of these, as the daily parade of desperation and diagnoses made evident, it was pain whose presence predominated.

What the majority of doctors see in a chronic pain patient is an overwhelming, off-putting ruin: a ruined body and a ruined life. "Chronic pain is like water damage to a house," Dr. Daniel B. Carr, then the medical director of the New England Medical Center Pain Management Center, told me. "If it goes on long enough, the house collapses." It is his job to rescue the crushed person within, to locate the original source of pain—the leak, the structural instability—and begin to rebuild, psychically, psychologically, socially.

"Some of my patients are on the border of human life." He sighed. "The mistake physicians make with chronic pain patients is that they assume that if they can't fix most of the patients' problems, they can't fix anything. They're too overwhelmed to find the treatable piece."

Dr. Carr's interest in pain began as an intellectual one. After training as an internist and an endocrinologist, in 1981 he published the landmark

study of runners that showed that exercise stimulates beta-endorphin production. He hypothesized that the increased endorphins lead to a runner's
high that temporarily anesthetizes the runner—the stress-induced analgesia of our ancestors running from the tiger. If the runner's high is an
example of how a healthy body successfully modulates pain, Dr. Carr began to wonder, then what abnormality leads to chronic pain? One way to
think of pain is to see it as the presence of a disease—a nervous system
gone amok—but another way to think about it is as *an absence of health*:
the failure of the normal controls that successfully modulate ordinary
pain.

Dr. Carr decided to do a third residency in anesthesia and pain medicine, and he became a founder of the multidisciplinary pain center at
Massachusetts General Hospital and a director of the American Pain
Society. Pain clinics are scarce: the time-consuming nature of patient care,
and the lack of quick moneymaking procedures on which insurance
reimbursement systems are based, means that these clinics tend to lose
money, and they maintain a precarious existence.

I had had pain for a few years when I was randomly offered a magazine
assignment to write about chronic pain. The assignment had been one of
several article possibilities: personal bankruptcy, a murder, a profile of a
celebrity I pretended to have heard of. My editor and I were at a Japanese
restaurant in midtown; I was poking at my sushi, thinking wistfully about
how hungry I always used to be, before I had pain, and how I used to love
being taken to lunch and ordering lots of courses. Through the glaze of
misery I heard the editor's idea. "Pain?" I said, waking up. "Does pain treatment even work?"

After I had finally gotten a diagnosis, I tried some pain treatment,
which mitigated but decidedly failed to resolve my pain. I had no confidence in any treatment methods because I didn't understand how they
were supposed to work, and I didn't want to understand—I just wanted to
be cured. But for the first time, in Dr. Carr's clinic, observing other patients' treatment, I began to wonder about the nature of pain itself.

Before going to the clinic each morning to observe Dr. Carr for my
article, I dressed carefully in a skirt and pointy shoes, anxious that the
patients not realize that I am one of them. Still, it surprised me that none
of them saw it, this scarlet *P* on my chest. I smiled tightly when the patients caught my eye. "Sounds dreadful!" I would say when they regaled

me with their stories. "Hope you get better!"—*I haven't.*—"Thanks for letting me observe!"

"If for some disease a great many different remedies are proposed, then it means that the disease is incurable," a character quips in a Chekhov play—a truth surely illustrated in the field of pain management. A pain doctor's kit has plenty of tools. There are drugs, such as antidepressants, antiseizures, anti-inflammatories, opiates, and opioids. (*Opioids* is the general term both for natural opiates derived from the opium poppy and for their synthetic counterparts, such as methadone and OxyContin, even though *opiates* is commonly—if incorrectly—used to refer to both.) There is also physical therapy, traction (to reduce pressure in the spine), chiropractic manipulation, steroid and other kinds of injections, surgery, and psychological treatments and techniques such as hypnosis, stress management, biofeedback, acupuncture, meditation, and massage.

Rarely do any of these prove to be a cure, but they can help modulate pain, offering patients "a toehold" to climb out of chronic pain syndrome, Dr. Carr said, "or at least slow the descent." Without intervention, the descent can be steep indeed. Most people with chronic pain sleep poorly (a problem exacerbated by opioid medications, which fragment sleep). Over time, sleep deprivation—a time-tested form of torture—can create the symptoms of mental illness. Yet insomnia can be treated with medication such as trazodone (which, unlike many sleeping pills, is not physically addictive, and the effects of which do not generally diminish over time). Many pain syndromes cause deconditioning and guarding behavior of the afflicted area, which can lead to muscle atrophy, which further impairs mobility and causes greater pain; physical therapy can intervene in the cycle. Pain can cause depression, which in turn causes more pain, yet depression can often be treated.

Dr. Carr's patients acquired their pain through all manner of diseases or accidents. They suffer from migraines, multiple sclerosis, rheumatoid arthritis, osteoarthritis, and fibromyalgia. And many people who suffer from chronic pain have no specific diagnosis at all. Back pain, for example, is one of the most common reasons for visiting a medical clinic, yet studies have suggested that for up to 85 percent of such cases, no definite diagnosis

can be made. People whose backs look normal on a scan can feel extraordinary pain, and people with scans that indicate problems often feel fine.
The back is too tightly wired to distinguish nerve from joint from muscular pain. This causes patients much unhappiness. What they don't realize,
however, is that it is not necessary to have a definite diagnosis in order to
get well; treatment options are sufficiently limited that a patient can
systematically work through each one.

Of all the patients of Dr. Carr whose treatment I observed, the last
patient on one day, Lee Burke, was perhaps the one whose story provided
the most insight into the current state of contemporary pain management
because her diagnosis and treatment turned out to be so simple, while the
fallacies that worked against the diagnosis being made earlier were so numerous and so revealing of the problems of pain treatment.

Seven years earlier, Lee told Dr. Carr, she had learned that she had one
of the most survivable varieties of brain tumor, a growth known as an
acoustic neuroma that nestled behind her left ear. The tumor was benign,
but its effects were not: as it grew, it threatened to squash useful parts of
her brain. The recovery period from the surgery to remove it was supposed
to be a mere seven weeks. Instead, she said, she awoke from surgery with
an unforeseen problem: headaches—lancinating, lightning-hot pain—
that knocked her out for periods ranging from four hours to four days. She
lost her job as vice president of human resources at a real estate firm. A
delicate-featured fifty-six-year-old woman in a blue cotton sweater that
picked up the blue of her eyes and the gray in her hair, she cried as she told
Dr. Carr how pain came between her and her husband when her headaches kept her in bed. She left him, and their money, and their million-dollar
condominium in downtown Boston.

"It was easier to be alone with the pain," she said. Like the wounded
animal that instinctively separates itself from the herd, many patients with
chronic pain are alone. "I couldn't hold anyone," another woman who was
suffering from a frozen shoulder explained to me. "My hands were full
with pain."

Because the head is the exclusive home of four of the five senses by
which the brain is informed of the outside world, it is commensurately
well protected by sensory nerves. Indeed, with the exception of the hands,
the brain devotes more space to processing sensory information from the

head than it does to the entire rest of the body. Damage to facial nerves thus has the capacity to cause great suffering.

Dr. Carr asked Lee to describe the headaches. Like most of the hundred-odd patients I observed in various pain clinics trying to describe their suffering, Lee seemed stumped by the question. Elaine Scarry characterizes pain as not only *not* a linguistic experience, but as a language-destroying experience. "Whatever pain achieves, it achieves in part through its unsharability, and it ensures this unsharability through its resistance to language," she writes, citing Virginia Woolf's famous observation that "English, which can express the thoughts of *Hamlet* and the tragedy of *Lear*, has no words for the shiver and the headache . . . [L]et a sufferer try to describe a pain in his head to a doctor and language at once runs dry."

Part of the curse of pain is that it *sounds* untrue to people who don't have pain. Patients grope at metaphors that seem melodramatic, both far-fetched and clichéd. "A hot, banging pain, like an ice pick," a homeless man described the diabetic neuropathy that scalds his thighs and feet as the small nerves die, deprived of oxygen by the disease. "It heats up and then sticks it in, again and again," he told Dr. Carr. "It holds my feet in the fire." He broke off, his face twisting into the particular stricken bewilderment that I observed on the faces of patients whom I watched in different pain clinics describe their afflictions: *What is tormenting me and why?*

"It's like being slammed into a wall and totally destroyed," Lee said. "It makes you want to pull every hair out of your head. There's nothing I can do to defend myself. It's like knives are going through my eyes." She started to weep again.

I felt the need to interrupt—to contradict or console. But Dr. Carr sat calmly as she blotted her face, his concentration fixed, his hands folded reassuringly across his lap, with the equable, impersonal kindness of a priest or a cop. Almost all of the patients during the long day broke down during their appointments. Perhaps because their lives echo the chaos in his own blue-collar Irish-Catholic upbringing as the son of an alcoholic bartender, he said, he isn't alarmed when patients scream at him. He is neither indifferent to emotion nor distracted by it; at all times, his focus is on the culprit—the shape-shifter, the pain.

Dr. Carr asked Lee to close her eyes, and he tapped her head with the stiff corner of an unopened alcohol wipe. Within a few minutes he had found a clear pattern of numbness that suggests that one of the main nerves in her face—the occipital nerve—was severed during her surgery. It was clear from their differing expressions that Dr. Carr regarded this as revelation—the demystification of her pain—and that Lee had no idea why.

I felt her bewilderment: *What was the connection between tapping with an alcohol wipe and the bottomless sorrow of her experience?*

Lee's voice became small as she asked, "If the nerve was cut, how could it cause pain?"

THE UNDEADNESS OF DEAD NERVES

How, indeed?

It is only recently that such phenomena have been understood. Doctors used to be entirely confident that severed nerves could not transmit pain—*they're severed!* Nerve cutting was even seen as the solution for many pain syndromes in the nineteenth and the first half of the twentieth centuries, a treatment no more effective than the old European practice of cauterizing wounds with boiling oil (standard until Ambroise Paré ran out of oil on the battlefield one day and noticed the next morning that the patients he had neglected to cauterize had fared better than those whose limbs had been helpfully scalded with boiling oil).

Americans are routinely schooled about many things, yet the inner workings of our bodies remain more remote than the turning of the planets. Certainly I had no model in my mind of the nervous system. I knew that severed nerves in the spinal cord cause paralysis. But I did not know that there are different types of nerves and that movement is enabled by motor neurons, whereas pain is transmitted by sensory neurons. Damaged or severed sensory nerves can cause only numbness, but they can also grow back irregularly and begin firing spontaneously, producing stabbing, electrical, or shooting sensations. Destroying sensory nerves as a treatment for pain usually makes sense only in the case of terminally ill patients who will die before the nerves begin to regenerate.

"Sensory nerves can come back," Dr. Scott Fishman quipped, "and when they do, they come back angry."

Indeed, nerve damage is now understood to be the cause of many chronic pain syndromes. The undeadness of dead nerves is at the center of the mystery of chronic pain—the ghost ringing the church bell in the empty steeple, signaling destruction on the land. Much chronic pain is now understood to be neuropathic—a pathology of the nervous system originating either in damage to the central nervous system of the brain and spinal cord or in damage to peripheral sensory nerves.

I took notes on science, medical terms, and studies in a pink spiral-bound notebook, which (unlike my green "Patient Interviews" or my yellow "Representation of Pain in Art, Lit, and Religion" notebooks) I presumed would be the boring notebook. In fact, I had allotted science my favorite color in order to offset its expected tedium. But the more I researched the science of chronic pain, the less dry and the more menacing it seemed.

Physical pain changes the body in the same way that emotional loss watermarks the soul. The body's pain system is not hardwired, but soft-wired (what neuroscientists call "plastic"), and it can be maladaptively molded by pain to increase its pain sensitivity. Ordinarily we think of neuroplasticity as being a positive trait: as the brain adapts to its circumstances and learns new things, new nervous pathways are laid down and old neural pathways disappear, the way the forest reclaims an untrodden path. But in the case of persistent pain, neuroplasticity is negative. The nerves in the spinal cord become hyperexcitable and begin spontaneously firing and recruiting other nerves in their service, and the whole system revs up to be increasingly responsive to pain, in a phenomenon discovered by the pain researcher Clifford Woolf and termed *peripheral sensitization* (when hypersensitivity occurs in the periphery of the body) or *central sensitization* (when hypersensitivity occurs within the central nervous system).

While the threshold to trigger the damage-detecting sensory neurons (nociceptors) is normally set by evolution at a relatively fixed point for all members of a species, peripheral sensitization and central sensitization lower that threshold, so that ordinary stimuli become painful. Central and peripheral sensitization routinely happen in a mild way after any injury, to protect the area. If you burn yourself, for example, an hour later a circle of redness will develop around the wound as the injured nerves transmit messages to the neighboring nerves, and the whole area develops an abnormal sensitivity. This heightened sensitivity serves the adaptive function of discouraging contact with the damaged tissue. If you take a bath, warm water that feels pleasant on most of your body will suddenly sting the burned area. To someone whose nervous system has been sensitized by a migraine, loud noise or bright light will hurt.

Normally, the wound begins to heal and the sensitization disappears. But in some chronic pain syndromes the sensitivity endures. Harmless stimuli—pressure or light touch—become painful, in a phenomenon known as *allodynia*. Ordinarily, light touch is transmitted by different nerves from those that register pain. In allodynia, however, the light-touch nerves change so that they function as pain nerves. To someone suffering from allodynia (which can afflict sufferers of the pain syndromes trigeminal neuralgia, postherpetic neuralgia, fibromyalgia, and peripheral neuropathy caused by injury or by a disease such as diabetes), tears can scald, a caress can feel like a blow, and the light pressure of a sock can feel like the hot iron shoes in which the wicked queen in "Snow White" was forced to dance until she died. Patients become, literally, afraid to move.

While allodynia involves harmless stimuli being misperceived as pain, chronic pain sufferers can also suffer from heightened sensitivity to painful stimuli, in a process known as *hyperalgesia* that involves an amplification of pain signals (in the periphery, or in the spinal cord, or in the brain itself). Hyperalgesia can endure long after its initial protective function has been served.

Pain begets pain. The longer that pain pathways relay pain messages, the more efficient those pathways become, causing greater pain to be transmitted, the way a stream carves a path through land, so that over time, it flows more quickly and turns into a river. Research by Allan Basbaum at the University of California, San Francisco, has shown that progressively deeper levels of pain cells in the spinal cord are activated with prolonged injury.

Hyperalgesia is a feature of many pain syndromes. Diabetic neuropathy, for example, can damage the nerves in one foot, causing local pain and numbness in it. Yet as the sufferer's entire nervous system is changed by pain over time, the other foot can become hyperalgesic as well, even though the nerves in that foot appear to be normal. Like the multiplying swarms of demons who slipped through the unguarded openings of the ancients' bodies to gorge on their blood and feast on their organs, the pain that pain spawns is ever more malign.

In short, I scrawled on the cover of the pink notebook, *"Bad, bad news."*

NEUROPATHIC PAIN SYNDROMES

Understanding chronic pain as a disease of the central nervous system sheds light on the riddle of chronic pain, solving the question of why, for many pain syndromes, there is no clear cause and why, even in pain syndromes where there is a clear-cut cause of pain, the cause bears no clear relation to the severity of the pain. Terrible osteoarthritis can be accompanied by mild (or no) pain, while mild degenerative osteoarthritic changes can cause crippling agony.

Ordinary conditions cause extraordinary pain—in some people. MRIs show only bones and tissue; doctors look at the patient's scan and say, "Your back looks fine, the swelling is gone" or "The bone's all healed," and they conclude that there is no reason for the patient still to be suffering. One study indicated that a full one-third of damaged disks looked normal on an MRI; another study indicated that nearly half of patients under sixty who had visibly degenerated disks on an MRI felt normal. The problem does not always lie in the tissue and bones; it can lie in the invisible hydra of nerves that MRIs often cannot detect.

Not all chronic pain is neuropathic. There is also muscular pain, nociceptive pain (pain that stems from tissue damage or inflammation), and psychogenic pain (physical pain that is caused, augmented, or prolonged by emotional factors). Pain-causing conditions usually involve multiple types of pain. However, many chronic pain complaints, like backache, that were once assumed to be wholly musculoskeletal, are now thought to have a hidden neuropathic component. Over time, neuropathic pain leads to musculoskeletal pain. Nerve pain makes muscles spasm, which in turn interferes with normal use of the area, which causes weakness and eventually atrophy. Changes in the person's mood and sleep and finally personality set in, and the original problem—the nerve injury—becomes harder to detect.

"There's tremendous ignorance about neuropathic pain," commented Dr. Clifford Woolf, a Harvard professor who is one of the world's foremost researchers of neuropathic pain. "Most doctors don't know to look for it."

Many unexplained chronic pain syndromes that appear not to be coupled with any nerve injury may be a result of a neurobiological amplification of pain signals that leads to central sensitization and hyperalgesia. With IBS (irritable bowel syndrome), which causes unexplained intestinal distress, for example, the abnormality may not originate in the intestines themselves, but rather in the person's central nervous system.

Another good example is fibromyalgia, a baffling syndrome that disproportionately affects women, the symptoms of which include chronic muscular pain, fatigue, depression, and heightened sensitivity to touch. Patients feel as if they have been "beaten up," as one patient put it, or are achy from a flu that never goes away. The disturbance appears to reside not in their muscles, but in their nervous systems. Fibromyalgia patients have been shown to have lower pain thresholds and altered chemistry in their spinal cords and in the parts of their brains involved in regulating pain. They also suffer from a dysregulation of the neurotransmitter dopamine (which is intimately involved in feelings of well-being) and a dysregulation of the neurotransmitters serotonin and norepinephrine (which are involved in both depression and pain modulation). The predilection to develop fibromyalgia is likely to be genetic.

Although fibromyalgia has been studied since the seventeenth century, it was not formally recognized as a disease until 1987, and many physicians continue to believe it is a psychological disorder. Of the dozens of women I saw in pain clinics during my research who were suffering from fibromyalgia, every one had had the experience of being disbelieved and being asked questions such as "Are you having marital problems?" in an insinuating tone, as if that were the cause of their pain. (And many were; chronic disease usually causes marital problems.)

Dr. Richard Gracely and Dr. Daniel Clauw have examined fibromyalgia patients and patients suffering from lower-back pain that has no identified cause. In one study, they attached a small device to the base of subjects' thumbnails that applied pulsing pressure at varying levels ranging from innocuous to painful. The investigators discovered that the subjects with fibromyalgia and back pain said they experienced mild pressure as painful, while the healthy control subjects experienced the squeeze as only slightly unpleasant.

Were those patients just—as British doctors like to say—moaners? Before the invention of functional brain imaging (a technique that allows researchers to take a video of sorts, or a 3-D movie, of the brain as it responds to pain), the question would have been unanswerable. Doctors' impressions of patients' credibility would have been mainly a reflection of their own personalities and whether they were inclined to believe or disbelieve patients. But in the Gracely and Clauw study, functional imaging was able to see that the patients were truthfully describing their experiences as the imaging documented activation in the pain-processing areas of the brain—activation that was not seen in the control subjects' brains until the pressure on their thumbs was dramatically increased.

What was the pain-processing circuitry in my brain like? I wondered when I read about the study. Was there a brain imaging study I could volunteer for?

SURGICAL PAIN SYNDROMES

Surgeons warn patients of many remote risks, from blood clots to the possibility of anesthesia producing a fatal reaction, but they often don't mention (and perhaps remain largely unaware of) the much more likely possibility of developing chronic neuropathic pain. One of Dr. Carr's patients was a wealthy man whose life was ruined by having a nerve nicked during plastic surgery to correct protruding ears. Another patient acquired chronic chest pain after being treated in a hospital for a collapsed lung, when a tube was inserted in her chest—one of the body's most nerve-rich areas. One poignant category of patients in pain clinics is that of those who have had surgery specifically *to treat* chronic pain, but instead, whose surgery worsened their pain, an outcome for which they say they had no warning. Pain following the common back surgery of laminectomy (which removes part of the vertebral bone and sometimes surrounding ligaments and muscles as well) is so common that it has a name (*post-laminectomy syndrome*).

The classic method of performing a thoracotomy (a chest incision that cuts through ribs to gain access to the heart, lungs, or other organs) carries a high risk of lasting pain. In one study, 30 percent of patients reported pain four years after their surgery. "If you ask thoracic surgeons," Dr. Woolf said, "they would say, these are big life-threatening situations—heart surgery or cancer. The fact that the patient has pain for the rest of his life is not important—they feel, 'I saved your life, what do you expect?' Pain is not seen as life threatening. And until patients have pain, they can't imagine what it's like—the way it's there all the time and makes you miserable."

A significant percentage of cancer survivors suffer from chronic pain, stemming either directly from their tumors or from their treatment (radiation and chemotherapy can damage nerves just as surgery can). Moreover, survivors often have difficulty finding doctors willing to prescribe opioids once their pain no longer enjoys the social sanctification accorded by malignancy.

A landmark 1997 University of Toronto study by Dr. Anna Taddio and others has troubling implications about the impact of pain on infants and children. The study compared the pain responses of groups of infant boys who were uncircumcised, circumcised with an anesthetic cream, and circumcised without anesthesia. Four to six months later, the group who had been circumcised without anesthesia had the lowest pain threshold, crying longer and showing more visible signs of pain at their first inoculations, providing evidence that there is enduring cellular pain memory when damage is inflicted upon the immature nervous system.

A CLASSIC MISINTERPRETATION

At some level, every doctor is familiar with central sensitization because they know that a patient who comes in with twenty years of back pain is more than twenty times less likely to get well than one who comes in after just six weeks (a fact I wish I had appreciated before my pain settled in).

"In our clinic, we're trying to undo eons of pain history—problems that began in the Mesozoic era," Dr. Carr commented. "The only real cure for chronic pain is prevention. But everything from physician and patient ignorance to managed care policies of *delay, defer, deny* means that by the time a patient gets to a pain clinic, it's late. Sometimes I wish I could send them back to their early doctors and say, 'Don't you see what's going to happen to this person if you keep letting this go?'"

Leigh Burke complained of pain for more than a year after the surgery for her brain tumor before she was referred to a cancer pain specialist and anesthesiologist whom she liked very much. Her records do not even note whether her occipital nerve was cut, and (since the risk of chronic pain is not an issue surgeons usually consider) her surgeon may not have noticed the dental floss–size nerve. At any rate, the Nice Doctor, as she thought of him, did not investigate the nerve; what were visible to him were severe muscle spasms in Leigh's head, neck, and shoulders.

It was a classic pain misinterpretation. He seized on muscular pain as the primary problem—the pain generator—rather than a secondary symptom, and he diagnosed tension headaches. He injected her forehead with

Botox—a preparation that, when injected into muscles in minute doses, essentially paralyzes them and thus prevents spasms for a few months. Although Botox is known mainly as a cosmetic treatment for reducing wrinkles, it is increasingly being used to treat a variety of medical problems, including headaches (even migraines).

He also prescribed migraine medicines and tricyclic antidepressants (an older form of antidepressants, which are considered more effective against chronic pain than the newer SSRIs, such as Prozac and Zoloft, but have more troublesome side effects). She tried range-of-motion physical therapy, stress-reduction courses, psychiatric treatment, yoga, and meditation. She also drank a dozen cups of coffee a day—an ill-advised treatment for migraines (small amounts of caffeine help headaches; large amounts produce dependency and can create rebound headaches). The Nice Doctor steered her away from opioids with warnings about their addictive qualities. Instead, she took dangerously large amounts of ibuprofen and Tylenol.

The Nice Doctor later explained to me that he felt comfortable with anti-inflammatory drugs and uncomfortable with opioids. Yet while large doses of the drugs are sometimes needed to treat inflammation, contrary to popular opinion, for long-term use, opioids can be a safer and more effective analgesic. Certainly, when I was overdosing on Tylenol, Advil, Motrin, aspirin, and Aleve, I would have been astonished to learn that. While anything over-the-counter seemed benign, I believed the rhetoric that opioids are a "gateway drug" that turn ordinary people into tragic statistics.

Anti-inflammatories are most effective at easing the pain of—*surprise*—inflammation, which comes from injury or inflammation-causing diseases such as rheumatoid arthritis. Tylenol, which works through an unknown mechanism, is not in fact classified as an anti-inflammatory. (The effects of its basic chemical compound were originally discovered when a pharmacist's mistake caused it to be accidentally given to a patient, whose fever was dramatically reduced.) It was introduced into the market in the 1950s, where it was a huge success, undermining aspirin's market domination. Although Tylenol does not upset the stomach, taking the maximum recommended dose longer than the short period the manufacturer recommends can cause liver toxicity, liver failure, and even death (risks that increase greatly when these drugs are consumed with alcohol, as I used to do). The most common cause of acute liver failure in the Western world is toxicity from acetaminophen (the ingredient in Tylenol). An often-fatal disease, liver failure annually affects two thousand people in the United States. According to a 2002 study, while a majority of the patients had exceeded the daily maximum recommended dose, nearly one-fifth had not. Three-quarters of the patients were women, although it is not known whether women are innately more susceptible to acute liver failure or are simply inclined to take more over-the-counter medications.

Aleve, aspirin, Motrin, and other nonsteroidal anti-inflammatory drugs (NSAIDs), as they are called, pose an even greater problem, causing stomach ulcers in as many as one-fourth of all patients who take them on a long-term basis. Each year 6,000 to 7,500 Americans die from gastrointestinal bleeding and related complications associated with taking NSAIDs.

"IT'S HARD WORK BEHAVING AS A CREDIBLE PATIENT"

Even as they endangered her life, the massive doses of Tylenol and aspirin medications failed to reduce Lee Burke's pain to a manageable level. Seven years—a biblical length of time—elapsed, during which she became increasingly disabled. She went from specialist to specialist—headache specialists, balance specialists, and behavioral pain-medicine specialists—and her worsening condition was met by skepticism, contempt, irritation, frustration, and pity.

Women report more frequent pain, as well as pain of greater intensity and duration, than men. They suffer disproportionately from pain-causing conditions, such as autoimmune diseases, migraines, headaches, musculoskeletal pain, and abdominal pain. In addition, they are more likely to seek treatment for pain than men are, and when they do, they present—or are perceived as presenting—more psychological symptoms. In medical literature throughout the centuries, the archetypal "problem patient" is a woman. Thus, a woman coming into the office of a male physician may find herself having inadvertently entered a highly coded complex social situation, the nature of which she may not understand and which may not serve her well.

A fascinating 2003 Norwegian study by Dr. Anne Werner, a sociologist, and Dr. Kirsti Malterud, a physician and researcher, focused on the gender dynamics between women with chronic pain and their physicians. Entitled "It's Hard Work Behaving as a Credible Patient," the paper detailed the ways in which women with chronic pain symptoms try to discern and comply with the hidden rules of the medical encounter in order to get the help they need. The women described struggling to present their pain in a way that others will feel is "just right": to make their symptoms "socially visible, real, and physical" and to achieve "a subtle balance not to appear too strong or too weak, too healthy or too sick."

The balance proves to be elusive. As in many other studies, the women provided accounts of how they were "met with skepticism and lack of comprehension, feeling rejected, ignored and being belittled," and continually "tested" and "assessed" for psychological factors. "How assertive can patients be without appearing too strong to pass as . . . ill?" the women wondered. Although they felt they needed to be assertive in order to get referrals, pain medication, sick leave, and treatment, some of the women were working to demonstrate "appropriate surrender" and to appear to follow the doctor's recommendations. Rather than confront their doctor with unmet needs, they often left him without saying why and paid for treatment themselves elsewhere. "You have to tread rather softly," one woman explained, "because once you antagonize them, it's not certain that you're any better off."

The women were also busy trying to achieve "appropriate appearance" because they felt—as in the case of rape—that their clothes and appearance were used to assess their credibility. "Comments such as 'You don't look ill' . . . or 'you are so young' made them feel irritated, sad and frustrated rather than flattered." They tried not to dress too attractively. They were concerned that if they exercised, their illness would not be believed. One woman felt she had tried too hard in a test of muscular strength and thus was seen as healthier than other patients who had tried less hard. Another woman discovered that spending time in the sun had given her too healthy a glow when the doctor greeted her by saying, "You're not ill!" She gazed at him in stunned silence, and he changed it to, "You certainly don't look ill!" The young women were told they were too young to have chronic pain; the middle-aged women were told their symptoms were merely menopausal.

Dr. Carr gave Lee a new medication—Neurontin—that has been found to be specifically effective against neuropathic pain. Invented as an antiseizure drug, Neurontin quiets the misfiring nerves responsible for neuropathic pain. He also told her to replace Tylenol and aspirin with Darvocet (an opioid) and Soma (a muscle relaxant).

When I called Lee four months after her appointment with Dr. Carr, she said she felt 50 percent better from a combination of Neurontin, Darvocet, Soma, and other drugs. The muscle spasms—so rigid that the Nice Doctor compared them to railroad tracks—had melted. She no longer needed a snorkel for her daily swim because she could move her head from side to side again. As with opioids, the side effects of large doses of Neurontin can be considerable. But while her headaches sometimes required so much Neurontin that she was too dazed to walk, Lee was glad to be able to sit up to watch television instead of simply lying prone in agony.

"Dr. Carr is my savior," she said. I recalled the way she left the appointment, clasping his hand as if she wanted to kiss it and looking at him with hope so intense it was hard to watch.

THE PARADOX OF PATIENTS' SATISFACTION WITH INADEQUATE PAIN MANAGEMENT

The outcome of pain treatment is rarely measured," commented Dr. Woolf. "The doctor hopes the patient has gotten better, of course, but often as not they simply got discouraged and went away."

He recalled a surgeon giving a talk about the success of the dorsal column stimulator—an electronic device implanted in the spinal cord on the theory that it interferes with the transmission of pain signals (a treatment I considered for myself). Dr. Woolf found that the surgeon's impressions were contradicted by one of his residents, who had actually communicated with the patients. The device was a *surgical* success, it turned out (it was properly implanted; the patients didn't suffer infections or blood clots, etc.). It just didn't help patients' pain—or at least not enough to offset the buzzing feeling patients describe as similar to having a bee trapped under their skin. Patients (such as a West Virginian coal miner with back pain whom I met) sometimes elect to have dorsal column stimulators eventually removed, but not necessarily by the same doctor.

Most patients avoid returning to doctors for whom they will represent failure, which would force them to confront not only the physician but also their own anger and disappointment. Fitting this pattern, I never let the orthopedist know I hadn't had a bicycle accident. Whenever I considered it, I pictured myself starting to yell, *I don't even own a bicycle*, and perhaps even bursting into tears, and who wants to make a call like that? After Dr. Carr gave her a new protocol, Lee Burke never spoke to the

Nice Doctor again, so he was left to assume that she was satisfied with her care and that she no longer consulted him simply because she no longer needed to.

Yet by the time she consulted Dr. Carr, Lee had been under the Nice Doctor's care for seven years. Why had she stayed so long if she wasn't improving?

Many studies document that most patients do not get good pain treatment. A 2005 Stanford University survey found that of the chronic pain sufferers who actually went to a doctor, fewer than half received adequate pain treatment, while the American Pain Society found that the same is true of cancer patients. A 2008 survey by researchers at the University of Pennsylvania and the National Cancer Institute found that more than a third of breast cancer patients who reported pain did not use medication to manage it. The primary reason patients gave: their health-care provider did not recommend pain medication. (This reason was followed by fear of addiction or the inability to pay.)

Why don't patients demand adequate pain treatment? A 2002 study by the U.S. Cancer Pain Relief Committee explored a more confounding barrier, which it termed "the paradox of patients' satisfaction with inadequate pain management." Although 43 percent of patients said that they had experienced moderate or severe pain in the previous three days, only 14 percent said they were dissatisfied with their pain management, and 77 percent said they were satisfied or very satisfied with how their pain was managed overall! The study's puzzling observation: "Recent pain intensity was not a significant predictor of satisfaction with pain management provided by the doctor."

Patients expressed resignation to their pain (commenting that they were "not one to take pills," "can stand pain," "hate to bother people," "have to live with it," "getting used to pain," "hurt a long time"). Many believed their doctor had done his or her best ("doctors have done all they can"). "Patients also expressed acceptance of their pain because it was chronic, implicitly endorsing the inability of doctors to manage this type of pain, through their maximally positive ratings," the authors observed. Willingness to take opioids greatly increased if the doctor or nurse explained that—when properly used—they were not addictive.

It had previously been demonstrated that by far the single most important factor in the successful treatment of chronic pain is confidence and trust in the provider. This study found that a primary care doctor or nurse *telling* the patient that alleviating pain was an important goal predicted roughly *as great a satisfaction as the patient actually sustaining relief within the past year.* In short, "inadequate pain management in the context of a caring or otherwise good relationship with the doctor can lead to inappropriately low patient expectations concerning pain relief," the study concluded—a conclusion echoed by the experience of Lee Burke. She said she never questioned the Nice Doctor's care because he seemed so empathetic.

When Lee's ex-husband—a malpractice lawyer—saw how Lee improved after Dr. Carr's treatment, he suggested that they sue the Nice Doctor. "But I would never do that," she said. "There were times I was in tears from the pain and he was in tears with me."

The drugs that ended up helping Lee—Neurontin, Darvocet, and a muscle relaxant—are extremely common. Apart from opioids, Neurontin is one of the most widely used drugs to treat pain, popular not only with pain specialists but also with primary care physicians because it has no risk of addiction. What prevented the Nice Doctor from thinking of these options?

My heart beat faster as I dialed the Nice Doctor's number.

I agreed with Lee that he was nice. He spoke about his concern for Lee and his frustration at the intractability of her condition. He also advocated the importance of a mechanistic understanding of pain and asked whether I knew the work of his Harvard colleague, Clifford Woolf. Contrary to Dr. Woolf's findings, however, the Nice Doctor believed that the pain of all the patients who had the type of tumor that Lee had should be similar, and in his experience most patients did, in fact, "respond to simpler, more holistic therapies." He was convinced that Lee suffered from tension headaches because she had such severe muscle contractions that even a light touch could make her wince.

Although Dr. Woolf and others had stressed that most doctors do not take account of neuropathic pain, it struck me as telling that even a pain doctor—confronted with a case in which there was a clear-cut cause for suspecting nerve injury—could still miss the diagnosis of neuropathic pain by focusing on secondary symptoms, such as muscle contractions, instead.

Because the Nice Doctor hadn't thought of Lee's pain as neuropathic, he had not considered Neurontin, and he feared opioids. "We don't always do patients a favor putting them on *high-dose narcotics*," he chided, assuming the particular intonations people do when borrowing language from the war on drugs. "If someone's dying of cancer, there's no drug we're afraid to prescribe. But when a patient is depressed or anxious, you're leery about narcotics," he said. "With Lee, I guess I'd have to say I was being cautious."

His voice changed—softened and quieted—as he got to the real point: "I was afraid."

Lee recalled that whenever the Nice Doctor sent her to other specialists, she would break down during the appointments in pain and frustration. "They all just figured I was a basket case," she said. "And I was. I was a basket case."

A 2004 study at the University of Milan School of Medicine asked 151 doctors to "tell us about an episode during your professional experience in which you found yourself in difficulty whilst confronting a patient who was in pain." The paper identified three modes of discourse in which the doctors talked about their patients: the biological perspective, the professional perspective, and the personal perspective. Many of the doctors did not talk exclusively in any of these modes, but fluctuated among them in discussing different patients or even in discussing one patient.

The biological perspective involves a "depersonalization" of pain—splitting off the disease from the suffering person. The doctor who assumes the biological perspective views the patient through the prism of pathophysiology. Yet such a mode collapsed every time that a simple biological model failed to explain a patient's pain—as it frequently did. In the personal perspective, the doctor becomes deeply identified with the suffering of the patient. But this perspective has risks: he may idealize her and turn her into a "hero patient." And when the doctor fails to be a hero himself by curing her pain, he may become a "hurt healer" and defensively distance himself from her, becoming upset and overwhelmed and even blaming her for failing to get better. Only the third perspective—the professional perspective—is able to reconcile science with compassion so that a patient's pain is seen as a biological phenomenon, but one that takes place in the context of the person's life, of which biology is only a part.

The Nice Doctor seemed to empathize with Lee, but in an excessively personal way that clouded, rather than clarified, his clinical judgment. He became overly focused on her psychic distress, trying to explain her pain through that prism: "Lee's pain seemed to be better at the times she was happier, was forming new relationships or helping others," he said. "And even though she was motivated and worked hard on stress reduction, the fact remains, she *is* a tense person."

THE SCAR HYPOTHESIS

W as anxiety, depression, or any other psychic problem the cause of Lee's pain? Or was her pain making her miserable?

It is generally estimated that between one-third and one-half of people who suffer from chronic pain also have a major depressive disorder. Conversely, pain is a frequent complaint in the psychiatric clinic: a Stanford University study of major depression found that almost half of those who are depressed also suffer from chronic pain. But the relationship between pain and depression turns out not to be one of those pointless chicken-and-egg questions.

A review study led by Dr. David A. Fishbain at the Leonard M. Miller School of Medicine at the University of Miami examined eighty-three studies that explored the relationship between the quality and extent of pain and the depths of depression among patients suffering from a variety of painful conditions (headache, spinal cord injury, cancer, angina, back pain, and so forth).

The majority of studies that tested what he calls *the antecedent hypothesis*—the idea that depression preceded pain—found it to be untrue, while all of the studies testing *the consequence hypothesis*, that depression follows pain, found it to be true. Moreover, the more severe the pain, the greater the depression. For patients who suffered from intermittent pain, the periods of depression echoed the periods of pain. The same was true of suicide: thoughts of suicide, suicide attempts, and completed suicides occurred far more frequently in those suffering from pain than in the general population and increased directly in proportion to the severity of pain.

Naturally, we might say: pain is depressing, disheartening, dispiriting. Who needs a study to understand that? But pain and depression turn out to be far more profoundly linked than is commonly understood: they are biologically entwined diseases with a common pathophysiology stemming from a common genetic vulnerability.

Chronic pain sufferers are more likely to have suffered from a depressive episode in the past and to respond to the onset of pain with a recurrence of depression. Dr. Fishbain analyzed studies that examined what he calls *the scar hypothesis*: that a genetic predisposition to recurrent depression is correlated with one for chronic pain. Depression is known to have a strong genetic component: sufferers frequently have family members or relatives who are or have been sufferers as well. And pain and depression are known to involve overlapping neural circuitry. Brain imaging scans reveal similar disturbances in brain chemistry in both chronic pain and depression.

There is increasing evidence that both conditions involve abnormalities in the neurotransmitters serotonin and norepinephrine, which play a role not only in mood disorders but in the gate-control mechanisms of pain. Increasing serotonin in rats engenders pain relief, while depleting serotonin increases their pain responses to electric shock. Pain decreases available serotonin (by increasing the rate at which it is reabsorbed), which weakens the pain-modulation system, creates more pain, and creates depression. Thus, we can see that anxiety and depression are not merely cognitive or affective responses to pain; *they are physiologic consequences of it.*

Pain causes depression just as reliably as difficulty breathing triggers panic. Thus the Nice Doctor's decision not to prescribe opioids for Leigh because she seemed "tense" makes no more sense than "not rescuing someone who is drowning because they're having a panic attack!" exclaimed Dr. William Breitbart, chief of the psychiatry service at Memorial Sloan-Kettering Cancer Center. "Serotonin facilitates descending analgesia" (the brain's ability to modulate pain in the spinal cord by stopping incoming pain messages), "and chronic pain uses up serotonin, like a car running out of gas. If the pain persists long enough, everybody runs out of gas."

Stressful events naturally enhance pain in those with a biological predisposition to it. "If we started putting sugar in the water, it would affect the diabetics first—pain patients respond to stress with increased pain," explained Dr. Scott Fishman, who trained as a psychiatrist as well as a pain specialist. But to make stress reduction a primary strategy for pain treatment is like counseling a drowning person to relax.

"Dr. Carr finally threw me a rope," Lee said.

OPIOID ADDICTION AND PSEUDO-ADDICTION

The misunderstandings that surround opioids have made doctors increasingly reluctant to prescribe them. In much of China and Africa, opioids are largely unavailable or prohibited. Opioids are stigmatized in the Muslim world on theological grounds; like alcohol, they are often considered a toxin that is prohibited by the Koran. Cheap opiates, such as morphine, that are no longer under patent are one of the few effective medical drugs that every country could afford. Yet the cultural acceptance of pain is such that few use these drugs. Most of the people in sub-Saharan Africa, for example, have no access to treatment for cancer (no chemotherapy, no radiation, no surgery), but if they had opioids, at least cancer sufferers could die without pain. And even in countries with high rates of infant mortality and obstetric complications, women could have access to painkillers.

In China, cultural taboos prohibit both opioids and the acknowledgment of the need for them. Decrying a nation of addicts, Mao banned opium (although he was not above growing and selling it to fund his army); today the cultural prohibition against opiates in China remains strong enough that their use is largely restricted to the elite—even for postsurgical pain. Surgeries in China are still sometimes performed using acupuncture alone, which sometimes controls pain and sometimes fails. Dr. Carr recalled observing some gruesome surgeries where the patients screamed in agony. Yet when he visited the patients in the hospital afterward, they assured him they did not suffer excessive pain during or after the operation. (Sometimes they had been given ketamine, a drug that affects memory, including memory of pain.)

Opiates are often portrayed as genies—trickster figures offering to do your bidding only in order to ultimately enslave you to theirs. Baudelaire lamented that opium was like a woman—"and like all mistresses, alas! prolific in caresses and betrayals." But in truth, opioids are neither the snake in the garden nor the Milk of Paradise. For a variety of reasons, as will be discussed later, the drugs do more harm than good for many people with chronic pain. They are much less effective against neuropathic than acute pain. A 2003 study led by Dr. Kathleen Foley at Memorial Sloan-Kettering Cancer Center in New York City found only a 36 percent reduction in pain among patients with chronic neuropathic pain receiving high-dose opioid therapy, and only a 21 percent reduction among patients receiving the low dose.

But if opioids are less efficacious for chronic pain than commonly believed, they are also less addictive. Studies of opioid addiction vary, but a recent analysis that appeared in *Pain Medicine*—of twenty-four studies involving more than twenty-five hundred patients with chronic non-cancer pain on long-term opioid therapy—put the average risk of addiction at slightly above 3 percent. But for chronic pain patients with no history of addiction, the rate was extremely low (0.19 percent).

The disease of addiction usually manifests itself early, when people are first exposed to addictive substances. Patients who have no previous history of drug or alcohol abuse are unlikely to become addicted to pain drugs, especially when they are elderly. It is undeniable, however, that if doctors started prescribing more opioids, the drugs would be more widely abused because some patients would conceal addiction histories or feign pain in order to solicit drugs for resale. A 3 percent abuse rate of a widely prescribed drug translates into a lot of addicts. The question for society, then, is not, *Does treating pain risk feeding addiction* (because it obviously does that) but, *To what extent should that risk influence pain treatment?* What are the moral implications of denying opioids to patients who are likely to benefit from them?

"Are we really going to allow the fact of substance abusers to deny others pain medication?" asks Dr. Daniel Carr. "Are we going to ban alcohol because of drunk driving or ration food because some people are overweight?" In *The Culture of Pain*, David Morris argues that withholding pain medication is nearly the moral equivalent of inflicting pain.

"We live in a medical society that would rather prevent one addict from being formed than treat a hundred suffering," Dr. Scott Fishman observes. "The war on drugs hurts the war on pain." Yet the eradication of pain is a more winnable cause.

Dr. Russell K. Portenoy, chairman of the Department of Pain Medicine and Palliative Care at Beth Israel Medical Center in New York City, pioneered the use of opioids to treat non-cancer pain. Dr. Portenoy recalls how, when he was a fellow being trained in pain management, it was widely accepted to treat cancer patients with high doses of opioids, while patients who did not have cancer but were just as disabled by chronic pain would not be offered opioids until many other treatments had failed. "Why is this treatment so accepted for one kind of pain and not the other?" he wondered.

One source of pervasive confusion about opioids lies in the difference between dependence and addiction. Everyone who takes opioids becomes physically dependent on them, such that abruptly stopping them produces withdrawal symptoms like trembling, headache, sweating, and nausea. But withdrawal symptoms can generally be avoided through gradually tapering doses. People with the disease of addiction, however, find themselves unable to taper their drug usage, not because of the unpleasant side effects of withdrawal, but because they experience an overwhelming craving. This craving differs not just in intensity but in character from ordinary withdrawal symptoms and stems from psychological, social, and genetic factors that are not fully understood.

Moreover, it requires a skilled physician to distinguish addiction from pseudo-addiction. Patients who are prescribed opioids that are inadequate to treat their pain may demand, beg, or even attempt to surreptitiously obtain more medication in a way that arouses fears of addiction in their physicians. Sometimes these behaviors lead to the patients' having their medication terminated, when in fact they should simply have been given a different or greater prescription.

Patients who admit to prior histories of addiction are rarely prescribed opioids. Yet the abuse of drugs, including alcohol, marijuana, and even opioids, can be a misguided form of self-medication or a manifestation primarily of addiction, but nonetheless driven by the stress or discomfort associated with pain. Dr. Portenoy tells the story of an alcoholic to whom he gave the benefit of the doubt. He made the right decision, for "it turned out the patient's pain was driving his drinking," and when the pain was

treated, he stopped drinking. But treating addicts requires greater moni-
toring; it is not only more time-consuming for the doctor, it is also risky.
In the current political climate, in which physicians have reason to fear
repercussions if a patient abuses drugs, many are increasingly unwilling
to try.

Perhaps the trickiest aspect of opioids is that there is no fixed proper
dose. Opioids have extraordinarily various effects on different people.
Dr. Portenoy explains that while most people receiving chronic opioid
therapy take a daily dose of less than 180 mg of morphine or its equivalent
(such as 120 mg OxyContin), he and other pain specialists have patients
who require the equivalent of more than 1,000 mg of morphine per day!

Dr. Portenoy says that many patients who take opioids have long periods of stable dosing but intermittently experience a flare-up of pain that
justifies an increase in the dose to maintain pain control (the medical term
for this is *titrating to effect*). As long as the balance between pain relief and
side effects remains favorable, he argues, the new dose should be continued. Over a long period of time, these events may lead to doses gradually
being adjusted upward to very high levels. Dr. Portenoy recalls a talk show
he was once on, in which he asked some elderly female patients of his to
join him; the elderly women explained blithely to the audience that they
were taking doses of opioids that would asphyxiate a football player. "There
is no ceiling dose on opioids," Dr. Portenoy says—a concept even many
physicians find difficult to grasp.

Once a person has become tolerant of the dangerous effects of an opioid, particularly respiratory depression, a high dose can be safely given.
(In this respect, the side effects of opioids are unlike those of other drugs,
such as Tylenol, where the liver never becomes tolerant of high doses.) If
a high dose of opioids were given to an "opioid-naïve" person, it would
put her in her grave (hence the high rate of deaths from accidental over-
doses of recreationally used opioids, like heroin).

In 2007, guidelines for primary care physicians were issued in the state
of Washington that warned them not to prescribe doses higher than 80 mg
of oxycodone or OxyContin for chronic pain. Patients who required
higher doses (as would be the case for most chronic pain patients) were
supposed to be referred to pain specialists. Yet the same state agency offers
a list of only fifteen such specialists. And—as recent prosecutions of physicians indicate—doctors who dissent have much to fear.

PROSECUTING PRESCRIBERS

The opioid backlash began in the late 1990s, when a rise in prescriptions of OxyContin led to an increase in abuse, particularly in small towns in Maine, Massachusetts, and Appalachia, where other recreational drugs were hard to come by. OxyContin is a new preparation of an old opioid, oxycodone (also used in Percocet), reformulated with a time-release mechanism designed to allow patients to avoid the typical peaks and troughs of pain relief associated with opioids, which had enslaved patients' schedules to the drugs' periods of peak efficacy. OxyContin's maker, Purdue Pharma, aggressively marketed the drug to ordinary physicians, claiming that OxyContin was less subject to abuse than other opiate drugs. But this turned out not to be true: addicts quickly learned that all they had to do to get high was to crush the tablets to destroy the time-release mechanism and then snort or inject the powder.

During the George W. Bush administration, the Drug Enforcement Administration (DEA) expanded the war on drugs by creating an action plan on OxyContin. Purdue was prosecuted, the company and its top executives pleaded guilty to misrepresenting their product and misleading physicians, and Purdue paid more than $600 million in fines. For the DEA, the addicts—often kids filching pills from their parents' medicine cabinets—were petty targets. But the prescribing physicians were not; if a criminal case is brought against a doctor, the DEA and local investigators are entitled to seize the physician's assets (on the grounds that they are drug profits). Moreover, the addicts could be compensated for their cooperation: if a physician is convicted in a criminal court, his or her patients may be able to win a civil case (with a lower standard of proof) against the physician for feeding their addictions!

It takes only a few lawsuits—or simply the threat of DEA oversight and regulation—to exert a chilling effect on prescribing practices. "Doctors feel damned if they do and damned if they don't," commented Dr. Scott Fishman. One day, brain imaging may develop to the point of being able to provide objective documentation of pain for each patient. But at the moment, a doctor can always be fooled by a patient who is feigning pain in order to misuse drugs. "You have to be willing to make mistakes," Dr. Carr said, "and you have to accept that some patients will take advantage of you, and your feelings will get hurt."

Hurt feelings are one thing; the threat of imprisonment is quite another. Of course there have always been physicians who actually *are* drug dealers—who sell prescriptions for money or sex and are appropriate targets for criminal indictments. But never before have physicians been held responsible for drug abuse that they did not know about or profit from.

The case of Dr. Ronald McIver, a sixty-five-year-old South Carolina pain specialist who received a thirty-year sentence for drug trafficking in 2005, is particularly striking. The government based its prosecution on a few patients who feigned pain to get prescriptions because they were addicted or wanted to sell the drugs. Dr. McIver took the precaution of requiring his patients to sign an opioids contract, stating, among other restrictions, that they would not ask for early refills of the medication and would bring their pills in at each appointment to show that they had the right number left. He became suspicious of two of his patients (one of whom he stopped treating after the patient altered a prescription to get an early refill) and wrote a letter to the state's Bureau of Drug Control asking them to investigate. Instead the DEA later used his letter as proof that he had knowledge of the diversion of pills he had prescribed!

After the verdict, for an article in *The New York Times Magazine*, Tina Rosenberg interviewed jury members who told her that they felt the dosing levels were too high. One juror thought his sister-in-law had become addicted to pain pills; another said that she had once been given opioids for a minor ailment, so she believed she knew what a standard dose was and Dr. McIver's dose was too high. None of the jurors appeared to grasp the idea that there is no ceiling dose for opioids. Still, they seemed shocked to find out that Dr. McIver had been sentenced to thirty years in prison (since they were not part of the sentencing phase of the case).

Since Dr. McIver did not profit from his patients' drug trafficking, the prosecutors had to come up with a motive to prove their contention that he intentionally prescribed drugs he knew would not be used for pain treatment. They proposed that he prescribed the drugs so that the patients would come to his office and then he could bill them for other treatments, such as injections and chiropractic adjustments. The fact that Dr. McIver's income was unusually low for a physician (indeed, his previous practice had ended in bankruptcy), because the procedures he performed were not, in fact, lucrative and he typically spent a full hour or more with patients, did not sway the jury.

Dr. McIver stated that his goal was to reduce his patients' pain to a 2 on a 10-point scale (with 10 representing the worst pain the patient can imagine) so that his patients could return to their previous levels of activity. The pain specialist who served as the government's expert witness at Dr. McIver's trial testified that he personally believed that 5 was a more reasonable goal. I wonder if the expert witness revealed to his own patients that he would be content to leave them halfway to *the worst pain they could imagine*. Had the expert witness ever experienced pain? Would he want to be cared for by a doctor who shared his philosophy?

Many of Dr. McIver's patients testified at the trial as to his success in rehabilitating them, such as a farmer and cattle rancher who, under Dr. McIver's care, was able to return to work by taking 1,600 mg of OxyContin a day. After Dr. McIver's arrest, the farmer's family doctor reduced his prescription to one-sixth of that—240 mg. He told Tina Rosenberg that he now gets three hours of sleep a night and can no longer stand for more than half an hour. He sold his cattle and stopped working, resuming his previous identity as a full-time chronic pain patient.

Dr. McIver also successfully treated a woman suffering from complex regional pain syndrome (CRPS, also known as reflex sympathetic dystrophy syndrome—an unusual, terrible disease of the autonomic nervous system) who had recently been addicted to crack cocaine. Under Dr. McIver's care, she did not become addicted to opioids, and her pain improved. But the prosecution presented the very attempt to treat such a person as an example of Dr. McIver's recklessness.

Along with a twenty-year sentence for drug distribution, Dr. McIver also received a concurrent thirty-year sentence for dispensing drugs that resulted in one patient's death. Yet the patient who died had suffered from advanced congestive heart failure, and there was no conclusive evidence that the stable dose of OxyContin he had been taking for many months had contributed to his death of respiratory failure. (Pain specialists say that a dose previously well tolerated would be extremely unlikely to cause respiratory failure.) Moreover, it is pain, not pain medicine, that adversely affects the heart.

Not all of the DEA's investigations and arrests of pain doctors are bogus: in some of the cases the doctors seem clearly to have been acting as dealers and writing prescriptions to patients they never saw. But in recent years there have been hundreds of investigations and dozens of arrests, and many of the cases seem to echo Dr. McIver's. Appeals of his case have been denied.

THE INVISIBLE HIERARCHY OF FEELING

Although affluent, educated patients are often able to find physicians willing to treat their pain for them, the most vulnerable members of society are not. "Pain is a good measure of our humanism," Dr. Daniel Carr says. "To value someone's suffering, you have to validate them as a person. We shouldn't be surprised that the least-valued members of society get the least pain relief. The deck is increasingly stacked against treating pain if anything about the patient's profile suggests their treatment course may be problematic. Poor people are more likely to sell their drugs. A lot of physicians feel, Why bother?"

Sex, race, and class adversely influence pain treatment. Many of Dr. Carr's patients would have—and have had—trouble finding another doctor to prescribe pain medication for them, because they have some social strike against them. Many are minorities, women, recipients of public assistance, workers' compensation cases, patients suffering from mental illness, patients with histories of substance abuse, or patients who fit several of these categories.

It has often been observed that male and female patients with complaints of pain are treated differently. Men are more likely to be given opioid medications, surgery, and complete exams, while women are given psychotropic medications for depression and anxiety. (One survey found that women with an identical complaint and diagnosis were 82 percent more likely than men to be given an antidepressant and 37 percent more likely to receive medication for anxiety.) Women tend to be either less

aggressive in demanding pain treatment or aggressive in ways that are
dismissed as mere hysteria. Dr. William Breitbart conducted a study of
women with HIV that found that they are twice as likely to be undertreated for pain as men are. Dr. Breitbart found that women's fear of being
perceived as demanding when asking for pain medication, as well as their
heightened sensitivity to disapproval, made them hesitant to report pain
to their physicians. He decided to design a course for female AIDS patients
on how to better communicate their needs to their doctors, and ("I swear
this is true," he says) some doctors he met when lecturing on this topic
responded with concern that the course would "teach a bunch of addicts
how to score."

Many studies have found that blacks are more likely than whites to
be undertreated for pain and denied opiate analgesics. Studies led by
Dr. Richard Payne, then the director of the Pain and Palliative Care Service at Sloan-Kettering, showed that minorities are up to three times more
likely than others to receive inadequate pain relief—and to have their
requests for medication interpreted as "drug-seeking behavior." A 2005
study at twelve academic medical centers in a primary care setting found
that although blacks had significantly higher pain scores, whites were
much more likely to have been prescribed opioid analgesics (despite the
fact that there were no significant socioeconomic differences between the
two populations, such as disability status, unemployment, income, or use
of illicit substances). Racial differences became even more pronounced in
the groups' comparative likelihood of receiving stronger and long-acting
opioids. The study concluded that racism—"systematic mistrust, bias,
or stereotyping phenomena" and "cultural communication barriers or
mistrust"—may cause physicians to discount blacks' pain reports. Other
studies have found that physicians perceived blacks as less compliant and
have documented unequal treatment of minorities in hospital settings.
Pharmacies in minority neighborhoods exacerbate the problem by failing
to stock adequate stores of opioids.

Historically, the unequal treatment of pain has been justified through
theories of pain sensitivity, by which certain groups suffered pain less than
others. This invisible hierarchy of pain sensitivity was believed to extend
from wild beasts to fair maidens and was organized by such attributes as

gender, race, social status, education, age, personality, obesity, and even hair and eye color. Countesses and criminals, saints and soldiers, slaves and "savages," responded to pain according to their fixed, true nature. Some of these theories still hold sway in the practice of pain today.

The second-century Greek physician Galen, whose theories shaped medicine up until the end of the Renaissance, linked personality to physical traits such as pain sensitivity or vulnerability to disease. He found that of the four "humors" (temperaments), pudgy, contented, phlegmatic types enjoyed a greater pain tolerance than did thin, irascible, choleric ones. In keeping with the Victorian love of classification schemas, nineteenth-century theories of pain sensitivity grew ever more elaborate. Such theories remained prevalent through the mid-twentieth century and are still not entirely extinct.

A colorful 1938 international bestseller about the history of anesthesia, *Triumph Over Pain*, by the German author René Fülöp-Miller, reflects many of the prejudices of the day, asserting that pain sensitivity is "a subjective matter, depending on personal characteristics, the outcome of heredity, environment, racial and social circumstances, varying with sex, occupation, age, climate, and individual temperament." The countryman is "less sensitive than the townsmen, and the mental workers more sensitive than the manual workers." The old are less sensitive than the young because "British and French investigators have proved that sensibility to pain diminishes with advancing years." The European is "at least twice as sensitive as the savage," and some European "races" are more sensitive than others.

Popular theories of pain sensitivity cannily valued the suffering of the elite while dismissing that of others as not only unimportant but nonexistent. "In our process of being civilized we have won, I suspect, intensified capacity to suffer," lamented Dr. Silas Weir Mitchell, a pioneer of neurology who documented the lingering effects of nerve injuries among Civil War soldiers. "The savage does not feel pain as we do," he concluded, echoing the belief of pain theorists through the ages: *they* do not—cannot—suffer as *we* do.

While fortitude manifested by soldiers and other manly men was a virtue, there was no bravery or endurance to speak of on the part of those who supposedly lacked the capacity to acutely feel pain. Poverty was a great anesthetizer, as was the criminal's lack of morals. Cesare Lombroso, an Italian criminologist, argued that in their insensibility to pain, "criminals closely resemble not the insane but savages. All travelers know that among the Negroes and savages of America, sensitivity to pain is so limited that the former laugh as they mutilate their hands to escape work, while the latter sing their tribe's praises while being burned alive."

Slaves' animal natures dulled them to pain, as did the supposed thickness of their colored skin (although the addition of white blood made mulattos more sensitive). "Negresses," an editor of a British medical journal stated matter-of-factly in 1826, "will bear cutting with nearly, if not quite, as much impunity as dogs and rabbits," while an 1856 article in the *Southern Medical and Surgical Journal* assured slave owners that "the Negro . . . has a greater insensibility to pain" and "suffers deeply, but not enduringly, from affliction." Lack of civilization was also believed to immunize "savages" from pain. "Savages . . . endure with comparative indifference inflictions which to most persons of the higher races would be terrible," wrote the British surgeon and pathologist Sir James Paget.

Theories of pain sensitivity set social expectations with regard to surgery, torture, and corporal punishment and were even employed to justify testing excruciating surgeries and medical experiments on criminals and slaves. The celebrated "father of gynecology," Dr. J. Marion Sims, one of the most renowned doctors of his time (whose statue can be found in Central Park today), honed his techniques on slave women. One of his greatest accomplishments was inventing a surgical repair for fistulas—tears in the vaginal wall caused by difficult labor. The tears allowed urine from the bladder to leak into the vagina, leading to incontinence and other problems, making such women outcasts. Sims obtained several Alabama slaves who had developed fistulas and kept them in a small hospital where he practiced, without anesthesia, procedures on them over the course of four years. It was not until June 1849, during *the thirtieth operation* on Anarcha, one of the slave women, that he succeeded in the repair. Moreover, during the last two of those years, anesthesia was already available!

The insensateness of "savages" was generally viewed much more favorably than that of slaves. Although Native American cultures placed a high value on pain endurance (many Native American puberty rites, for example, involved physical mutilation), whites attributed such endurance not to cultural conditioning but to innate character. Although this myth helped justify torture and slaughter, it also won a certain admiration for Indians. While Indians were sometimes seen as brutish, they were also viewed as innocents. According to the theory of the noble savage, indigenous peoples were untroubled by pain because, like animals, they had tasted less of the fruit that exiled Christians from the natural world. Lacking knowledge of good and evil (lacking even self-consciousness to properly clothe their bodies), they had evaded Adam's curse and legacy: suffering pain.

White children were subject to similar debate. One strand of Victorian thought was that since children were not yet fully civilized, they lacked developed capacities for suffering. Another strand of thought viewed children as delicate creatures, more like women than like animals, who required special protection from pain. The increasing prevalence of the latter belief contributed to the decline of corporal punishment and child labor during the century. Since the development of the intellect was thought to yield greater pain sensitivity, there was even concern that education itself might create excessively sensitive children and should be curtailed, especially in the case of young girls.

Of all sensitive civilized Victorian creatures, however, the most sensitive of all was thought to be the fair-haired, fair-skinned upper-class lady. From ancient times it was believed that the same strong physique that made men hunters and warriors also shielded them from the pain of wounds—a protection not shared by the weaker sex. Belief in the exquisiteness of female pain sensitivity reached its zenith during the nineteenth century. As spiritual creatures, women were expected to suffer from their earthly embodiment; indeed, suffering was considered positive evidence of their spirituality.

"With her exalted spiritualism" a woman "is more forcibly under the control of matter; her sensations are more vivid and acute, her sympathies more irresistible," wrote the British surgeon John Gideon Millingen in 1848. The masculine and feminine ideals in regard to pain were not just different, but opposite from each other: men were admired for stoicism and bravery, while women were to *cultivate* hyperalgesia (abnormally heightened pain sensitivity). In an era whose seminal work was Darwin's *On the Origin of Species by Means of Natural Selection*, Victorian society nonetheless favored women who seemed particularly unsuited for corporeal life, especially in regard to reproduction.

Medical texts treated menstruation in well-bred women as something that required bed rest. Childbirth was thought to be "exceedingly painful . . . especially in the upper walks of life." City-dwelling women were deemed more sensitive than countryfolk, fair hair trumped dark hair, and of course fair skin outranked all other pigmentation. Even Sir James Young Simpson—the doctor who discovered chloroform and was the first obstetrician to use anesthesia during labor—was convinced that "women in a savage state . . . enjoy a kind of natural anesthesia during labor"!

Pain sensitivity was considered so reliable a reflection of social status that it was regarded as a proof of rank—an idea starkly expressed in the Hans Christian Andersen fairy tale "The Princess and the Pea," variations of which are found in classical India, East Asia, and other cultures. Indeed, the tale appears in enough forms that a standard classification system of mythology and folklore labels these stories the "Princess and the Pea" type. In an Italian version of the tale, "The Most Sensitive Woman," three exceptionally delicate ladies compete for the hand of the prince. One suffers from sleeping on a wrinkled sheet, another is pained when her comb pulls a hair from her head, and the third—the most sensitive of all—is injured by the fall of a jasmine petal onto her slender foot.

In the 1835 Andersen version of "The Princess and the Pea," the queen places a pea under twenty mattresses and twenty eiderdown quilts to test whether the bedraggled young woman who shows up at the castle one stormy night is a real princess. The result: in the morning the princess declares herself grievously bruised, thus proving herself fit (albeit not in the Darwinian sense!) to be the prince's mate.

The previously incontrovertible fact of female pain sensitivity came to be debated at the close of the century, when some theorists suggested that women could actually bear *more* pain than men, a point they defended from an evolutionary perspective. "Women, upon whom nature imposes the painful and arduous task of childbearing, can, in general, bear pain better than men," asserted *Triumph Over Pain*.

PAIN THRESHOLD AND PAIN TOLERANCE

onfusion about pain sensitivity continues, and many of its myths
still exert a pernicious influence on patient care by justifying dis-
criminatory treatment. Is there actually an invisible hierarchy
of feeling? Or does the curse of *'etsev* and *'itstsabown* afflict all mortals
equally?

Pain sensitivity is measured in three ways. The first measure is on a
cellular level, where the *nociceptive threshold* marks the point at which a
thermal (burning or freezing), mechanical (pinching or pulling), or chemical (poisonous or acidic) stimulus is sufficient to trigger the peripheral
nerves (nociceptors) designed to sense cell damage. Because it is hardwired by evolution, the nociceptive threshold is common to all members
of a species and can be altered only by disease processes, such as leprosy
and diabetes, that eat away the peripheral nerves, causing local areas of
numbness (called peripheral neuropathies).

A second measure of pain sensitivity is called simply the *pain threshold.*
The pain threshold is a function of consciousness; it is the point at which the
brain processes information from the nociceptors and perceives a stimulus
as painful—for example, the sensation of pressure turns to the sensation of
crushing pain or the sensation of warmth turns to the sensation of burning.
Although it is not as uniform across a species as the nociceptive threshold,
the pain threshold is also fairly similar from individual to individual.

The third measure of pain sensitivity—*pain tolerance*—accounts for
the variability of what we can endure. Pain tolerance is commonly

measured in experiments, for example, as the point at which a subject declares a painful stimulus unbearable and asks for it to be discontinued. Pain tolerance depends not only on the temperament of the individual but also on the circumstances of the pain. Not surprisingly, participants in pain studies have no particular motivation to suffer for the sake of an experiment, so their tolerance tends to be low; by contrast, the study's conductors are very motivated to sacrifice in the service of their own work and therefore tend to discover that their own pain thresholds are high.

Yet the very participants who are quick to find a mild heat stimulus unbearable in a laboratory would respond quite differently if they had a compelling reason (or, indeed, any reason) to endure it—say, if they were rescuing their cat from a fire, or fire walking in a Hindu rite or a Western team-building exercise. Even in an experimental context, pain toleration varies with circumstances; subjects asked to hold their hands in icy water will endure it twice as long if they are not alone.

Is pain tolerance affected by gender, race, age, ethnicity, weight, or educational level? Are whites more sensitive than blacks, women than men, the slender than the stout, the fair-haired than the dark-haired, the young than the old, the educated than the ignorant? Clearly, different cultures respond differently to pain. A well-known study of housewives in the late 1960s found that in the United States, what were then known as "Yankees" (white Protestants of British descent) had the highest pain tolerance, followed by first-generation Irish, Jews, and, lastly, among those studied, Italians. (Interestingly, another paper found pain tolerance markedly increased for Jewish subjects with the presence of a non-Jewish, as compared with a Jewish, investigator.)

But perhaps the Italians being studied simply expressed more pain because their culture permits greater expressiveness, and since expressing pain can ease it, perhaps they actually suffered less. Indeed, a recent study by British researchers asked volunteers to hold their hands in painfully icy water; one group was allowed to continually swear aloud with a curse word of their choice, and the other had to repeat a non-swear mantra. The people who were allowed to swear were able to keep their hands in the water longer, and they perceived it as less painful. The testers theorized that the swearing induced a fight-or-flight response (release of stress hormones), which reduced fear of pain and therefore pain perception.

A benchmark 1972 Stanford University study, led by Dr. Kenneth M. Woodrow, of more than forty thousand patients belonging to a large

HMO found that age, sex, and race do modify pain tolerance. Older men's pain tolerance was two-thirds to three-fourths of that of younger men's. In women, the decline was less pronounced, however, and even the oldest men had a higher pain tolerance on average than the youngest women. Pain tolerance, in general, varied less among women than men. Whites showed more pain tolerance than blacks, and blacks showed more tolerance than Asian Americans. Another study found Hispanics to be more sensitive to pain than non-Hispanic whites.

The Woodrow study made no claims as to whether the differences in pain toleration between ethnic groups are culturally or biologically determined. But the more that subjective differences in pain sensitivity are studied, the more frequently they appear to have a biological basis. Although the data is complicated and debated, numerous studies suggest (irritatingly) that nature may indeed be sexist and females simply have lower pain tolerance than males. Perhaps as an adaptive response to males as warriors and hunters sustaining more acute injuries than females, there seem to be differences in male and female pain-modulatory systems, with males enjoying more robust pain modulation. Female hormones are a potential mediator of the sex difference in pain sensitivity. Certain phases of the menstrual cycle are associated with a lower pain threshold.

There are interesting differences in male and female opioid receptors. (The differences are also present in male and female rats.) There are three types of opioid receptors, most notably *mu* and *kappa*; most opioid drugs such as morphine target mu receptors. Few drugs that target kappa receptors have been developed, because early trials found them ineffective. The research, however, was conducted largely on men, and it turns out that women are more responsive to kappa-receptor drugs. One study of a rarely prescribed kappa-receptor analgesic (nalbuphine) on postoperative pain in men and women who had their wisdom teeth removed found that the drug had opposite effects on the two sexes, ameliorating female pain and exacerbating male pain. Studies of mice suggest that the sex differences in the analgesic effect of kappa opioids could be traced to one gene, known as melanocortin-1 receptor, or MC1R.

The common mu-receptor analgesics, by contrast, are less effective in women than in men (and less effective in female rats than in male rats). A 2003 study by Dr. M. Soledad Cepeda and Dr. Daniel Carr of postsurgical pain following general anesthesia found that "women have more intense pain and require 30% more morphine [on a per-weight basis] to achieve a similar degree of analgesia compared with men." The study advises that "clinicians should anticipate the differences in opioid requirement to avoid under-treatment of pain in women." So although women are less likely to be prescribed opioids, they actually require more. There is also some limited evidence that women respond differently to nonsteroidal anti-inflammatory drugs (NSAIDs): although the drugs act equally on inflammation in both genders, men receive more analgesic benefit from the drugs than women do (a finding that may provide clues to why women suffer more from chronic inflammatory conditions).

Even the far-fetched Victorian notion that hair color affects pain sensitivity turns out to have a grain of truth in regard to fair-skinned redheads. A certain type of opioid pain medication that acts on kappa receptors (pentazocine) was found to work dramatically better for red-haired women; it turned out that the same gene MC1R that accounts for women's responsiveness to kappa opioids is also responsible for red hair and fair skin pigmentation. Interestingly, common opioids work less well in redheads. Redheaded women need an average of about 20 percent more general anesthesia than dark-haired women. They also derive less analgesia from novocaine and are more likely to avoid going to the dentist.

Puzzlingly, studies prior to Dr. Woodrow's agreed with the Victorian notion that the old are less pain sensitive than the young. But those studies employed thermal pain (heat or cold stimuli applied to the skin), whereas the Woodrow study employed mechanical pressure on the Achilles tendon (which produces a deep pain). Aging, it turns out, has contradictory effects on pain: sensitivity to cutaneous pain *decreases*, while sensitivity to deep pain *increases* (which is more clinically relevant because it more closely resembles the pain produced by disease processes and injuries than does a superficial stimulus). This finding may be of great value in developing analgesia for elderly populations.

Although Galen believed that fat, phlegmatic types had diminished pain sensitivity, the contrary seems to be true. Unsurprisingly, obesity creates pain-causing conditions, such as greater rates of degenerative arthritis, because of the extra weight that joints must support. (Degenerative arthritis, also known as osteoarthritis or wear-and-tear arthritis, involves a deterioration of the cartilage that cushions the bones at joints, which results in pain, stiffness, and inflammation.) But do the obese also suffer from lower pain toleration? Do painful stimuli actually hurt them more?

Many studies have shown that the obese *report* more pain in labora-tory pain-toleration studies. But does this reflect a difference in their bod-ies' innate pain sensitivity? A 2006 Ohio State University study attempted to answer that question by measuring the muscular response to electrical stimulation of a nerve in the legs of patients suffering from osteoarthritis of the knee. The obese patients reported no more pain than non-obese people (and rated their pain in a similar fashion in questionnaires). But their ankles demonstrated a greater muscular pain reflex. When all the volunteers were given a pain-toleration training session that included a progressive muscle relaxation exercise, both groups reported less pain and showed diminished pain responsiveness. But the obese continued to show greater pain sensitivity.

The view that children were not sensitive to pain continued to hold sway through the first half of the twentieth century. Many in the medical profession held that infants felt no pain at all and that young children were simply not developed enough to suffer. Until the late *1970s* (this is not a typo), most surgeries in the United States and around the world were per-formed on infants with little or inadequate anesthesia (although they were paralyzed with a neuromuscular blocker) because general anesthesia was believed to introduce unnecessary risk. Pain medication was also with-held from infants and young children during recovery from surgery, can-cer, and even severe burns.

Even after the practice was recognized as harmful, anesthesiologists and hospitals resisted change. As late as 1987, an editorial in *The New En-gland Journal of Medicine* still found it necessary to argue that the evidence was "so overwhelming that physicians can no longer act as if all infants were indifferent to pain." Finally, a study conclusively demonstrated that babies who were operated on without anesthesia were more likely to die! By contrast, those given anesthesia recovered more quickly from surgery and suffered fewer complications.

Although pain generates less lasting *emotional* reaction in infants and young children than in older children and adults (hence children can emit bloodcurdling screams of pain at one moment and then laugh the next), *physiologically*, young children are much more adversely affected by pain because the nervous pathways that conduct pain develop earlier than the brain's ability to modulate pain. While the ancient Assyrians were con-cerned enough about pain to asphyxiate their baby boys to the point of unconsciousness before circumcision, many infants today continue to be circumcised without anesthesia, even though the practice has been shown to have long-lasting detrimental effects.

A doctor who worked for the French pain-treatment charity Douleurs Sans Frontières (Pain Without Borders), found that physicians in Africa had to be trained to recognize pain. A pediatrician at a good hospital in Mozambique, for example, assured the French doctor that none of his patients had pain. He took him to the children's ward to prove it. "You see," he said, "none of the children are crying or fussing. They are lying quietly in their beds." The French doctor had to explain that it is natural for children to cry and move about and that *not* crying can be a sign of terrible pain. Daniel Carr recalled a paper submitted to *Pain*, a professional journal he edits, in which a Chinese physician argued that children in China recovering from abdominal surgery were not given—and did not ask for—pain medication and concluded that Western children are wimps.

The Victorians were also right that race affects pain sensitivity—but in the opposite way from what they believed. African Americans are more hampered by chronic pain; they report suffering greater pain severity and disability in connection with a variety of pain-causing conditions. Moreover, this phenomenon holds true over a wide variety of age-groups and populations, including young children.

Part of the reason is now thought to lie in ethnic differences in pain-modulation systems. Although it has been extensively documented that African Americans have lower pain tolerance than whites in laboratory studies, the relevance of the finding has been unclear. Most of the studies relied on healthy volunteers, often college students. Acute pain and chronic pain are known to involve different physiological mechanisms: the nervous system of a healthy person may differ profoundly from that of someone with chronic pain. Moreover, the psychological experience of suffering from chronic pain is utterly unlike that of the test of acute pain in a lab, where subjects are explicitly reassured that they will not be hurt (and ethical guidelines require that tests be discontinued prior to tissue damage, even if the subject does not request it).

A 2001 study led by Dr. Robert R. Edwards of Johns Hopkins School of Medicine tested pain tolerance in a chronic pain population of blacks and whites. His team tested 337 patients with a painful arm tourniquet procedure. African Americans showed dramatically less arm pain tolerance (whites tolerated the pain for an average of nearly nine minutes, and African Americans lasted five) *and* their increased sensitivity was found to correlate with their reports of higher levels of chronic pain as well as greater pain-related disability.

Why? Another study found that a subgroup of African Americans had significantly lower beta-endorphin levels in response to stress, which would lessen the ability to modulate pain. An alternative explanation may involve differences between black and white Americans in their central nervous systems in relation to cardiovascular and hormonal responses to stress. Pain causes the release of the stress hormone adrenaline (epinephrine), which has a variety of effects, increasing heart rate and blood pressure and intensifying the experience of pain; African Americans have been shown to have greater vascular and hormonal responses to stress than do whites, which might create more pain. Moreover, African Americans suffer from greater levels of daily stress, which may lead to greater levels of daily pain. A 2005 study at the University of North Carolina at Chapel Hill found changes in African Americans in pain-regulatory mechanisms involving blood pressure and the stress hormones cortisol and noradrenaline.

The pharmacological implications of genetic differences among ethnic groups is an emergent area of research, as drugs have traditionally been tested exclusively on Western populations. Research done on genetic samples from Tel Aviv University, for example, recently discovered that many Ethiopian Jews have a gene variation that makes them metabolize opioids and some other common drugs more quickly than other Jews, thereby putting them at risk for greater side effects.

Although the Victorians were wrong more often than they were right about the *sequence* of the links in their great chain—and Anarcha, the slave on whom J. Marion Sims honed his surgical techniques, may have been more sensitive to pain than he—the concept of a continuum of pain sensitivity turns out not to be entirely specious. But the social and moral implications of the metaphor of the chain and the algorithm employed in the calculus of suffering certainly were: while the difference in pain sensitivity between a fair maiden and a wild beast is significant, beasts nevertheless feel pain and suffer from it, and among humans, the differences are modest. With respect to pain, humans are more alike than different—and in need of treatment.

INDIVIDUAL PAIN SENSITIVITY

If certain groups are more likely to develop chronic pain, what about certain individuals? Most pain does not become chronic pain—why does some of it? Are some people genetically at risk for pain in the same way others are at risk for cancer or obesity? If so, how can we identify them and try to prevent the development of a chronic pain syndrome?

An article by Dr. Robert R. Edwards hypothesizes that individual differences in pain sensitivity and pain modulation place individuals at varying risks of suffering severe acute pain following an injury and also of suffering chronic pain. Although most studies focus on pain sensitivity, another important factor is how well an individual's nervous system modulates pain. When repeated painful stimuli are administered close together in time, their effects become additive: each successive shock hurts more than the last as the nervous system becomes increasingly sensitive. But this effect is checked by the body's own pain-modulatory capacities—the robustness of its descending analgesia (the brain's ability to temporarily switch on pain-inhibiting mechanisms). In chronic pain patients, those capacities are reduced. In fibromyalgia patients, for example, the pain caused by successive noxious stimuli increases much more rapidly than in normal individuals. And while both high pain sensitivity and low pain-modulatory capacities increase an individual's risk of developing acute and chronic pain, pain modulation seems to be the more significant factor.

Innate pain sensitivity not only makes the development of pain syndromes more likely, it also reduces the efficacy of opioid analgesics to ameliorate the syndromes (in mice as well as humans). Patients who suffer from postherpetic neuralgia (recurrent herpes that causes itchy, burning pain) also have low pain thresholds in areas of their bodies unaffected by the neuralgia, and they have been found to derive less analgesic relief from opioids than those with normal pain thresholds. Moreover, treatments that do not involve drugs (physical therapy, talk therapy, meditation, and so forth) have also been found to be less successful on pain-sensitive people.

Pain sensitivity may reflect the influence of countless factors, ranging from cultural training to personal history. Brain imaging has shown that the psychological tendency to "catastrophize"—to embroider pain with fear and anxiety—results in enhanced central nervous system activity and more pain and anxiety. Early exposure to pain has been shown to lower pain thresholds by damaging the undeveloped nervous system. Emotional trauma has also been shown to affect pain sensitivity: victims of childhood sexual abuse, for example, have higher rates of chronic pelvic pain as adults because the trauma seems to alter the way they process pelvic sensation.

There also appears to be an important—if largely unknown—genetic basis for variations in pain sensitivity. In addition to the opioid-receptor genes, there is promising research on a lesser-known gene that encodes an enzyme (catecholamine-O-methyltransferase, or COMT) that appears to modulate pain. A 2005 study published in *Human Molecular Genetics* identified three variants of the COMT gene associated with differing degrees of pain sensitivity in the laboratory, which turn out to be predictive of the chance of healthy women developing myogenous temporomandibular joint disorder (a common musculoskeletal condition involving pain and inflammation of the joint that connects the lower jaw to the skull, often called TMJ or TMD).

Another recent study concerned a gene called SCN9A that is involved in the functioning of nociceptive neurons. Severe mutations of SCN9A are known to produce both extreme pain syndromes (when they increase neuronal activity) or, in other cases, complete congenital analgesia (when they block it), but the new study showed that much smaller, more common mutations were predictive of pain scores among patients with osteoarthritis, sciatica pain, and phantom limb pain, and even affected the pain sensitivity of healthy women to a heat stimulus in a lab setting.

If individuals at high risk for chronic pain could be identified through genetic tests, many pain syndromes could be prevented through aggressive early intervention. For example, pain-sensitive individuals are more likely to experience severe pain during an initial outbreak of herpes zoster. And higher pain ratings, in turn, have been shown to be predictive of the development of postherpetic neuralgia many years later. Yet an immediate antiviral drug treatment for herpes zoster can prevent the development of the syndrome.

Knowledge of genetic vulnerability to chronic pain might influence choices about surgery. With certain surgeries, nerve-sparing techniques are available, although not always practiced. With other surgeries, such as plastic surgery, knowing the likelihood of chronic pain might make the risks outweigh the benefits. Greater pre- or postoperative analgesia might be employed, or more intense follow-up conducted.

One of the most common general surgeries is a technique for hernia repair that involves severing the ilioinguinal nerve in the groin. The surgeon does the procedure and declares it a success; the patient goes home, and the surgeon never sees him or her again. But a large-scale Danish survey of prior scientific studies found that 10 percent of the patients developed moderate to severe chronic pain subsequent to the operation, and up to a quarter of the patients said that the pain restricted their daily activity. A British study found that 30 percent of the men reported chronic pain persisting more than three months after the operation. There are alternative surgical techniques that preserve the nerve, but doctors don't understand the importance of using them, and patients don't know to demand them.

THE CELLULAR SECRET OF THE
CHRONIC PAIN CYCLE

The gap between what's going on in the lab and among practitioners is enormous," Dr. Clifford Woolf commented, in his soft-spoken way. "Pain management now is on the level that treatment of TB once occupied—driven by desperation on the part of the patient and the clinician." A South African emigrant who trained as a neurologist, he is a tall, fine-boned man with a shaved head, a gentle manner, and a vaguely melancholic air. He gives the impression of being attuned to suffering. Although he does no clinical work, when he talks about pain patients, he conveys a sense of deep feeling. He hunched his shoulders against the rain in his black leather jacket as we walked toward the neuroplasticity lab he directs at Massachusetts General Hospital, curiously located in the Charlestown Navy Yard.

"This is the new frontier of medicine. What we're learning is that chronic pain is not just a sensory or affective or cognitive state. It's a biologic disease afflicting millions of people. We're not on the verge of curing cancer or heart disease, but we are closing in on pain. Very soon, I believe, there will be effective treatment for pain because, for the first time in history, the tools are coming together to understand and treat it."

In the harbor, hulking relics of yesterday's battles still float, but inside the lab is a vast landscape of test tubes containing rat DNA, and delicate machinery with which to interpret it. The critical tools of modern pain research are the increasing sophistication of functional imaging techniques in recording pictures of brain activity (fMRIs), the completion of the human genome project, and new "gene chip" technology derived from the computer world—plastic detectors coded with an array of DNA sequences that can detect which genes become active when neurons respond to pain-causing stimuli. "In the past thirty years of pain research, we've looked for pain-related genes, one at a time, and come up with sixty," Dr. Woolf said. "In the past year, using gene-chip technology, we've come up with fifteen hundred." He looked more cheerful. "We're drowning in new information. All we have to do is read it all—to prioritize, to find the key gene, the master switch that drives others.

"The psychological element to pain clinics"—teaching people how to cope with their pain—"is an admission of how poor the treatment options are. Although we know chronic pain is a disease, there's no diagnosis or treatment protocol for it as a disease now." Among practitioners, he added, "there's this amorphous notion that pain is one thing and can be treated as one glob of problem." With most problems, such as lower-back pain, it is not possible to say whether the pain is neuropathic, arthritic, or muscular-skeletal in nature. "Is the pain 25 percent peripheral, 25 percent central, 25 percent inflammatory, and 25 percent muscular? Or are the joints diseased but the nerves normal? There is only symptomatic rather than mechanistic treatment, yet the symptoms all overlay."

He mentioned a grim truism in analgesia research known as the "30 rule"—that the existing pain drugs generally reduce pain by 30 percent in 30 percent of people—"and before we start treating them, we have no idea who is going to respond or not." His aim is to "push the idea that there are distinct pain generators, and what we need to do is to identify them in each patient—to find the fingerprint of the underlying neurogenetic mechanism in each patient and see which one is actually operating. What is the damage to the central nervous system and how can it be repaired? What are the nervous pathways? What genes are switched on and off?"

Descriptions of the quality of the pain, such as "burning" or "aching," do not actually reveal neuropathology: burning pain in one patient appears not to have the same mechanism as burning pain in another and does not necessarily respond to the same treatment. "Right now we can only deduce backwards who is suffering from what by how they respond to the treatment," he said, "if they find a treatment they respond to." Pain patients typically have to try many drugs to find one thing that works—if they find anything.

Much of the lab's work uses rats to try to identify the cellular mechanisms of neuropathic pain. On the table the day that I visited, a graduate student was measuring pain responses in a plump white creature. First an electric shock was applied to the sensory fibers of a rat's paw, and the firing response in the neurons of the spinal cord was measured. Then a burn injury was made elsewhere on the paw. When the same electrical stimulus was applied to the original sensory nerves, there was a much greater neural response. Moreover, the rat's other paw became more responsive to the pain stimuli as well. The rat's nervous system had undergone what Dr. Woolf termed a central sensitization. The nerves in the spinal cord became hyperexcitable and began spontaneously firing. This state of hyperexcitability causes the neurons to die—a phenomenon called *excitotoxicity*. It turned out that after a major injury to a peripheral nerve, *a quarter of the cells in the spinal cord died from excitotoxicity*: not only the injured neurons die, but the adjacent ones as well. Dr. Woolf believes that excitotoxicity is a critical feature of neuropathic pain because—bad luck—many of the neurons that die are *inhibitory* ones, whose function is to dampen pain.

"The loss of the normal brakes in the nervous system that inhibit pain signals creates disinhibition—a persistent amplification of pain," he said. "If we could identify the missing inhibitory signals, perhaps we could introduce them as a drug."

Terrifyingly, it is not only the spinal cord but also the brain that can be pathologically reordered by pain. Dr. Woolf bred a particular strain of rat to be prone to pain sensitivity. Then he injured the rats' sciatic nerves. Ten days later, when he cut open the rats' brains, he could discern the imprint of the nerve injury: corresponding maladaptive changes in the way the rats' brains process and generate pain. "In animal models, anytime there is an injury to a major nerve branch, this nasty cortical reorganization occurs," he said.

What about humans? Work done by Dr. A. Vania Apkarian at Northwestern University found that chronic pain causes degeneration in parts of the

human brain in a way that he speculates is due to "overuse atrophy"—
death of neurons owing to excitotoxicity and inflammatory agents (as had
been previously found in the spinal cord). He also found that chronic pain
appears to diminish cognitive abilities and interfere with parts of the brain
(specifically areas of the prefrontal cortex) that are involved in making
emotional assessments, including decision making, and in controlling
social behavior.

One of Dr. Apkarian's studies contrasted brain images of normal subjects with those of twenty-six patients who had suffered from unrelent-
ing chronic back pain for more than a year (with the typical pain patient
having had pain for five years). Back pain is the most common pain syndrome next to headache: a quarter or more of Americans report suffering
from back pain in the prior three months, and for a quarter of those, the
pain becomes severe and chronic. The scans revealed that chronic pain
had *dramatically reduced the gray matter of the patients' brains.* (The
amount of gray matter in certain areas of the brain is correlated with intelligence; it contains neurons that process information and store memory.)
While normal aging causes gray matter to atrophy by half a percent a year,
the gray matter of chronic pain patients atrophies dramatically faster: the
pain patients showed losses amounting to between 5 and 11 percent, *the
equivalent of ten to twenty years of aging.*

Normal aging processes differ from the process associated with chronic
pain, in a particularly disturbing way. Where aging causes atrophy in
many regions of the brain, chronic pain specifically atrophies those parts
of the brain whose job is to modulate pain (the thalamus and parts of the
prefrontal cortex). Both neuropathic and inflammatory pain were associated with decreases in gray matter density, but neuropathic pain had a
distinct and much greater impact on the brain. The loss in brain density
seemed related to pain duration, with 1.3 cubic centimeters of gray matter
being lost for every year of chronic pain. When asked, Dr. Apkarian estimated that the chronic pain patients would lose roughly twice as much
gray matter per year as the normal subjects.

Here, finally, I realized, is the secret of the chronic pain cycle, why
it worsens over time without new nerve or tissue damage: *pain causes
changes in the brain that diminish the parts of the brain charged with modulating pain, which results in an increase in pain, which further atrophies
the brain* . . . and so forth. "As atrophy of elements of the circuitry [of the

brain] progresses, the pain condition becomes more irreversible and less responsive to therapy," the study ominously concluded.

If my own brain had lost 1.3 cubic centimeters of its gray matter for each year I had pain, then it would have lost . . . what percent by now? How many extra years had pain aged my brain? The thalamus and prefrontal cortex—the parts of my brain that were supposed to modulate pain, the parts of my brain with which I was trying to understand pain . . .

I couldn't bear to complete the calculation.

THE WONDERFUL DREAM THAT PAIN HAS
BEEN TAKEN AWAY FROM US

How can such a syndrome be prevented? Dr. Woolf has some ideas about molecular agents he believes may be critically involved in inciting or sustaining neuropathic pain. For example, he said, in animal models there are certain abnormal sodium ion channels that appear and become activated only in the damaged sensory neurons. There are also sodium channels involved in inflammatory pain that help determine the excitability of nerve fibers or pain fibers in the vicinity of the damaged tissue. If the critical molecular components in different types of chronic pain could be identified, then an antagonist might be found and introduced as a drug.

Would "the wonderful dream that pain has been taken away from us," which was trumpeted at the invention of anesthesia, finally, then, be true? Would such a drug help all the people who already have this pain—or only prevent others from developing it? Can the cortical reorganization be reorganized, the gray matter un-atrophied, the damage to the central nervous system repaired? After all, neuroprotective drugs can't protect neurons that have already died, and neurons cannot regenerate. What about Lee Burke, and the babies circumcised without anesthesia? What about me?

Dr. Woolf looked at me and hesitated, as if wondering just how unwelcome the news would be. "We don't really know," he said tactfully. Another pause. "Not in the present state, no." But even if the damage cannot be undone, he pointed out, treatment might still help suppress the abnormal sensitivity. "But obviously it's going to be much easier to prevent the establishment of abnormal channels than to treat the ones already there." He rested his head against his hand. "Obviously."

I glanced out the window and tried to make out the shapes of the ships in the harbor through the rain. But just then pain radiated down my shoulder and into my hand, so swiftly I dropped my pen on the tabletop. I thought of the Righteous Sufferer.

Head pain has surged up upon me from the breast of hell . . .
A demon has clothed himself in my body for a garment . . .

I asked about pain's relationship to meaning.

Dr. Woolf blinked, surprised, and then scrunched up his face as he recalled a lecture given to the Harvard Medical School by Divinity School faculty on the religious meanings of pain.

"Imagine how foreign that point of view was to me," he said, shaking his head disapprovingly at the memory.

"But pain feels meaningful," I suggested timidly, "like a riddle or a dream."

"That's crazy," he said forcefully. "That's like the myths about TB we were talking about. Chronic pain is not some"—he searched for the right word—"*code*. It is a terrible, abnormal sensory experience, pathological activity in the nervous system."

Could these science terms, still so foreign in my mouth, become mine? Could the demon that clothed itself in my body turn into excitotoxicity and overuse atrophy? Cervical spondylosis and spinal stenosis and impingement syndrome—if I truly believed that's what it was and that's all it was—would be far less alarming than a curse, a punishment, a private sorrow, a symptom of aloneness, an inexplicable blight, or any of the myriad unhappy ways I understood and experienced and expressed my condition.

Would it also be less painful?

Seven years later, Dr. Woolf—newly appointed director of the neurobiology program at Children's Hospital in Boston—was replete with good news. His group had recently discovered a drug combination they are working on to develop into a pain-specific local anesthetic—an anesthetic, that is, that would act only on pain nerves and not affect the motor and autonomic nerves the way the current ones do. Such an anesthetic could potentially allow a person, for example, to go to the dentist and eat a pastry afterward, because the mouth muscles would be unaffected, or enable a woman to feel no pain during labor yet still register other sensations in her uterus and retain command of the muscles needed to focus her pushing.

The common local anesthetic lidocaine works by generally depressing the activity of all neurons. But by combining a derivative of lidocaine with capsaicin (the substance that makes chili peppers burn your mouth by binding to the pain receptors that detect burning), Dr. Woolf was able to target the lidocaine derivative into the pain neurons through the channel opened by capsaicin while leaving the other neurons unaffected. His work has been done on rodents, but he has licensed the idea to a pharmaceutical company that is preparing to begin human trials.

Most of Dr. Woolf's lab's work of recent years, however, has focused on decoding the genetics of neuropathic pain. "It is clear that pain is a complex disease, involving lots of different genes. We've been able to identify several key players," he said, sounding—in his low-key way—distinctly pleased. "It looks like about 50 percent of variation in neuropathic pain sensitivity is heritable," he told me.

Some pain research has focused on obscure pain-related genes, looking at interrelated families in Saudi Arabia or Pakistan. Such work has led to the identification of the genetic mutations responsible for the rare, bizarre disease *congenital insensitivity to pain*, which is marked by the inability to feel physical pain. Dr. Woolf's group has focused instead on the common genes found in different variants throughout the population. He recently identified a gene that produces an enzyme called GCH1 (GTP cyclohydrolase), which is a key modulator of pain sensitivity; one variant of this gene is significantly protective against the development of neuropathic pain.

Can the action of the pain-protective gene variant be copied and introduced as a drug for those who lack it? (Enroll me in that trial!) The gene variant inhibits excessive production of a substance called BH4 (tetrahydrobiopterin), which plays a critical role in pain sensitivity and persistence, with greater amounts of BH4 causing greater sensitivity to pain. Fifteen percent of the population has the lucky gene variant that most strongly limits BH4 production and makes people less susceptible to developing persistent neuropathic pain—and makes healthy humans significantly less sensitive to acute pain in lab experiments.

Dr. Woolf has identified a gene substitute—an agent that inhibits the production of BH4—which he is attempting to develop into a drug. Of course, there can be a long road between discovering a substance that does the job molecularly, so to speak, and turning it into a drug (the substance may be unstable or toxic, or it may dissolve too quickly in the body, or someone else might own the intellectual property!). But the first step has been taken.

Pain Diary:

I Try to Understand Science

BAD NEWS
nociception
pain-sensitivity gene
hyperalgesia, allodynia
central sensitization, peripheral centralization
excitotoxicity, overuse atrophy
cellular pain memory
cortical reorganization
gray matter shrinkage, neuronal loss, atrophy of the circuitry
the pain that pain spawns is ever more malign

GOOD NEWS
developing pain-nerve-specific analgesia
pain-protective gene
agent that mimics pain-protective gene action
hope agent can be turned into drug
the wonderful dream that pain has been taken away from us

IV

FINDING A VOICE:

Pain as Narrative

FINDING A VOICE

P hysical pain has no voice, but when it at last finds a voice it begins to tell a story," Scarry writes, expressing the paradox of the relation between disease and the narrative it inevitably becomes. Pain has no voice. Why, then, does it seem to speak?

When Hippocrates instructed physicians to treat the patient rather than the disease, it was because physicians did not understand disease. Now that science has shown that pain is a biological disease, to treat it otherwise would seem to do the sufferer a disservice: to personalize it, to see it as a state of being (which is what it feels like) rather than a state of the nervous system.

Yet, as lived experience, the disease of pain turns into the individual suffering of illness, an understanding of which requires studying the patient as well as the disease. Recall Foucault's neat formulation that modern medicine began when the doctor switched from soliciting an illness narrative—"What is the matter with you?"—to asking the medical question "Where does it hurt?" Alas, that insight does not finally or perfectly illuminate pain. For better and for worse, the nature of the person in pain bears on the nature of the pain itself.

What story, then, does pain tell?

INSPIRATION

The pain specialist was half dreading his first consultation in the hospital that morning. *So grim.* The patient was a middle-aged train conductor who suffered from multiple sclerosis. He had fallen from a train one day (MS affects balance) and sustained such severe injuries that his legs and one arm had to be amputated. He was now suffering from the onset of phantom limb pain.

"And he still had MS?" I said without thinking when the doctor later told me the story, as if the universe—having stolen three of the patient's limbs—would at least recoat the myelin on his aberrant nerve cells.

The doctor recalled how when he walked into the room, the patient was lying in bed reading. "Hey, Doc—have you read this book?" he said, showing him Rachel Naomi Remen's *Kitchen Table Wisdom*, a book of medical stories. "Some of these people—the things they've been through, the way they cope—it's incredible."

The doctor did a double take. The patient—*holding the book with his sole remaining limb*—was being inspired by the characters, most of whose medical adversities were less grave than his own. The patient had no idea that his capacity for inspiration would inspire the doctor, such that years later the doctor would tell the story to me and I, too, would feel a quickening (although I had read *Kitchen Table Wisdom* myself and felt only alienated by its stories of ennobling illnesses).

"I always think about that," the doctor told me. "Why? Why do some people do so well with intractable pain problems while others fall apart with ordinary ones? I've had patients with nonspecific lower-back pain give up—go on disability, become depressed, turn into full-time chronic pain patients—while others with more serious conditions are resilient."

"These lectures—" He made a dismissive motion with his hand about the lecture he and I had just attended about a gene that may or may not play a role in a type of pain.

Is the mystery of resilience a matter of genetics, character, temperament, will, luck? he mused. How can a physician (not a priest, not a magician) help patients who are broken by pain metamorphose into the train conductor whose empathy for the suffering of others is so great he momentarily forgets about his own?

"If we knew the answer to that," he said, "we would truly know how to heal."

SUFFERING

Nociception
Pain
Disability
Suffering
Pain Behavior

If pain worked the way it should, these things would reliably follow one another: nociception (the impulses transmitted by nerve cells that detect tissue damage) would cause pain. Pain would cause disability. Disability would cause suffering. Suffering would predictably cause certain pain behavior, so that you could accurately assess how much a person is suffering from the person's words and actions.

Yet none of this is true. Nociception can cause pain—or not. Certainly, the quality of pain bears no clear relation to the nociceptive input. Pain can cause disability—or not. But the most mystifying relation is that of pain to suffering: there are those who appear to suffer greatly over modest pain and those who appear to suffer far less from great pain. Pain behavior cannot be assumed to provide an accurate guide to the internal experience of suffering. The train conductor, balancing the book of inspirational stories in his one hand, provides a dramatic illustration that extraordinary nociception, pain, and disability do not necessarily occasion extraordinary suffering or pain behavior that demonstrates such suffering.

Sufferers experience their suffering as stemming from something outside them, Dr. Eric J. Cassell writes in *The Nature of Suffering and the
Goals of Medicine*. Yet "the factors that convert even severe pain into suffering depend on the particular nature of the individual . . . [T]he pain is
the pain that it is and the suffering takes the form it does in part because
of the contribution of meanings of the patient. Same disease, different
patient—different illness, pain and suffering."

I had seen this myself in patient after patient. The assignment I had to
write about chronic pain should have taken a month or two, if I dallied. I
wasn't being asked to *write a dissertation*. Yet seven months later I was still
visiting pain clinics around the country, following the director of each
clinic and observing each one's interactions with patients. Eventually I
observed several hundred patients.

After my article was published, in 2001, I decided to write a book because I wanted to answer one crucial thing: *Why do some people get better?*
How did the outcomes match the doctors' original predictions? Was there
a recipe for healing, and if so, could I employ it for myself? Why was a
West Virginia logger I met, who can no longer work owing to a back injury, suicidal? Yet Holly Wilson—paralyzed from a spinal cord injury—
did not seem even mildly depressed. Holly had been paralyzed in a cruelly
ironic way: a surgeon accidentally damaged her spinal cord during a
minor surgery to remove a bulging disk in her neck.

"I had this neck pain that radiated into my arm," she explained of
her original condition. "I thought it was the worst thing! I complained
about it constantly—I couldn't wait to have the surgery. I had no clue what
intractable pain was like." Now she suffers from the intractable pain, common with spinal cord injuries, that she experiences as coming from her
paralyzed body, which she calls her "shadow." She is loathe to take opioids in the doses required to control her pain. "I like to be clear-headed.
Clear-headedness is more important to me than lack of pain." She tried
a spinal cord stimulator, but it made her pain worse. She told me the
case settled out of court for a sum that is insufficient to cover a lifetime of
medical expenses, and now—ten years later—she fears running out of
money.

I kept her hour after hour, interviewing her—watching her face, the
way she laughs, the way she holds her head. But behind all my questions I
had only one question: *Why haven't you despaired?* She has pain; she has

disability; she describes her pain and disability vividly. Why don't they seem to cause her greater suffering?

One part of the answer lies in her relationship with her husband. "He's always there for me," she said. "I'm sure—I'm 99 percent sure—he's never going to leave me." Another part of the answer seems to lie in her relationship with her doctor, Scott Fishman. Although he had not yet been able to adequately control her pain, he was always trying—he always had a plan, six months ahead, of treatments to try. Whenever he heard about experimental treatments, he would find out whether they were suitable for her. "I'll call anyone in the world about Holly," he told me. Dr. Fishman's care for her—and her belief that he was always thinking of her—helped to balm the psychic scar of the fact that the surgeon never personally apologized to her for it or came to visit her in the hospital after the surgery. But Lee Burke had a good relationship with the Nice Doctor—indeed, his empathy blinded her to the failure of his treatment.

"I don't really know," said Holly when I asked her directly how she combats despair. "I'm not going to say that I've never thought of ending my life because I have and it would be easier for me, but I would never do that to my family. I know I could never do that to my family because my father did."

P ain upsets and destroys the nature of the person who feels it."
Aristotle's epithet seems all too true: pain fills consciousness,
blotting out the components of which the self is made. Yet such is
pain's peculiar relationship to meaning that this loss can take startlingly
different—indeed, opposite—meanings.

Suffering is sometimes described as a state that poses a threat to identity. While some pain poses a grave threat, other pain paradoxically strengthens the sense of self. Chosen pain—the pain of childbirth, a tattoo, an athletic feat, an act of bravery on the battlefield—can be *integrative*, strengthening integrity. For religious devotees and participants in the mourning and coming-of-age rituals common to most cultures, pain's dislocation of self is valued as a means of reshaping that self according to the religious ideals of the community. In a secular context, hazing rituals use pain to create "brothers" rather than discord. The pain of S and M fulfills deep erotic desires. The pain of self-mutilation may accomplish relief from a greater psychic pain or a sense of emptiness or numbness.

Chosen integrative pain differs profoundly from unchosen *disintegrative* pain: pain that cannot be reconciled with one's sense of self, but undermines and destroys it, as the pain of surgery differs from the pain of disease, even when they result in the same tissue damage. The pain of surgery can be integrative because it furthers the goal of survival, whereas the pain of the progression of a disease brings us closer to the self's dissolution. The pain of childbirth differs from the pain of miscarriage. Some women today elect to forgo anesthesia in childbirth and say that they are glad that they did.

"One word frees us of all the weight and pain of life: That word is love," Sophocles wrote in the fifth century B.C.E. Sean Mackey, chief of the Pain Management Division at Stanford University and the director of Stanford's Neuroscience and Pain Lab, recently showed that the pain of which Sophocles spoke can include physical pain. Dr. Mackey was struck by the parallels between the experience of early romantic love and the experience of addiction. Early romantic love involves overwhelming cravings for and emotional dependency on the beloved, obsessive thinking, a sense of energy, euphoria, and intensely focused attention, and piercing pangs of withdrawal. He wondered if both addiction to opioid painkillers and romantic love activate similar opioid brain systems. If so, does romantic love confer analgesia?

He and his colleagues recruited Stanford students who identified themselves as being in the first nine months of passionate romantic relationships. The students were asked to bring photographs of their beloved as well as of an equally attractive acquaintance. The students were then given a painfully hot stimulus while their brains were scanned and they were told to focus on a photograph of their lover or a photograph of their acquaintance. Love ameliorated the pain. When students were given a moderate-intensity pain stimulus, looking at a lover's picture caused a 46 percent greater reduction in pain, as compared with looking at an acquaintance.

When competing with a high-intensity pain stimulus, however, love's powers began to wane, reducing the students' pain by only 13 percent. But the more passionately in love the students were, the more analgesic benefit they received. Students who said they spent more than half of the day thinking about their partners experienced more than three times the analgesic benefit than that of those who were less preoccupied with their partners. The imaging revealed that the photographs of their lovers activated brain regions involved with opioids as well as those involved with dopamine. (The dopamine regions are also activated in people with addictions.)

The study seems to raise the intriguing question of whether the effects of love could be nullified by giving the subject a drug that blocks opioids, such as the drug naloxone. Could naloxone be the romantic antidote that would close the wound of Cupid's arrow—a condition whose pangs have tormented unrequited lovers from the beginning of time?

It is not only love, but community that balms pain. Researchers at Oxford University recently discovered that rowers who trained together were able to tolerate twice as much pain as rowers who trained alone. The rowers did a training session alone and a training session as a team; after each session their pain threshold was measured by seeing how long they could bear a blood pressure cuff squeezing on their arm. The men's pain threshold generally increased after exercise, but it increased far more significantly after group training sessions than after single sessions, suggesting that for humans, it is not only running from a tiger that produces the flood of endorphins of descending analgesia, but also communal activities (a phenomenon that may shed light on the embrace of pain during religious rites).

In his book *Disease, Pain and Sacrifice*, the psychologist David Bakan refers to integrative pain as *telic centralizing*: pain that is interpreted as consistent with one's *telos* or sense of purpose. Sacred pain is telic centralizing; secular pain is *telic decentralizing*. Torture maims the victim's sense of self; thus "whoever was tortured, stays tortured" after wounds have healed, as Jean Améry wrote about his torture by the Nazis. The Nazis arrested and tortured him, hanging him by his arms, and then sent him to Auschwitz. He survived torture, but not the memory of it, and eventually he committed suicide.

Torture involves the deliberate creation of suffering, which may or may not involve physical pain. "Waterboarding"—favored by the Spanish Inquisition, the Khmer Rouge, and the Bush administration—simulates drowning in such a way that it creates the overreaching desperation to make the torture stop, which is torture's hallmark. Confusion about the distinctions among tissue damage, pain, and suffering underlay the Justice Department's argument that "the waterboard, which inflicts no pain or actual harm whatsoever, does not, in our view inflict 'severe pain or suffering.'"

Rape is torture, even though it does not necessarily cause significant or enduring tissue damage. The torture of starvation only intermittently causes hunger pains. The torture of prolonged sleep deprivation or sensory deprivation (used by the British on IRA prisoners until the technique was outlawed) does not cause any tissue damage, but it can produce psychosis and long-term psychological damage. The forced lobotomies in the Soviet Union and America in the first half of the twentieth century involved little pain. And, of course, psychological tortures—such as the torture of knowing one's loved ones are being tortured—require no physical pain at all.

Context stamps pain like a coin. Torture in one context may be part of an occasion for rejoicing in another. I heard a lecture on pain and suffering once in which the speaker showed a photograph of a Hindu devotee during the festival of Thaipusam with hooks in the flesh of his back connected to ropes that followers were *tugging on*, like the reins of a horse (a festival I would later witness). "You see, the man's face is in repose," the lecturer commented. "The piercing does not cause him suffering, because it strengthens, not weakens, his sense of himself and his bond with his community." If the devotee is in pain, that pain is telic centralizing.

But for a Western person (like me) for whom pleasure and well-being are central, is physical pain inevitably disintegrative and telic decentralizing? Does faith play any role in shaping the experience of pain today?

THE RISKS OF RELIGIOUS BELIEF

In recent years, a number of studies have attempted to quantify the effects of religious belief on pain, health, disability, depression, and mortality in the context of chronic disease, with surprising results. A 2005 study led by Dr. M. Ojinga Harrison at Duke University Medical Center examined the role religion plays in modulating pain in African American patients with sickle-cell disease.

As a group, African Americans are strikingly religious: historically, the church has played a central role in helping its members cope with their plight, and a high proportion of African Americans continue to attend church and describe their faith as central to their lives. Sickle-cell disease has no cure. Despite recent advances, the lives of those afflicted by it are punctuated by disabling episodes of severe pain, lasting from a few hours to several days, which often require hospitalization and intravenous pain medications. But studies of sickle-cell disease have found that the frequency of pain crises is associated not with the severity of the disease but with the emotional state of the patient—with depression, anxiety, and other negative emotions correlated with greater pain. Those who attended church once or more per week were found to have both lower levels of psychiatric disturbance and the lowest scores on pain measures.

Larger studies have found that—for unclear reasons—people who attend religious services live longer and are generally healthier, less depressed, and less likely to be disabled. A famous nine-year analysis of more than twenty thousand adults in the United States, led by Robert A. Hummer at the University of Texas at Austin, found an astonishingly strong statistical correlation between churchgoing and mortality: Christians who attended church once a week lived an average of six years longer than non-attendees, while those who attended more than once a week lived an average of seven years longer. Even the timing of death seems to be influenced by religion: the devout are less likely to die before important religious holidays. African American Christians who attended church once a week lived eight years longer, while those who attended more than once a week lived fourteen years longer!

What about the devout who do not attend church? Curiously, "private religiosity" (prayer, Bible study, or self-described "intrinsic religiosity") does not appear to yield any of the dramatic benefits of church attendance. Indeed, private religiosity turns out to be associated with both negative and positive health outcomes and both worsens and ameliorates pain and depression.

It appears that the concept of private religiosity is too broad and that, from a health perspective, there are helpful and harmful forms of faith. Some of the benefits of churchgoing are thought to stem from *cognitive reframing*—the ability to reinterpret pain and illness as potentially furthering spiritual health even while they threaten physical health. But while some people believe that illness draws them closer to God, others may interpret it as God's punishment or abandonment, or they may begin to question God's very existence.

An intriguing study published in 2005 in the *Journal of Behavioral Medicine* tried to distinguish "positive religious coping" (strengthening faith) from "negative religious coping" (struggling with faith), among 213 cancer patients with advanced multiple myeloma, at a particularly difficult juncture—shortly before undertaking a painful, debilitating, risky treatment regimen (high-dose chemotherapy and stem cell transplantation). The patients described themselves as having high levels of religious faith and relying heavily on their faith to cope with the crisis of their illness. But the study found that patients who employed "negative religious coping strategies" had significantly greater pain, depression, distress, and fatigue, while (in contrast to the findings of some other studies) positive religious coping yielded little to no benefit compared to those who were not religious.

Critically, however, it is not known whether religious conflict causes poor health outcomes, or whether poor health creates religious conflict. Or, perhaps, the two unhappily feed upon each other as pain and suffering create doubt, and doubt fosters further pain and suffering.

THE PHOENIX

I f suffering occurs when there is a threat to the integrity of the person or a loss of a part of the person, then suffering will continue if the person cannot be made whole again," writes Eric J. Cassell. Chronic pain poses a particular challenge, for "in acute illness the threat is perceived as distinct and limited, whereas in chronic illness the threat is ongoing, long-lasting, global (encompassing all aspects of the person's life) and incapable of direct resolution."

How can wholeness be restored?

"Most doctors are not up to the task of chronic pain," John Keltner told me. Preparing himself for the task has been a process of extraordinary length—and one, in his mid-forties, in which Dr. Keltner is still immersed. Blessed with a patient wife, he began as a resident in anesthesia and pain medicine at the University of California at San Francisco (following a Ph.D. in physics), where he trained primarily in procedural pain interventions—injections and the like. Frustrated with their limitations, he decided to focus on trying to understand pain in the brain, and he moved his family to England to work on functional brain imaging at Oxford University. After two years, he decided he wanted to bring some of the academic insights into his practice, and (despite the lack of a trust fund to assist two decades of higher education and training) he embarked on another residency in psychiatry at the University of California, San Diego.

"You want to take advantage of all the physical tools that treat the body, but the part of pain pathology that continues to be less fully understood is the mindful part. Chronic pain is a devastating disease, a devastating diagnosis. Most people—including most doctors, who were trained in physical medicine—are stuck in the paradigm that the physical aspect of pain is the important one. Our understanding of the mind—of perception, cognition, belief—is not very far along."

Dr. Keltner pointed out that the mind is a new field. Psychiatry is little more than a century old, and neurology, in the contemporary sense, only half a century.

"I have this faith—and at this point it is only faith," he said, "that at the end of the day, mental therapies have the potential to be stronger interventions than physical interventions. My instinct is that ultimately there is more power in treating the mind, teaching the mind, healing the mind.

"Most doctors are normal people dealing with people whose lives are shattered. My patient isn't saying, *I have repetitive strain syndrome*, he's saying, *My life is ruined.* He's a butcher who can't chop anymore. I have an anesthesiologist with a pain that radiates down her arm who can't do her job anymore. We're taking a history and getting their rating of pain, but what they're really saying is, *I'm losing my fiancé, I'm losing my house, I'm losing everything*, and we ignore that. We need to treat all those other things as well: to help them figure out a way to be—to address the total human experience of being incapacitated. How can we create an AA for pain?"

Although most physicians speak in a quick, efficient style, Dr. Keltner often pauses for long moments in the midst of a conversation, as if grappling with the issues anew. Dressed in rumpled, graduate-student-type clothes, he has an intense gaze, bright blue eyes, and a boyish air of physical vitality.

"Like all chronic disease, chronic pain involves a bifurcation," he said. "There is the normal state, where you used to live, and you are conditioned to that state. Then you face a debilitating circumstance that lasts for months or years. When you're in that second state, you hold on to expectations of that first life: you mourn that first life—you want it and want it a million times over. But people have to let themselves die and lose their old expectations. If they let it die, they can rise like a phoenix from the ashes and can have a new life. The doctor has to help them die and be reborn with a vital, rich life."

THE FEARED-FOR SELF, THE ACTUAL SELF, AND THE HOPED-FOR SELF

Currents of hidden feeling complicate doctor-patient relations in every field of medicine, but the one between a pain doctor and his or her patient is especially fraught. Observing patients' appointments in a dozen pain clinics around the country, I was struck by the intense intimacy of the rendezvous, as the patient (usually female) waited half undressed, with her enormous hopes, offering her pained body to the stranger (usually male) who, like a savior, is vested with the power to ease suffering—or to fail.

The pain doctors I observed were excellent. I had selected them because I wanted to see how effective pain treatment could be; I had plenty of information from patient histories as to how it could fail. In the several hundred appointments I observed over the years, I never witnessed a doctor stumped by a case. Not only had the patients not tried everything—even the ones who had seen dozens of doctors—but frequently they hadn't tried the most obvious treatments. The doctor concluded the appointment satisfied. There were protocols to try, reasons for hope. When the doctor left the room, I stayed behind to talk and was startled at how often the patient's perspective was different.

There were two particular questions I always asked. The first was, "What do you think your diagnosis is?" The second was, "Do you think your doctor wants you to get well?" More often than not, these questions revealed that the appointment had—in a fundamental sense—failed. The patient did not understand the diagnosis. The patient did not believe the diagnosis. The patient was not certain that the doctor cared whether she or he got better—and on that lack of certainty, everything somehow foundered.

I'd have to resist the impulse to hurry down the hall after the doctor and drag him back. During each appointment, I had heard the doctor explain the diagnosis, explain the treatment plan, and then ask—as is customary—whether the patient had any questions. But the intense emotions that pain evokes interfere with patients' abilities to absorb biomechanical explanations—or even to be interested in them. (Prior to being given an assignment to write about pain, I had never informed myself even at the level of looking up my symptoms on the Internet, because at every minute I was busy trying—and failing—not to think about pain.)

Patients have only one question in their minds, sometimes voiced, sometimes not.

"Do you think I'll get well?" Elena asked the pain doctor. Elena had developed complex regional pain syndrome (also known as reflex sympathetic dystrophy syndrome), an enigmatic dysfunction of the autonomic nervous system that afflicts a limb like a fairy-tale curse, causing it to slowly wither.

The syndrome usually begins in one limb with an injury of some kind, yet the injury can be as significant as surgery or as small as an injection. For unknown reasons (perhaps owing to a genetic vulnerability), the autonomic nervous system that controls temperature, blood flow, hair growth, and sweating goes crazy. The afflicted suffer from burning and shooting pains; the limb becomes swollen and discolored, purple or rose, and the skin becomes too painful to touch. Hair grows rapidly or stops growing; sweating increases or ceases; the nails become disfigured, cracked, and brittle; the skin becomes dry or eerily shiny; the joints stiffen; the muscles go into spasm. In its most severe form, the changes become irreversible as the bones soften and thin, the muscles atrophy, and the limb becomes fixed in a furled position, as useless as a relic. The disease sometimes claims the opposite limb as well, or spreads to other parts of the body. Its course is unpredictable. Occasionally the progression can be halted by early treatment, although it sometimes disappears with no treatment at all, and sometimes all treatment fails.

The doctor was one who prided himself on his honesty, in contrast to what he thought of as the showmanship and empty promises of sham medicine. He had told me how enraged he was when he saw advertisements for products or services that professed to "cure" the syndrome, because they were all either useless or dangerous. Elena asked about the most dangerous of all, one that could cure or kill: a medically induced coma. Patients are given doses of the drug ketamine, an anesthetic and hallucinogen (whose street name is Special K), so massive that they lapse into a coma for five days, where they are often tormented by hallucinations. The treatment has not been approved in the United States, but patients go to Germany or Mexico for it.

Ketamine blocks pain receptors; massive doses of the drug shut down the nervous system, and for unknown reasons, when it restarts, it sometimes functions normally again—a process analogized to rebooting a computer. But sometimes people wake and find that while their pain is gone, they no longer know how to walk and talk. In 2008 a New Jersey woman went to Germany to undergo the treatment and emerged paralyzed from the neck down. Her husband told a reporter that her pain had been so terrible that if they had to do the treatment again, they probably would.

In one sentence, the doctor dismissed the idea, saying it was dangerous. "We'll try to get you sorted out," he told Elena quietly.

She looked at him agog. She was a middle-aged mother of five with no previous health problems, and the syndrome had begun nine months ago when one of her daughters had slammed a door on her hand. But instead of healing, the injury had metamorphosed, so that she was unable to continue work as an administrative assistant. She needed her hand back. *He would try to get her sorted out?* She held it up for emphasis; it looked swollen and mottled, like a dying guinea pig.

"Do you *think* it will?" she asked, the anxiety level in her voice rising.

It was clear to me that the question was not a medical, but a personal one. She didn't want an analysis of the odds; she wanted the doctor to show that he had a personal investment in her and was willing to verbally bet on her, as it were. She wanted to know that he saw the disease that was stealing her hand as *wrong*, that he could picture her the way she used to be, and that he believed she could be that way again. In asking about the ketamine coma, she had been conveying that the disease was killing her old self and that she was willing to risk dying in order to regain it.

Pain, it has been said, fragments the sufferer's sense of self, creating a feared-for self, an actual self, and a hoped-for self, each of which the doctor must address. Having spent a few weeks following this doctor, I knew he was personally invested in all his patients' treatment. But in addition to a penchant for clinical speech, he has a shy manner. His warmth seemed to disappear beneath his beard as he told her, "We don't know who will respond to the treatment and why. The only critical factor that we've identified so far in limiting the disease is keeping the limb mobilized." He went on to talk about nerve blocks (injections of local anesthesia that temporarily block pain). The blocks do not directly treat the condition, he said, but the temporary suspension of pain they create allows the patient to be able to endure physical therapy—and physical therapy alone can sometimes prevent irreversible atrophy . . .

But she had stopped listening. Although she made a follow-up appointment, it was clear that she would not return. She did not do physical therapy. She told me she wanted to try the ketamine coma but did not have the $50,000 it can cost. Instead, she sought holistic treatments, which failed to arrest the progression of the disease. The critical initial window of time elapsed, and the hand turned into a withered claw, never to be used again. She lost her job and, with it, the family health insurance. Her feared-for self became her actual self.

I puzzled over her story for a long time. It seemed like a parable of the failure of pain medicine, whose lessons were not fully clear to me. So often, I felt that the treatment failed because the patient didn't "buy" it. But in this case, was there anything the doctor could have done? What he had to sell (a treatment that might not work) was not very attractive, and he was honest about that. Was he too honest? Or was the problem that he had failed to use his powers (the strength of his personality, charm, empathy, expertise, or authority) to persuade her that, inadequate though it was, *this treatment was her only hope.* I thought about the alternative practitioners I had observed. I had been struck by how little they offered in the way of sound treatment, but they all possessed some kind of personal power; they knew how to evoke belief, and their patients actually followed their suggestions.

The last time I called to check in on Elena, her husband told me she didn't want to come to the phone.

THE RUSTLING OF STRANGE WINGS

A 2005 Stanford University survey found that people in pain ranked the two most effective treatments as prayer and prescription drugs. I puzzled over this pairing when I came across it. Prayer? *Prayer?* Most of those who used prayer relied on it in combination with drugs, and ranked them together.

I added prayer to the questions I was in the habit of asking patients after observing their appointments. Would they like their doctor to pray with them or for them?

Most patients said yes. Their doctors' reactions were almost comically different. "Seriously?" several doctors asked. An orthopedic surgeon recalled how, once—just as the anesthesiologist was about to put his patient under to begin a laminectomy—the woman had asked them to pause and join her in a prayer. The three men—poised, focused, and energized to perform the task they had trained so many years to master, cutting through the layers of soft tissue to excise the bony lamina—froze. They eyed one another uneasily.

They could close their eyes perfunctorily for a moment, but the specter of another realm intruded unsettlingly upon them. Of course, they didn't believe prayer affected surgery (after all, presumably she had prayed to God to cure her pain without surgery). But what if, inexplicably, the prayers now worked? What if an angel floated into the room during the operation and stood there shimmering? Would they

freeze in wonderment, fumbling with their scalpels, and let the patient perish? Or would they be able to ignore the rustling of strange
wings?

"The anesthesiologist finally mumbled, 'I guess we could have a
moment of silence,' " the surgeon recalled. "Then the patient prayed aloud!
For, like, *six minutes*, while we're all standing there in the OR, waiting to
do our job. I prayed to regain my concentration."

He glanced at me anxiously. "You wouldn't want your doctor to pray
with you, would you?" he said.

I assured him I would not. I pictured myself feeling suspicious that the
doctor was displacing his responsibility onto the type of intervening God
I didn't believe in (and felt relieved not to believe in, lest I be angry at His
failure to cure me and therefore accentuate my pain through *negative religiosity*). Yet why—I wondered—was it so important to me to feel that my
doctor truly *wanted* me to get well?

I recalled an interaction I had once had with a doctor whom I was seeing for a medical problem unrelated to pain. The doctor had made a small
gesture—one that he no doubt forgot minutes after it happened, but which
was of great importance to me.

I had gone to the clinic early in the morning for a test that would reveal
whether the treatment I had undergone with this doctor had succeeded. A
technician performed the test. As I was leaving the clinic, I glimpsed the
doctor across the reception desk, on the far side of the room. He held up
his hand, crossing his fingers. He was wishing me luck, reminding me that
the treatment was over, my fate was now up to chance, for—powerful
though he was in my mind—he did not possess the kind of power that
determines lab results. But he was also telling me that he hoped that chance
went my way.

I had previously undergone treatment with other doctors; each time
the treatment failed, I had switched doctors again. At the end of my initial
consultation with one of them, I had asked whether he was optimistic or
pessimistic about my case. "Pessimistic," he replied immediately. "You'd
need to be lucky." The way he said it made it clear that he thought it was
unlikely. After all, had I been lucky in that respect, I wouldn't be seeing
him. When the treatment failed, I associated my unluckiness with his pes-
simism and found yet another new doctor.

I had asked the nurse to leave the result on my voice mail later that day so I could listen to it alone. The treatment had failed again. I lay down on my bed, too disappointed to cry. I closed my eyes, and the image of crossed fingers came to mind—a stay against the darkness. I suffered from that failure in many ways, but I did not suffer from loss of faith in my doctor.

GHOST OF A MEDICAL MEANING

When the doctor explains to the patient what's wrong, he imagines that she is a blank slate—baffled by her pain and waiting for an explanation that she will wholeheartedly accept, since he, not she, has the correct information. If she had any interpretation of her pain before, she will naturally immediately relinquish it in the face of his overwhelming expertise.

Yet by the time the patient comes in, she has a long, intimate relationship with her pain, developed over months or years. Her perspective—the personal, radically subjective experience of pain—bears no relation to the scientific perspective, the objective, biomechanical view. She and the doctor do not speak the same language. The patient knows pain intimately—its taste, texture, and quality—and in one sense she is the only one who can know it. But from a physician's perspective, she knows nothing about it.

One of the doctors I observed kept a yellow plastic skeleton in his office. As he earnestly explained to patients their problems, he would point helpfully to the skeleton. The patients would look at him with the same baffled horror I recalled having as they realized that he thought there was an analogy between *it* and *them*.

While the doctor uses medical science to understand pain, the patient has constructed a personal narrative, one that weaves religious, mythical, and psychological elements with fragments of science, like a spider's web, suspending the patient above the abyss. Some of these narratives relieve suffering; others add to it.

In her memoir of rheumatoid arthritis, *Out of Joint*, Mary Felstiner writes of her fantasy of an Angel of Anatomy that descended on her after the birth of her beloved daughter Sarah, sparing her daughter and settling on her. The fantasy was inspired by something she had once read, to the effect that there is a higher incidence of the onset of RA following child- birth. The fantasy seems positive, turning her disease (about which she had no choice) into the necessary consequence of a joyful choice—the price of having a child. She also imagines that the Angel of Anatomy will spare her other diseases, since in having RA, she's done her share.

But most medical fantasies are not positive. Olive, who had come to a pain clinic I was visiting, had developed chronic burning pain in her breast following a mastectomy. Speaking with her afterward, I came to see that she and the doctor had very different interpretations of this pain. A forty-seven-year-old executive at a financial firm, she was used to making data-driven conclusions. In regard to her body, however, she had taken a ghost of medical fact and perverted it to torture herself with.

She had read that women who had babies had a reduced risk of breast cancer. When she was younger, she had terminated two pregnancies. If she had had a baby instead of an abortion, she reasoned, she wouldn't have had the cancer. (In fact, she had had the abortions in her thirties, and the dramatic reduction in breast cancer occurs only in women who have a baby before age twenty; having children after age thirty actually *increases* the risk.) The cancer turned out not to be an enduring punishment, after all, though; it went into remission. But she was left with an eternal reproach—the pain. The pain was a punishment for the abortions. If it weren't a personal punishment, she wondered, why did she, in particular, have pain from her mastectomy when other women had none?

Had she and the doctor been communicating well enough that he had ferreted this out of her, he could have given her the medical explanation. Indeed, a significant percent of women used to complain of chronic pain following radical mastectomies. Their pain was often interpreted as a psychological phenomenon: they were just "missing" their breasts. But in the early 1980s, Dr. Kathleen Foley at Memorial Sloan-Kettering Cancer Center in New York identified the pain as being caused by the severing of a major thoracic nerve during surgery. The technique is often performed now in such a way as to spare the nerve, but in Olive's case the nerve had been damaged. And apparently Olive was part of the fraction of the population that has a genetic predisposition for developing chronic neuro-pathic pain.

But that conversation with her doctor never occurred. Although the pain medication he prescribed eased her pain, it failed to address the suffering that arose from her mistaken understanding.

THE DIFFICULT PATIENT

When Sean Mackey, director of Stanford's pain management clinic, was considering what kind of specialist to be, he noticed the way other physicians were always carping about chronic pain patients. The patients threatened suicide, misused opiates, treated the doctor distrustfully, failed to adhere to their treatment plans, and then blamed the doctor when they didn't work. The doctors felt irritated, defensive, and frustrated in return and wished they could wash their hands of them.

"The more I heard, though, the more I realized that the difficulty of difficult patients lay not in the patients themselves," Dr. Mackey told me, "but in the feelings they evoked in their physicians—and the physicians' lack of training to handle those feelings." He decided to specialize in pain medicine.

Dr. Mackey is one of those people who makes one reflect on how unfairly nature distributed energy and optimism, for he—radiating well-being at dawn rounds—seems to have captured the lion's share. Tall and robust-looking, he has thinning strawberry blond hair, freckles, and a happy, joshing rapport with the residents. He possesses a Ph.D. in engineering as well as an M.D. (which he somehow managed to obtain simultaneously, in two unrelated programs), and he brings to medical encounters an engineer's rational, data-driven approach along with an air of straightforward goodness. I found keeping up with his clinical schedule emotionally, as well as physically, exhausting; I periodically excused myself and wandered down to the cafeteria to get tea, but mainly to get away from the patients and their suffering.

I once read a paper entitled "Dealing with Difficult Patients in Your Pain Practice," which provides advice for physicians. The paper cites a large study at a primary care clinic that treated patients for a range of problems. The study found that physicians rated more than 15 percent of patients to be "difficult" and had trouble working with them. The less empathetic the physician (as measured by empathy testing), the more likely he or she was to perceive encounters as difficult.

These problems are hugely magnified in the specific case of chronic pain patients, where pain causes psychopathology, which in turn hampers effective pain treatment. About 30 to 50 percent of chronic pain patients suffer from some kind of psychopathology, such as depression, anxiety, personality disorders, and substance abuse disorders (which the majority developed *after* developing pain). These problems can doom the treatment: untreated or undertreated psychopathology has been found to be *the most important factor* in unsuccessful pain treatment. Such patients not only report more pain and show more disability than other patients, they also benefit less from interventions such as pain medication, nerve blocks, and physical therapy than other patients. They describe themselves as "broken" by pain and feeling tormented, worthless, isolated, and unable to cope.

In response, Dr. Mackey and his colleagues developed what they called the Stanford Five, a list of points that they trained their residents and fellows to ascertain about every patient.

1. Patient's belief about cause of pain (cancer, muscular strain, etc.)
2. Meaning of pain from patient's perspective (association of pain with ongoing tissue damage, sinister ideas of pathology)
3. Impact of pain from patient's perspective (has it disrupted their social, vocational, recreational activities?)
4. Patient's goals (to be happier, to be less depressed, to go back to work or school)
5. Patient's perception of appropriate treatment (including whether the patient wishes to be referred to other specialists)

At first these questions struck me as rather prosaic, but over the weeks during which I observed appointments at Dr. Mackey's clinic—his own appointments and those of the residents he was training—I decided that they are genius. If a doctor doesn't know what the patient believes to be the problem, he can't try to persuade the patient of an alternative explanation. If he doesn't know the impact of the pain, he can't help minimize it and formulate functional goals for the patient. If he doesn't know what kind of treatment the patient is looking for, he can't either offer it or explain why he isn't offering it. Patients who come in wanting drugs or injections are unlikely to follow an order for physical therapy unless the doctor works hard to persuade them of its necessity. Likewise, patients who want MRIs or referrals to other specialists are going to be dissatisfied with their treatment unless they receive them.

Finally, it is essential to discern the meaning of the pain from the patient's perspective; in particular, Dr. Mackey focuses on the patient's interpretation of his or her pain and whether the patient harbors what he terms "sinister ideas of pathology." A patient who believes that his or her pain signifies a terrible disease that is causing ongoing tissue damage is going to experience the pain as worse than a patient who understands that—although chronic pain feels like an alarm bell—it is often a false alarm, signifying only that the alarm system is broken.

Ed, a young telemarketing manager, came to Stanford complaining of pain running into his testicles following a hernia repair operation. The pain was so severe he could barely sit down, yet he had refused pain medication. The resident probed his reasons why and elicited Ed's belief that medication would "mask" the pain and that, then, the pain might be getting worse without his knowing it. The resident explained that pain is a perception, so it can't secretly worsen without awareness. Conversely, if the medication mitigated his pain, he would not be deluded by the drug— he would genuinely have less pain.

"I don't want to cover up the pain. I want the problem cured," Ed said sharply.

"The problem is the pain," the resident said. "The nerve was damaged or severed during the hernia surgery. Your only symptom is pain, and so the only treatment is pain treatment."

When the resident left the room, Ed told me, "The doctor doesn't understand my problem."

George was another Stanford patient who had resisted treatment based on a misunderstanding about the nature of pain. Ten years earlier, he told the resident, he had broken his neck in a recreational game of football. Although he had been lucky to escape paralysis, he suffered from chronic neck pain, which interfered with his concentration in his job as an engineer. Taking opioids made him feel fuzzy. He was considering quitting his job and going on disability. The resident told him to stay in his job, explaining that "studies show that people's pain gets worse, not better, when pain causes them to quit their jobs." The resident suggested adding to his drug regime an antidepressant, Cymbalta—the first drug specifically approved to treat a type of neuropathic pain (diabetic peripheral neuropathy).

"I'm not depressed—I'm *in fucking pain*," George said. "It's *normal* to be depressed when you're in fucking pain. What should I be doing? Partying?"

"You won't be taking the antidepressants for your mood, but for their analgesic effect," the resident countered.

George seemed skeptical. When the resident left the room, I asked if it would make a difference to him to know that there is some evidence that antidepressants mitigate pain in rats as well as humans.

"Rats!" he said, sounding impressed. When the resident came back, he asked for a prescription. It had not been enough for him to be told that antidepressants effectively mitigate pain in humans, because he believed they worked in the wrong way. But to work for a rat—that was really working.

WHEN PAINKILLERS CREATE PAIN

I f only the answer to pain treatment were as simple as prescribing opioids for all patients—removing the social biases that prevent physicians from prescribing to certain groups, the myths that have led to bad public policy concerning them, and the taboos that prevent patients from demanding them. But in truth, opioids are overprescribed as well as underprescribed, and in the course of my research I observed patients who were helped and patients who were harmed by them.

There is no simple formula to determine who is appropriate for chronic opioid therapy. Rather, the drugs have to be carefully scrutinized to see the role they play over time in the complex course of an individual's life. The standard medical guideline for chronic opioid therapy is to evaluate not whether the drug reduces a patient's pain but whether it makes the person more *functional*. Thus opioid therapy is considered inappropriate for someone who says her pain has improved, but who sits around all day in a daze, while the therapy is considered successful if it enables her to return to work. The degree of relief the drugs bring to each individual has to be balanced against the adversity of the side effects.

Many of the patients I observed in pain clinics were in such agony that there was no issue of whether the drugs would interfere with their normal lives, because they no longer had normal lives. But what about people who are not in such desperate straits?

"If a house is on fire, you have to douse it even if it ruins the furniture," said Ari, a thirty-seven-year-old Israeli artist and professor in Chicago. "But what if your pain is not a fire, and you don't want to ruin your life to treat it?"

Seven years earlier, Ari had begun taking methadone because he decided, "My life is not good and I need to make some fundamental change. I just can't do it with the pain." Ari had been in treatment for depression since he was seventeen. Curiously, his emotional distress had always been accompanied by unexplained physical pain. When he tried to describe his "dis-ease" to his psychiatrist, he said he felt as if his "skin were so sensitive that the air hurt." The doctor emphatically assured him that his pain was a manifestation of his emotional blocks and would resolve naturally when he broke through.

By his early thirties, though, he felt he had accomplished many of the goals of psychotherapy, but the pain remained. "I began to say to myself, Fuck. I've done so much work in therapy, and I've made so much progress, but no matter whether I'm depressed or engaged, whether I'm frustrated and alone, or in bed with a woman I desire—whatever—I still feel like shit," he said. "I was more and more aware of the discomfort as *embodied*—as physical, as concrete.

"Pain is this huge presence. You try to ignore it, but it's always there, tearing you away from the moment," he added, his expression darkening at the memory. He has large, lucid, hazel eyes, close-cropped dark hair, a beard so short it might be carelessness at shaving, and the kind of tall, lanky body that causes his pants to slip from his hips as he stands. He is skittish about making eye contact, often looking away distractedly or fiddling with his iPhone.

He consulted with a neurologist who diagnosed him with migraine headaches and also with fibromyalgia, based on his diffuse muscular pain, tiredness, and depression. The neurologist prescribed methadone. Although methadone is supposed to be taken in a steady dose, perhaps because he resented his dependence on it, Ari took it haphazardly.

"Methadone really changed the way I thought about mind-body stuff," he said. "I would start to have classic depressive thoughts—like *my life is terrible*—with no awareness that they were coming from my physical state. Then I'd realize I was two or three hours behind in taking my pill, and my body felt like shit." Within twenty minutes of taking a 2.5 mg pill, he would feel pain's grip loosen and his body and mood unclench.

At first he found it "revelatory" to be in the world again without pain. He would go to a party and be struck that he could fully engage in conversations. But after six years on methadone, he began to reevaluate. "I realized I had lost access to parts of myself that were valuable to me. Opiates wrap a warm blanket around you when you want to be sheltered from the elements. When does encountering those elements become necessary?" Coddled in a pleasant, fuzzy, pain-free haze, he felt he could not become the artist he hoped to be. He also began to wonder if the drug was contributing to his clinical depression and sense of constant exhaustion. (It probably was. Opioids can cause depression. They also interfere with the architecture of sleep, making it less restful.) But because his body had become accustomed to the drugs, when he finally stopped taking them, he was tormented by insomnia that was still troubling him a year later, at the time we spoke.

Ongoing opioid therapy is usually resorted to only when the more benevolent options have failed. But Ari had never systematically tried the mainline treatments for either migraines or fibromyalgia. Fibromyalgia is characterized by distributed "tender points"—muscle knots that radiate pain when touched and can be treated by trigger-point injections (in which dry needles or ones containing local anesthetic or a steroid are inserted into muscle knots in order to get the spasms to release). He had not tried daily aerobic exercise, or even a simple but effective treatment of taking two twenty-minute hot showers a day and stretching under the running water.

"My doctor never suggested any of these things," Ari said. When I asked why he—an intellectual, a college professor—did not take charge of his medical care, even to the extent of researching the side effects of methadone, he paused and gazed off into the distance.

"My energies have been split between these radically different types of healing and modes of addressing human trouble," he said. At times he was convinced that his pain was simply a manifestation of his inner troubles, "a basic discomfort in the world" that he had tried to treat with a multitude of approaches: the traditional talk therapy approach, the psychopharmaceutical approach, the approach of meditation and mindfulness, the approach of acupuncture/chiropractic/bodywork and "releasing energy," the approach of trying to find greater satisfaction in work and love, etc., etc.

"I have a problem with faith with respect to Western medicine," he said dolefully. "I alternate between 'fuck those people' and 'okay, I need help.' Perhaps if I had more faith, the application of effort would yield benefit, I would put in more, and it would work better and I would be healthier . . . Do you believe in medicine?" he asked abruptly.

"I'm trying," I decided.

Ari is unusually attuned to his psychological state, so he was able to see that although the drug had initially helped him, it came to impede his life. But many people are unaware of the damage narcotics cause to their lives.

Marc—the sixty-eight-year-old owner of a horse farm in Virginia—suffered from scorching pain in his legs and feet for eleven years. It was diagnosed as an idiopathic peripheral neuropathy—a diagnosis that means simply "a pathology of the nerves of no known origin." He did not understand that sensory and motor nerves are different and that a pain problem like neuropathy is a sensory nerve problem that does not affect motor function, so he was haunted by fear that pain was damaging his legs and he would become crippled or even paralyzed, like Christopher Reeve. He began taking OxyContin. He noticed that he felt more energetic when he took OxyContin, which seemed to confirm his hypothesis that it was the pain that was weakening him (rather than the simple fact that—as the Greek warriors who took opium before battles knew—the drug can be stimulating).

The drug also made him disinhibited—impulsive and loopy. He was a self-made man, driven and disciplined, and with the disappearance of those qualities, so went the life he had constructed. He wrecked Lexuses. He quarreled with people and was unable to recall the quarrels. He abruptly abandoned his new wife, with whom he had been very happy, rushing through divorce proceedings, and then he just as abruptly reversed course to reunite with her.

He switched to methadone (which many pain specialists regard as more effective for neuropathic pain), but it had the same psychological effects. "I lost friends, relationships, business opportunities—I lost ten years of my life," he said. But like many people, he had had such searing experiences with pain that he had developed a horror of it and believed that his pain had to be completely medicated away, regardless of the damage to his life.

After he had had pain for more than a decade, he had a surgical procedure on his heart called a cardiac ablation. While he was in the hospital recovering from complications, he realized his pain had changed. He was accustomed to being aware of the precise moment in each day that his medication wore off and he needed another pill. But this time, that moment failed to arrive—he found he was able to reduce from eight methadone doses a day to two to alleviate the lingering discomfort. "Just as mysteriously as it came, it mysteriously went away," he said with wonder. He felt as if he had woken from a dream and returned to his former self. If only his decade could be returned to him!

What was the connection between the heart procedure and his leg pain? A cardiac ablation attempts to cure abnormal heart rhythms by destroying the section of tissue causing a signal in the heart muscle to misfire. Had the procedure somehow reset his nervous system as well? Marc asked his doctors for an explanation, but they had none.

It was as the Righteous Sufferer said:

> *My illness was quickly over, [my fetters] were broken . . .*
> *The relentless ghost . . . returned [to] its dwelling.*

Many people are unable to go off opioids, because their nervous systems are accustomed to the drugs. As soon as they try to reduce their dose, they feel terrible "rebound" pain (which they do not understand is actually being caused by the drug and which they misinterpret as a sign that their underlying chronic pain is unendurable). For others, though, simply taking opioids causes neurological changes over time that worsen pain.

Jose, a building superintendent in his early sixties, had come for a consultation because his pain had steadily worsened. The year before, he had injured his back while installing an air conditioner. He went to see his primary care physician, who gave him Percocet (oxycodone with acetaminophen) and then, when that ceased to control his pain, OxyContin. But the pain—which had been localized at the base of his spine—began to spread until his entire torso was affected. The doctor escalated the dose; the pain escalated in turn. The doctor ratcheted up the dose once more, to no avail, and finally referred him to the pain specialist he was seeing that day.

There is increasing evidence of a long-suspected condition known as *opioid-induced hyperalgesia* in which some patients (and animals in laboratory studies) on chronic opioids become dramatically more sensitive to painful stimuli (hyperalgesia) or experience ordinary stimuli as painful (allodynia). This opioid-induced enhanced pain sensitivity appears to be distinct from patients' original pain problems; it is often located in other parts of their bodies and has different qualities. In short, for these patients, opioids enhance the same kind of pathological pain sensitivity that is at the root of much chronic pain.

Jose did not want to hear that he needed to withdraw from the medication. As soon as the doctor began to talk about tapering down, he stood up, crossed his thick arms across his chest, and muttered, "It hurts me to sit too long." The doctor continued to talk. Jose shifted his weight from one leg to the other in a way that conveyed he wanted to leave.

I saw the doctor hesitate. Should he try to convince him? The next patient was probably waiting. He let him go.

SINISTER IDEAS OF PATHOLOGY

Studies suggest that one of the best predictors of whether a patient will adhere to a treatment plan is the patient's relationship with his or her doctor. In a good relationship, the patient and the doctor collaborate to create a wellness narrative: a story he or she can use to get better.

"I'm so tired of feeling like hell, trapped in a bad body," Danielle Parker told Dr. Russell Portenoy, the head of the pain medicine service at Beth Israel Medical Center in New York. "I've been feeling like a victim for a long time." She crossed her legs, leaned an elbow on them, and propped her chin on her hands, so that strands of shiny blond hair fell forward over her shoulders. She was wearing tight black jeans and a small, shimmery top that exposed her delicate collarbones.

She had been seeing Dr. Portenoy for a year at that point. Her pain had begun at the gym four years previously, she told me later. It was just after her thirtieth birthday; she was living on the Upper East Side, working as a freelance writer and in the bloom of health. She loved sports: tennis, parasailing, running, yoga. One day she was finishing her weight-training routine at the gym when a trainer approached her and asked if he could help with her workout. He was a large, muscular, 250-pound former military man from South America; she had a petite, 98-pound body. He asked her to lie on a mat to help stretch her out. First she lay on her back, and he stretched her legs. Then he asked her to turn over onto her stomach. But instead of the usual stretch, he grabbed her torso and, without explanation or permission, did a chiropractic maneuver of some kind on her upper back. She heard a popping noise and screamed in pain. "Oh my God, what did you do?" she cried.

"It was a horrifying, traumatic moment. In a split second my life changed," she recollected for me later. "I went from being a healthy person to a sick person." When she was twenty-five years old, her mother had been murdered in Arizona. The injury "felt like the physical manifestation of what I went through when I lost my mother. First someone took my mother away from me, and then another person took my health."

The injury had herniated a disk in her neck and destabilized her spine. A disk herniation (sometimes also referred to as a "slipped disk") occurs when there is a rupture in the outer, fibrous ring of the disk, causing the soft inner material to bulge outward. It causes pain in several ways. The inner material of the disk is itself irritating to the nerves and causes inflammation. The material can also get wedged against a nerve root, causing nerve compression, resulting in pain and numbness (if it compresses a sensory nerve) or a loss of mobility (if it compresses a motor nerve).

She stayed up all night after the injury, sleepless with pain and fear. Her entire upper body was paralyzed by muscle spasms, such that she was unable to turn her neck or torso. Although she regained mobility after three months of physical therapy, the pain remained. She had had many injuries in the past—from sports, gymnastics, dancing—and they had all healed. But this one did not. "I developed a disease of pain," she says. "My brain reads pain on a constant basis."

Dani began a medical journey in which she would see eighty-five doctors and spend a six-figure sum. When, after years of freelance writing, she finally landed a good full-time job at a magazine, she found she wasn't able to sit for enough hours to perform her responsibilities there. She continued to freelance when she felt well enough, scheduling periods of time to lie down during her workdays. Although her husband was supportive, she felt isolated. Because the pain built throughout the day, she stopped going out at night. Her friends didn't seem to understand her situation. When she tried to explain "my neck is on fire," they'd respond, "you look normal." She felt a burning, stabbing, tingling pain, as if "someone was lighting fires in my neck." When she typed, pain shot down her arm, making her fingers tingle, and she had to stop and ice.

"It's like being in a long war with my body. I became very despondent. I realized, *Oh my God, my life as I know it is gone.*" When her husband asked her what she was going to do that day, more often than not her answer was, *I'm going to see Dr. So-and-So.*

As often happens with back pain, the original problem leads to new ones as the injury distorts posture and prevents exercise. A few years after the incident she herniated two disks in her lower back. The neck pain "switched off, and the back switched on." She redoubled her effort to find treatment. She saw chiropractors and acupuncturists. Since there was no way to know what type of pain she had, she tried all the different classes of pain medications. She tried OxyContin, which made her break out in hives and itch all over. She tried Celebrex, but she believed it caused her to gain weight and she felt she had lost enough of her body as it was. Physical therapy seemed dull and futile, although she tried it on and off numerous times. She saw Dr. Portenoy, who prescribed Percocet and Klonopin, an antianxiety drug that can also quiet misfiring nerves.

"Am I taking too many opiates?" she asked Dr. Portenoy, looking at him intently. "Am I addicted?"

"You are not addicted; you are physically dependent," he reassured her. "It is totally different."

Her husband touched her thigh. I felt a pinch of envy and wondered what it would be like to have a partner who attended doctors' appointments. Her feet, I noticed, were clad in stylish high-heeled black boots: a token of her former self—the blithe young woman who had no need for sensible shoes. I wondered if she realized how they distorted her posture, so that wearing them actually made it less likely that she would regain that self.

Dr. Portenoy had sent her to see the clinic's psychologist—as he did most of his patients—but she said she had stopped going. "I don't want to talk about pain all the time," she said. "I want a break."

"It's fine if it's a break, but you need to get back to it," he said.

"You always emphasize the psychological," she said accusingly. She glanced toward her husband, a nice-looking music executive.

"I think Dani should go back to the psychologist," he said, looking directly at Dr. Portenoy. Dr. Portenoy urged her to go on Wellbutrin, an antidepressant that is sometimes used for patients with pain because limited evidence suggests that it can help alleviate nerve pain and because it does not usually cause sleepiness or fatigue. Unlike Zoloft or Prozac, Wellbutrin acts not only on the serotonin system but on the norepinephrine one as well, both of which play a critical role in the brain's pain-modulatory system.

"I don't like the label of antidepressants," she said. "I feel uncomfortable with the association of being on that type of drug."

"You'd be using them for the analgesic effect," Dr. Portenoy said, but he made no attempt to explain how they worked.

"You love to focus on the psychological," she said again.

"My note says that your pain is multiply determined: neuropathic, muscular-skeletal, and psychological," he replied. But in attributing three major categories of causes to her pain and weighing none more heavily than the others, it sounded like he simply didn't know.

"I can feel my back swelling up!"

"I'm not seeing swelling or feeling heat. You have perceptions of your body that no one else does. You can get misconceptions that can frighten you." Dr. Portenoy's tone was clinical—not accusatory, but not warm either. He was trying to dispel (as Sean Mackey describes it) sinister ideas of pathology. But the message did not seem to reassure her.

"You think my disease is now chronic pain," she said flatly.

"Exactly," he said, sounding pleased that she understood. "The last time I saw you, we talked about a lot of strategies. Where do you want to go?"

"I've been doing the quintessential thing of doctor shopping." She sighed. "Getting eighteen different opinions."

"No one can tell you it's time to stop looking," Dr. Portenoy said, "but I think it's in your best interest to stop looking."

She asked about a steroid injection, but Dr. Portenoy said he couldn't recommend one—by this point her pain was too diffuse to know where to put it. He recommended trying a new anti-inflammatory drug, a low dose of an antidepressant, and a return to physical therapy and to seeing a psychologist. But Dani seemed disinclined to do any of these things. The appointment was at an impasse.

"You look a lot better," he concluded. She had a fresh, wholesome girl-next-door beauty; despite her dark, sophisticated New York attire, she looked positively perky. The invisibility of her pain seemed to both flatter and disturb her. She put her lips together and smiled, a suspicious, quizzical smile. "But," he added, showing his experience as a practitioner, "this isn't to say you aren't miserable."

"I sometimes felt that my husband and Dr. Portenoy were ganging up on me," she told me later. "I kept feeling like, *Is anyone really hearing what I'm telling you? I'm not freaking out, I'm in pain. Somebody, please help me . . .*"

THIS CURSE THAT I'M LIVING WITH

The neurosurgeon John Loeser says that if a doctor does not believe his or her patient, the appointment will necessarily be a failure.

Dr. Portenoy was an agnostic when it came to Dani's pain. "I don't know what her pain comes from," Dr. Portenoy told me in his even, well-modulated voice at the end of the day as we walked out of the hospital. Of modest height and build, he has rust-colored, gray-flecked hair, with a beard, large glasses, and the serious, impassive, yet attentive demeanor of a psychiatrist. "She has disk herniations, but many people have herniations. Her pain may be partly neuropathic. Or it may be largely muscular. Or it may have been primarily psychological—depression and anxiety feeding muscular pain. If you ask me if a single incident could cause chronic pain for the rest of someone's life, I'd say yes—absolutely. Whether Dani is that person, I don't know."

Dani had sued the gym and the trainer, and that suit was still pending. Sometimes, Dr. Portenoy pointed out, chronic pain patients do not get better until their suits are concluded, because the necessity to prove their pain provides a conscious or unconscious disincentive to get better. But winning a suit does not always provide the imagined satisfaction. Daniel Carr recalled a patient of his whose lower back was crushed owing to a defect in the installation of the seat of his new car. During the years the patient was fighting his suit, he endured the pain by fantasizing about reparation: how the law would come down on the car company and compensate him for his suffering. But when the big check finally arrived and he truly understood that he could not buy the only thing he really needed—his old body—he ended his life.

Three years later, when I checked in with Dani, she was worse. She was still trying lots of therapies. She received injections of Demerol, morphine, and Valium in her lower back. She took Klonopin and Vicodin. The Vicodin helped her pain, Klonopin helped her sleep, but nothing really helped. Her weight had dropped, and she felt weak and depressed. "I feel like I'm deteriorating," she said.

Although she told me that her lawsuit against the gym settled in her favor, the resolution did not provide the expected catharsis. "I felt victimized that I didn't get to go to court and tell them what that bastard did to me," she said, but her lawyer had advised against it, on the grounds that juries—especially after 9/11—were not always sympathetic to chronic pain. But at least the settlement money could help pay for her treatment.

"There are cures for much more serious diseases," she said wistfully. "I imagine a lot of pain patients die depressed and lonely—not able to live life as before." She asked about other patients I had interviewed. "I bet you won't find one person who is all better," she said. She keenly felt "the domino effect of what it does to a person's life. You lose friends; you lose co-workers; you lose everything. I felt like I was being stabbed in the heart when my mother died. Now I'm being stabbed in a different way—lying in bed, screaming in pain, being knifed over and over. Pain killed me. There was a different Dani before the injury."

She felt she had exhausted Dr. Portenoy's repertoire. She recalled how one day she went to him and said, "I can't live like this. When I think of living for the next fifty years in pain, I don't want to do it."

The detachment she felt in his clinical manner gave way to a shared sadness and failure. "I saw a glimpse of his humanity. For once, he seemed like he was really sorry. He had a tear in his eye." But she felt like they were talking about a patient with a terminal disease, for whom nothing more could be done—a message other doctors reinforced. She went to a surgeon and begged him to operate on her, but he declared her condition nonoperable. (Disk herniations do not usually require operations, because the fluid is eventually reabsorbed by the body.) Although she was lucky the surgeon was so honest, as back surgeries often worsen the original problem, she understood the word *nonoperable* to mean that her condition was hopeless, rather than simply that an operation wasn't necessary.

"I told the surgeon that I really want to have a baby, but I'm in so much pain I can't imagine carrying a child. I asked him if he could give me a referral, and he said, 'No—you've tried everything. You're going to have to learn to live with the pain.' It's disgusting to be told you have to live with pain. It disgusts me!" she reiterated, as if trying to remind herself to reject that kind of thinking.

She enrolled in a treatment program of Dr. John Sarno—the famous back pain guru whose book I had read at my friends' beach house long ago. But she felt skeptical of his theory of TMS (tension myositis syndrome), according to which repressed negative emotions cause pain and muscle tension, and when you let go of the emotions, the pain disappears. "It's ludicrous for some doctor to say it's completely in your head—it makes you feel crazy. There is a physical root. Moreover, he had my husband convinced. Danielle's gone through trauma—let's blame it on Danielle's mother's murder."

The loss was compounded by the fact that the crime remained unsolved and Dani felt she needed to stay actively involved to bring attention to the case. The details were all so devastating. The last place her mother was seen alive was a convenience store. The store's security tape might have captured the killer, but, she told me, the detective assigned to the case took the day off after the murder and the store erased the tape.

The simple causal link Dr. Sarno was making between Dani's pain and her mother's murder seemed illogical; she hadn't developed pain until four years later. And she felt her fragile mental health was caused by—rather than the cause of—her pain. "If you're in goddamn pain all the time, of course it's going to mess you up," she said.

Dr. Sarno instructed her to write in a journal, she said, to explore childhood trauma, but she couldn't think of any—she felt she had a wonderful childhood. She wrote poetry about the loss of her mother, but it just made her cry. "Bringing back her murder, I'd get more pain. Negativity is part of pain."

Dani recalled the way in which Dr. Sarno bristled when she questioned him about his methods, and he insisted that she quit PT, which he told her is harmful because it focuses on the body instead of the mind, which he considered the root cause of pain. She replied that she had muscle spasms and needed the relief provided by the massage technique her physical therapist employed, but he told her, "If you can't follow the program, you're out." She wondered if that was how he achieved his vaunted high success rate: from kicking the failures out of his program.

"I'm sure there are some patients who actually have TMS and are helped," she said, "but his program made me worse."

In talking to me, Dani struggled to come up with a positive narrative—one that reconciled pain with her self-image. "I believe there are a lot of people who wind up crazy. But I'm a fighter, a survivor—that's part of the story, too. I have this curse that I'm living with, but I'm learning to live with something that most people would consider unlivable." Still, she added, her "greatest wish in life is to have a solution—I pray every day."

A PARTNER IN WELLNESS

Dr. Portenoy had no doubt that seeing doctor after doctor was not helping Dani. But although she half agreed with him, pain kept pushing her on.

Eight years after the initial injury she and her husband were on vacation in Aspen, Colorado, when she noticed a sign in the lobby of the St. Regis Resort for the Aspen Back Institute. "I've already been to eighty-four doctors," she told her husband. "Might as well make it eighty-five." The institute's website described it as "a unique, non-surgical oasis for injured backs and bodies" and sported testimonies from celebrities, athletes, and businessmen who had been reunited with their golf games.

The founder, Clint Phillips, had trained as a chiropractor in South Africa and had come to Aspen (of all places) to pursue his passion for rugby. With his earnest gaze and his chiseled jaw and shoulders, Clint looks like someone who could inspire people to work with him for many reasons. "Back pain is so misunderstood," he says in his seductive South African accent, looking directly into the camera on the website's video. "Let me teach you the secrets that doctors don't know or that they won't tell you . . ."

Dani decided to test Clint by not telling the full story and seeing what he could discern. When he felt her back, he was able to pick out the muscles in spasm and show her that they were trigger points (muscle knots that are tender to touch and refer pain to other areas). She was astonished; she felt that her pain was speaking to him directly. Many of the fancy physicians she had consulted hadn't even bothered to examine her. And when she worked with a physical therapist, they had always focused on one area at a time (perhaps for billing purposes) rather than developing a comprehensive rehabilitation program.

Dani extended her vacation so that she could work with Clint for a full three weeks. He came up with a stretching and strengthening program to keep her muscles out of spasm. Each morning, he would work with her and talk to her for an hour. He showed her how, when she wore high heels, it threw her posture out of alignment and strained her back muscles. Although her relationship with Clint is neither mystical nor romantic, the language she uses to describe it borrows from both arenas in attempting to capture its singular importance. "I think he's a miracle worker. I knew it in one session with Clint—I knew he was the one for me. He represented hope and healing."

Although she knew that Dr. Portenoy cared about her, the way that Clint related to her felt essentially different. Dr. Portenoy had never suggested that she was fabricating her pain, but neither had he reassured her of his belief. Clint's faith in her, on the other hand—his understanding of her feared-for self and her hoped-for self—felt tangible. Clint seemed like a healer in the ancient sense of the word: one invested with "a particular potential for witnessing suffering—a charismatic authority," as the sociologist Arthur Frank puts it. "I had met a lot of doctors before," Dani said, "but I had never met a healer. He said he was going to treat the body *and* the mind; he spoke to me about the devastating emotional impact of pain."

Dani found the way Clint spoke of the importance of the mind much more persuasive than the way Dr. Sarno had done, because Clint's philosophy involved attention to the body rather than denial of it.

"He breaks the pain cycle, and then he asks, 'How are we going to get rid of these pain behaviors and change how you respond to pain?'" she told me. "Instead of reaching for that pill, you go for a walk, go for a bike ride, move around." He told her, "You're going to feel discomfort. Don't let your mind focus on it when you feel an unpleasant sensation." He didn't use the word *pain*. "In the past, I used to panic as soon as I felt a zing," she said. "Now I try to focus on something else. I don't talk to people about my condition anymore. If someone says, 'How are you?' I say, 'I'm great,' deflect the question, and ask about them."

After seeing Clint in the morning, she worked with his physical therapists in the afternoon. They massaged her neck and taught her ergonomics and isometric exercises to strengthen her neck and build up shoulder strength. They stressed the importance of posture. Clint explained how the head is like an eight-pound bowling ball, and if you carry it forward, it pulls on all your neck muscles, causing them to spasm. Dani attributed the fact that she can now sit without pain to having strengthened her stomach muscles enough to hold her back in place.

In the afternoon each day in Colorado, she went for a hike. Then she went on her first bike ride in years. She had to walk partway, but on the second day, she made it the whole three and a half miles. She had developed a fear of the gym from her injury, but soon she was doing one-hour circuit training with Clint's wife, Jade. She recalled how Clint constantly said, "Dani, you're a young woman, you have a good body." He called the troubles with her body *issues* rather than *problems*. "I was made to believe that I had a bad spine—a defective spine with defective disks that the MRIs showed. But the spine can heal itself with the proper posture and exercise," she said. He kept telling her, "You're not sick, you can live a normal life."

He enticed her into trusting her body again. He didn't order her to stop taking pain medication, but he suggested that if she could start cutting down, she would be more attuned to her body's response and that she needed to be able to feel her body again. By that point she was taking six Vicodin ES a day—a substantial dose.

"I was so dependent. I used to walk around all the time with a pillbox. By 1:30, if I hadn't taken my Vicodin, I'd start craving it," she said. "I don't know if my pain was real or if my body was generating pain because it craved medication." When she finally stopped taking the pills, she realized how they had been affecting her cognitive abilities. By the end of the day, she often found herself watching TV because she didn't have the concentration to read. The six tablets of Vicodin ES she was taking contained 4,500 mg of acetaminophen (the ingredient in Tylenol), which upset her stomach and put her at risk for liver and kidney disease (above 4,000 mg per day—or 2,000 mg per day for a person who drinks alcohol—can lead to potentially fatal liver damage).

"We're going to have a party where we burn all the chronic pain books and flush the meds down the toilet," she said.

Although the Aspen Back Institute is expensive, it was a fraction of what she had spent pursuing futile treatments in previous years. In just three weeks of her program she felt the beginning of "a new identity." The biggest change, she said, was simply "to realize I'm a normal person—there is nothing wrong with my body." But "letting go of the emotions of pain is traumatic. If you have pain for eight years, then you become a pain person. I took a twelve-mile bike ride around Manhattan yesterday. I feel great; I feel like an athlete in training. The mind is such a powerful thing."

She feels that traditional doctors partner with patients in sickness, whereas "with Clint you feel you have someone dedicated to your wellness. Clint looks you in the eyes. He's *in it* with you," she said. When she left Colorado, she said, Clint was worried that she'd revert to hanging out in bed and watching TV, so he scheduled conversations with her. He told her she didn't need PT—the label would only remind her of being sick (although, of course, the exercise regime he prescribes is a form of physical therapy). She decided instead to rejoin a normal gym.

Like Dr. Sarno, Clint used cognitive reframing, preaching a shift in narrative from sick to well. But unlike Dr. Sarno, he did not insist that if you believed his theory, you could make your pain simply melt away. Rather, Clint's narrative used belief to make its premise true by transforming the body physiologically, as well as psychologically, through exercise.

Physical therapy is the most effective treatment for most back pain. Strengthening the muscles that stabilize the spine can relieve pressure, and muscle growth has been hypothesized to actually stimulate nerve growth. Most important, physical therapy intervenes in the cycle of chronic pain. The body is designed only to respond to acute pain. Muscles contract rigidly around an injury to hold it in place and protect it from further damage. But when pain persists after the original injury has healed, that protection mechanism becomes maladaptive. The contracted muscles clamping down on nerves cause pain, and muscles atrophy from disuse and become another source of pain themselves.

But physical therapy does not appeal to most people. It's boring, it sometimes hurts, and it usually takes an extremely long time to work. Repeatedly I had observed doctors recommending physical therapy only to discover, when I followed up with the patients, how few people dedicated themselves to it. (Then again, my own initial attempt had been halfhearted. But yours, reader, if you have pain, should not be! Truly, if you take any advice from this book, take this one.)

Chronic pain patients have low rates of response to a placebo because they expect to be in pain. Without belief—and the initial rush of analgesia that a placebo creates—it is difficult to invest in a treatment that requires great effort before yielding any results. Clint used his charisma to make

Dani believe that his particular program of physical rehabilitation could work, so she applied herself to it in a way that she had never done with physical therapy, and she began exercising constantly. The rapidity of her improvement initially may have been the endorphins of placebo as well as exercise, but its initial success conferred on Clint a gurulike status and kept her committed to the program when the placebo disappeared. Her faith also enabled him to change her perception of pain, persuading her that the lingering sensation in her back should be reframed as discomfort.

"I'll get little twinges now and then," she said matter-of-factly, "but that's just because my body is used to producing it. I will follow my wellness program like a bible." We had been talking for several hours at this point, in a café in midtown Manhattan. "I want to move around—we've been sitting a long time," Dani said. "Not because I'm in pain," she added quickly, "but just because I want to move." She was excited to go across the street to Bloomingdale's and shop for her new favorite thing: cute workout outfits.

"I think I got a little too confident," she told me when I talked to her next, a few years later. When she feels better, she is tempted to slack off on her exercise routine. "I think, I'm better now, I can just live my life." Then the pain crashes in again. "I need to honor my body by having an ongoing commitment to wellness, the way some cancer patients need to take ongoing medications."

She found it hard to wean herself entirely from Vicodin; she liked the feeling of knowing that when she was in pain, there was something she could do about it instead of just feeling victimized. But she also found herself periodically slipping back into a dependency she dislikes. She found Klonopin even harder to quit. When, at a doctor's advice, she simply stopped taking it, she suffered from such severe withdrawal symptoms she ended up in the emergency room, her heart racing, her blood pressure soaring. (Withdrawal from benzodiazepines, such as Klonopin, Ativan, and Valium, can include panic attacks, anxiety, hallucinations, and life-threatening seizures.) She wishes that the doctor who first prescribed Klonopin had informed her that benzodiazepines are more addictive than opiates, and that they impair cognitive abilities and memory.

She is no longer completely convinced that her body is entirely normal, as Clint says. If it was, why did she develop such excruciating, protracted pain from a single injury? "There are people with disk herniations who have no pain," she said soberly. She puzzled over whether there is something about her body and its genetic makeup that makes her vulnerable to chronic pain. "That's the missing piece of the puzzle." But talking to me, she said, made her recall how terrible she used to feel. Now, when she complains of setbacks, it is in the context of something wondrous: "I expect to feel well. And when I don't, it's usually my fault because I have not been following my program."

"That's great!" I said. "You can be a star patient in my book—one who stopped being a pain patient. I don't have as many as I would have hoped . . ."

I had certainly seen many improvements over the years. The ones who didn't take active steps to treat their pain usually worsened over time, although some got worse despite their efforts and some also improved with no particular effort. Just as there is a chronic pain windup, for some patients, there can be a chronic pain wind down over time. But not that many people had been cured.

"Except for you," she said. "Your book includes the story of how you cured your own pain?"

"Oh, no, no. But my pain improved . . . And I developed a good understanding of pain, which in a way makes it less painful by making it less sinister seeming."

"But you have an inspirational story?"

"It's not that kind of book," I said unhappily.

"You need to focus on curing yourself!"

I had reduced my pain, but I had never fundamentally shifted my narrative. "Build . . . an illness narrative that will make sense of and give value to the experience," the medical anthropologist Arthur Kleinman enjoins. When I first got the results of my MRIs, I had resolved to take control of my situation. I felt I was suddenly seeing things clearly: the nature of my pain, the nature of my relationship with Kurt. I made a slew of doctor's appointments, left Kurt, and ordered a special pain diary from the Arthritis Foundation to document my quest for healing. I loved reading pathographies—first-person accounts of illness. Perhaps I could write one.

The pain diary had an uplifting title printed on its glossy cover, *Toward Healthy Living: A Wellness Journal*, but I added my own title: *Pain's Progress*. When I was eleven, I had been taken with *Pilgrim's Progress*, and for a year or so, I had seen my life through its story. Perhaps it could be my model: my pain the burden on the pilgrim's back as he struggled up the Hill of Difficulty or descended into the Valley of the Shadow of Death. Soon I, too, would arrive at the Delectable Mountains.

But my tale was not turning out like the pilgrim's. I hated to reread it.

Pain Diary:

I Wish for More Betterness

"Even comparatively well-adjusted patients can have the idea that their pain physician should be able to eliminate all of their pain and that failure to do so is tantamount to withholding treatment," the article "Dealing with Difficult Patients in Your Pain Practice" warns physicians. "Some of the primary tasks a pain physician faces as a healer are to foster realistic expectations for treatment success . . ."

The only thing I had wanted from a doctor was a cure. The first seven doctors I brought MRI films to were not inclined to offer this, and neither, I realized ten minutes into the consultation, was the eighth. I had gone to see a rheumatologist (a doctor who specializes in arthritis, autoimmune diseases, musculoskeletal pain disorders, and the like) who had sent me to the Jock, a physiatrist—another specialty I had never heard of, which focuses on rehabilitation. The Jock, as I thought of him (a short man in his early thirties, with an aggressive manner and an alienating buzz cut, whom I dismissively pegged as a former hockey player), was talking to me about the same treatments other doctors had suggested: physical therapy, steroid injections, anti-inflammatories, more physical therapy. I tuned out as he detailed them, because I felt that he was fundamentally talking in the wrong way.

There were two modes of discourse in medicine, I had recently realized. There is the Cure Mode, the one I had always been in before, in which the doctor said things like: take this and call me if you don't feel better, and we'll give you something else. "I hate to see it drag on like this," my primary care physician would say of an ordinary cough that had lasted what I now saw was a paltry few weeks, sounding impatient not with me, but with the cough. Then he would scribble a prescription that would put an end to it. This was the way I liked to interact with doctors: problem, solution, gratitude.

But there was another mode, I now realized: the Treatment Mode. In the Treatment Mode, appointments were long, and they involved an unknown number of follow-ups and referrals to multiple other health-care professionals. Conversation centered on *improvement* and *reduction* and *management*, as in, "the goal is to reduce your pain to a manageable level."

That was not my goal! I appreciated that the cure for my pain must not be obvious, or the other doctors would have thought of it, but I still felt that if the Jock had realized that *I was only interested in the cure option*, he should be able to come up with something else. I wasn't asking him to think outside the box: the Treatment Mode simply was not my box.

"Could surgery fix my problems?" I liked the idea of that—cutting out my pain like a tumor.

"Not with a multilevel problem. Surgery can't fix degeneration of the cartilage, and you can't go through at every single level and shave off all the bone spurs—and we don't know which ones are causing the pain, anyway. Now, if the stenosis progressed to the point of impinging on the cord itself, and you were losing function, we'd go in there and open it up . . ."

The old image of myself as a skeleton came to my mind. *This is an example . . .* the doctor was saying to the eager young students.

"So you'll give physical therapy a try?" he said.

I frowned. "I told you, I already gave it a try."

I had stopped in at the physical therapy department in the basement of the hospital after a previous consultation, and I didn't want to go back. There were old people, and young people whose bodies had been made old with disease, humbly trying to make a little progress—to stretch or strengthen or unshrivel. I didn't want to work *with* a broken body, I wanted my old, true body restored. Just yesterday (okay, a few years ago), I had had a good body—not especially strong, but at least smooth and sleek. I wanted the Jock to reassure me that we agreed on the same goal.

"If I did physical therapy, would I be able to canoe?"

"Hmm. We have to see how your shoulder progresses," he said, and began to discuss rotator-cuff disease. "Is canoeing important to you?"

"Critical," I said with great feeling. Despite my lifelong dislike of canoeing, the idea that I would never be able to change my mind and take an interest in it suddenly seemed terribly sad. "And kayaking," I added, for good measure.

"Paddling is hard on the rotator cuff. We'll have to see."

"If I did physical therapy, how long would it take?"

"You should see improvement within three or four months."

"But when would it be normal? When would I be able to canoe?"

He demurred.

"I want to set *a definite date*. I'm not doing PT without a definite date."

"I can tell you in my experience that once these things become chronic, they rarely *if ever* go away," he snapped.

I began to weep. As I left, everyone stared: the receptionist, the nurses, and the other patients in the waiting room. I went to the bathroom and ran cold water over my face, but tears kept burbling up through my eyes.

"He said that it couldn't be normal," I complained to the rheumatologist who had referred me to the Jock.

"He did?" the rheumatologist replied.

I nodded, tears beginning to well again at the memory of the pronouncement.

"I am very surprised. I don't know why he would talk to you like that." He looked genuinely perturbed. "In fact, I am going to call him and discuss it with him."

I sniffled and nodded.

"He says he didn't say that," the doctor said when he hung up. "He said he is optimistic about your case." He waved his hand optimistically. "And so am I."

So there it was. I had manipulated the senior doctor into criticizing his junior colleague so that the junior doctor would say what I wanted to hear. The absurdity of the Bargaining Mode was suddenly clear to me.

"I know it might not get totally better," I said in a small voice. "I just want to make some improvements."

The rheumatologist nodded affirmatively. "Absolutely. You can definitely make improvements. Let's walk down to physical therapy." As we walked, he began explaining how strengthening muscles can stabilize joints and compensate for nerve damage. I had heard it before, of course, but this time I began to listen.

AT THE WILL OF THE BODY

I had been struck by how the rheumatologist talked to the physical therapist—respectfully, deferentially, as if the therapist were in possession of knowledge and skills he didn't have. There is a body narrative, I tried to tell myself: the physical therapist directs the body narrative, just as a psychotherapist tries to improve a psychological one and a religious counselor fosters a spiritual one. A person must be patient with a body narrative. A person must try every single thing with an optimistic—not desperate—attitude, hoping it will help but not being devastated if it doesn't. Ten treatments that each result in a 5 percent reduction in pain can collectively cause a 50 percent reduction . . . that kind of attitude.

As I did the exercises and built up muscle, the image of the skeleton receded. I still resented physical therapy—I wanted to punish my body for hurting me, not coddle it!—but I did it. I read Arthur W. Frank's memoir of his illnesses, *At the Will of the Body*, and I tried to accept his idea that we are at the will of—not at war with—our bodies, regardless of whether our bodies are the way we want them to be. Disease is natural, as is death; our bodies have not betrayed us by sickening.

At the rheumatologist's suggestion, I wore a big white cushioned brace, known as a cervical collar, around my neck that held it upright. It was extremely noticeable. When people asked, "What did you do to your neck?" I couldn't think of an answer.

"I didn't do anything." *It got bad on its own.*

"Were you in an accident?"

"No." The silence was awkward. I experimented with adding, "It's a treatment for a type of arthritis."

"Arthritis! But you're so young! How did you get that?"

It's a punishment for my sins. "Bad luck, I guess."

"Did you have an accident?"

"It's congenital."

"Does it run in your family?"

"No."

I wanted to take Vioxx or Celebrex—anti-inflammatory drugs known as "super-aspirin"—which, unlike aspirin and Aleve, are designed to protect the stomach. But my insurance wouldn't pay for them, so I took Aleve until the lining of my stomach wore away and I became chronically nauseated. A camera was sent down my throat to photograph the dilapidation, and lots of expensive stomach work later, Vioxx was approved. I puzzled about this: the insurance mastermind with the incorrect calculus. Since such a large percentage of people who take anti-inflammatories do end up with stomach problems, why wouldn't my insurance company, Oxford, pay for Vioxx in the first place? Was its CEO planning to cash in his stock before everyone's stomach problems set in—or would he move to another company where they had been paying for their customers' stomachs all along?

Then, in 2004, people who were at risk for heart attacks and strokes had a higher rate of them on Vioxx, and the drug was removed from the market. The media coverage presented this as a good thing, which infuriated me. They were at risk! My drug! What the fuck. I called the pharmacy the minute I finished reading the article to see if I could get a refill, but the recall had already taken effect. I had nine remaining pills. I called a friend who took the drug and asked if she had any leftovers.

"Oh, no. Haven't you read about it?" she said. "Vioxx is dangerous."

"Do you still have any?"

"I would not be comfortable sharing them with you," she pronounced primly.

I switched to Celebrex, which was good, but not as good for pain relief (and poses some cardiovascular risks for the same population as Vioxx did). Moreover, although evidence is mixed, one study found that taking COX-2 inhibitors (the category of drug that include Celebrex and Vioxx) for two or more years reduced the risk of breast cancer by 71 percent. And breast cancer, unlike heart attacks and strokes, is a disease for which I am actually at risk.

I tried a stronger anti-inflammatory in an injection of cortisone—a steroid—into the inflamed tendons of my shoulder. Steroids, which reduce pain and inflammation, are more effective when injected directly near the afflicted nerves than when they are taken orally and diffuse through the body. Then a pain specialist recommended a steroid injection directly into the vertebral space of my neck. Unfortunately, the space between the vertebrae is small, and when I was getting the injection, the needle accidentally punctured the membrane that surrounds the spinal cord. I thanked him, got in a cab, and scheduled a blind date for three days later—the time the steroids were supposed to take effect. I imagined how much prettier I would look by then, my head on top of a pain-free neck.

I did not know that the spinal cord (like the brain) is always bathed in fluid, which is held in by the dural membrane. This fluid rises up the spinal column to the brain, where it cushions the brain from the skull and keeps the brain at a certain pressure. In the days after the procedure, the hidden puncture in my dural membrane caused the fluid to slowly leak out of the hole, so that the pressure in my skull changed and my brain no longer floated in the right way. When I moved my head, my brain sloshed around, causing *excruciating pain.*

It was the worst headache I have ever had or imagined: the kind of headache that makes one long to be beheaded. I was supposed to be writing an article about vampires, but instead I lay perfectly straight in bed, with the crimson curtains drawn, staring into the shadows. Every time I turned my head, my brain thumped sideways and I wished I were dead.

After three days, I stumbled back to the hospital. I had never felt so thankful to have faith in a doctor. A short, ethnically Chinese man from Malaysia who had done his medical training in England, Dr. Ngeow had a large, saintly sort of presence, upon which it was impossible to project malevolence or carelessness. (And a dural puncture actually is just a risk of the procedure—not a failure of skill—but without his saintly personality, I'm sure I wouldn't have seen it that way.)

He offered a solution: a "blood patch." He would pump a syringe of my own blood into the hole in my spinal cord until it clotted and patched it up. In the hours while we waited to get approval from my insurance provider, as the Oxford doctor failed to return Dr. Ngeow's call and then disappeared for a long lunch and then went into a meeting ("a doctor who keeps banker's hours," Dr. Ngeow fumed), we chatted about translations of the New Testament.

When the approval finally came, he withdrew some blood from my arm and pumped that blood into the dural space (with a splitting, violating, penetrating pressure). Then I lay prostrate on a hospital bed, feeling like a vampire enlivened by blood, rising from the dead. Once an hour, a nurse came and raised the headrest of the bed a few inches, as the fluid regenerated, rising up the spinal column into the skull, until at the end of the afternoon I was sitting up, my brain buoyed, images of the vampire dispelled, and my thoughts returned to normal.

They did not stay normal, however, because over the next month the steroids slowly diffused through my system and made me crazy. I suffered from a side effect called disinhibition, which was like being drunk in a way that I was never drunk: aggressively. I told an editor his publication sucked. I told an American Airlines representative she was scum. I would wake up the next day and recall fragments of what I had said the day before and blanch in shame. At that time I was in the habit of going out every night. I didn't want to stay home until I was no longer crazy—I wanted to avoid being alone and in pain and to avoid thinking about the future and how I would be older and still alone and in more pain. But each time I went out, I alienated someone else.

In the steroid state of mind, social occasions struck me as opportunities to air old grievances—grievances I had successfully kept to myself, but suddenly felt compelled to expound upon at great length. When I went to dinner at the house of an old boyfriend and his wife, I was reminded of their wedding years before, where I hadn't been allowed to bring Kurt, on the grounds that they didn't believe I would marry him and didn't have room for stray dates. So I went alone, and the groom's family came up to me and said, "This must be *so* weird for you," and I had to smile blithely and say, "Why, no," instead of, *You are making it weird right now.*

It had all happened years before, and the groom had been right: I hadn't married Kurt, so if that was the selection criterion for their guest list, he had selected correctly. And it was their wedding, so the guests were theirs to select. But under the influence of the drugs, those things only irritated me more. And it suddenly seemed urgent to communicate to them the full extent of that irritation.

When the drugs wore off, I found these conversations impossible to retract, because the feelings I had expressed were ones I actually felt—but shouldn't have shared.

In the years that followed, I tried to stay clear of invasive interventions and to focus instead on treatments that had no side effects. I counseled myself in a chirpy, women's-magazine be-your-own-life-coach manner on the value of small Lifestyle Adjustments, such as replacing my heavy leather Coach handbags with nylon fake Prada ones from Chinatown. I was chary about medical expenses, shunning treatments that insurance didn't cover, and avoiding doctors who were out of network, because the reasonable and customary charges Oxford covered were not reasonable or even customary. Yet I had two savings accounts: one to save money to buy an apartment (a goal I never got closer to realizing as my savings grew incrementally while the price of real estate in New York City grew exponentially) and the other for a rainy day.

One day it occurred to me that my priorities were absurd. *It was raining.* This was my body—my permanent residence! As long as I didn't go into debt (or perhaps even if I did), I should spend all my resources trying to shore up the house of my soul—the only place we ever truly dwell.

I began having weekly massages and taking Pilates lessons to supplement physical therapy, and I found an osteopath who told me she was manipulating my spine into a better place and that it would stay that way. Did it? Who knew. The important thing was to keep trying things and stay positive. I set a timer and took twenty-minute showers while stretching under the running water. I used heat therapy with an ingenious product called ThermaCare, pads that adhere to your neck or back that interact with the air in some way that makes them stay hot for hours. I love ThermaCare. I bought carts full in fear that one day Proctor and Gamble would callously discontinue it and I would be left with—what?—only a few years' supply. But sometimes the depth of my feeling for the product depressed me, and I thought, *How did my bodily welfare* (which turns out to be the same as my welfare) *come to depend on* ThermaCare?

The treatments were all so modest, I felt that none of them addressed the depth of my despair. In being grateful for them, I was aware that I was conceding (to myself, to the universe) that there was no cure. Sometimes I'd hear patients talking about magical cures—urging me to try this healer, this diet, this technique—but I didn't believe they would help me. I'd think of the joke in which a patient consults a doctor about a problem. "What do you think I am? A magician?" the doctor declares, throwing up his hands. So the man goes to see a magician. "What do you think I am?" the magician says. "A doctor?" Just because Western medicine was failing me didn't mean alternative medicine would not also fail.

But failure was not to be dwelled on. I did exercises in chronic-pain self-help books on cognitive reframing to learn to avoid *catastrophizing* and *Cassandraizing* and told myself they could make a difference. The voice of doom, for example, that says *I will never get better* could be reframed as *I feel optimistic about my treatment.*

How optimistic? Every birthday I wished for my pain to go away, and every year that wish had not been realized. I had other wishes, of course, involving love and work, but each year when I stared at the melting candles and compared them with pain, there was no comparison. People who spend their lives wishing for things that don't happen are pathetic and should get a grip, I decided, so one year I resolved to wish for something I wanted, but that was likely to come true—something, in short, that would not excessively tax the Wish Fairy. I settled on long life for my cat, Cambric.

On my next birthday I woke bedraggled with pain, while Cambric was as healthy as ever. I refocused my birthday wishes on my affliction.

MORE BETTERNESS TO GET

The fetters of my pain loosened; the relentless ghost returned to its dwelling. When I first got the results of my MRIs, I assumed I was condemned to ever-worsening pain. The diagnosis had seemed so devastatingly definitive, substantiated by films that revealed the truth of my diseased skeleton beneath the cloak of flesh. But I was wrong. Although I do have cervical spondylosis and spinal stenosis and other degenerative conditions, I now understood that the course of chronic pain is unpredictable. There are people whose MRIs show significant problems who feel fine, and there are others who appear to have normal films whose lives are besieged by pain.

My pain was getting better. *Better and better*, I told myself. I was getting stronger through physical therapy and could open jars and pick up things that used to be impossible. I took note of other small markers of progress: how I used to be pained by riding in a bouncing taxicab, or having my hair blown dry in a salon, when the brush would pull the hair taut, then release it in a way that jangled my neck and caused a small, evil sensation. But none of the treatment I tried was transformational in the way that Dani's was, and although I was getting better all the time, somehow there was always more betterness to get. I wasn't aware of being in pain all the time, but whenever I thought about whether I had pain, I always did. There were pain-free moments owing to my being preoccupied—happily or unhappily—with something else, but I was never able to "catch" a pain-free moment and enjoy it, which meant that, in some sense, I was always in pain.

Although my shoulder improved through physical therapy, my neck improved less, and over time, a new pain developed on the right side of my face and forehead, like a snake that slithered up behind my ears and struck behind my eyes. It was diagnosed as an occipital neuralgia, which meant, I discovered, a problem with the nerves that supply the eye area, for which there was no good treatment (except for a major surgery that attempts to decompress the blood vessels that cluster behind the eye and has a high rate of complications and a low rate of success).

The occipital neuralgia caused muscle spasms, which triggered migraine headaches, so I got Botox injections every three months at the New York Headache Center to paralyze the muscles in my face, as well as to treat the spasms in my neck and shoulder caused by the problems in my spine. A 2005 study found that three Botox injections cut the frequency of migraines by 50 percent or more for the majority of patients. I tried to be grateful that the treatment helped me, which it did (and, unlike other medications, did no harm), rather than disappointed that I wasn't among those it cured. I liked going to the Headache Center. I liked the neurologist, Alexander Masukop; the nurse practitioner, Lynda Krasenbaum; and the waiting room, where I would admire the stylish Upper East Side women who looked to me like the worried well, which is what I aspire to be.

I felt jealous of everyone who didn't have pain, which—it seemed to me—was everyone else. At a department store one day, all the clothes my friend Amanda tried on draped perfectly on her voluptuous body, whereas on me—still underweight from nausea—they hung as on Raggedy Ann. Sitting across from her at tea afterward, I thought how once, I would have envied her breasts, but now I only wanted her neck. I wanted to reach across the table and snatch it and place my own head upon it.

But what would I do with Amanda's head? She has her own sorrows; even in the fantasy I didn't feel good about sticking her with my neck. I paused, trying to think of a solution, until she looked at me quizzically—*Hello?*—and we resumed analyzing the bounty of the after-Christmas sale.

A HUNDRED BLESSINGS

Since I do not believe in a god who should come to my aid or a goddess who should have compassion for me, pain did not make me suffer from negative religiosity. Nevertheless, I was filled with telos decentralizing thoughts.

Over the years, pain undermined my sense of myself as a lucky person. I had always placed great emphasis on luck: in my *telos*, luck was what substituted for the idea of an intervening creator. The street always had two sides: the sunny and the shadowed; the blessed and the blighted; the one who has, to whom all will be given, and the one from whom all will be taken. Luck, for me, had the erratic character of an ancient deity, a necessary protection that could be lost at any moment.

Most people internalize their luck—it becomes *them*—something they feel they deserve, as one always deserves to be oneself. Yet because it's luck, it can change at any moment. Suddenly you'll find yourself exiled to the shadowed side of the street. The coin had flipped my way again and again. Good (compared to most) historical period. Good (qualification, qualification) country. Good birth family. Good body: good heart, good kidneys, good lungs, and then . . . The toss was unfavorable. In the Book of Life, a small genetic error had been made. The vertebral passage that held my spinal cord was too narrow. The cartilage—which usually lasts most of a century—had begun to degenerate after only three decades.

The answer to *why me?* seemed plain: bad luck. And this was an answer I found devastating, since I don't believe in fate, but I do believe in luck. I felt as crushed and blighted as if the fates were actively smiting me. Our bodies are the landscape in which our lives take place; pain was my landscape now. I felt like a cartoon Eskimo lying on a shrink's couch complaining, *I always feel cold* and *I don't want to build an igloo—I belong in Key West.*

A friend told me about a self-help exercise she was trying in which she had to think of a hundred blessings she had received from her newly ended marriage.

"Were there a hundred blessings?" I asked. *You are, after all, divorcing.*

"Well, that's the work of it," she said, "to think of a hundred. That's how you experience the blessing—by thinking of it."

"How many have you thought of so far?"

"A number," she said, lifting her chin slightly. "Half a dozen at least."

Although I could see that the kind of person who thinks about catastrophes in terms of blessings is, in fact, blessed, I couldn't think of a single blessing associated with pain. The next time I saw her, she had found true love and was basking in new blessings, while my pain remained the same.

Blessings, blessings . . . Would pain make me more sympathetic to people with health problems, or less, because I was preoccupied with my own? Perhaps pain would inspire me to take better care of myself—unless I felt too wretched to bother. I thought of a Zen tale about a boy who is given a horse. How lucky he is, the villagers say. We'll see, the Zen master says. Then the boy falls off the horse and breaks his leg. How unlucky he is, the people say. We'll see, the Zen master says. Then war comes, and the men go off to die and the boy stays safely behind . . . We'll see, we'll see, we'll see.

But to see pain as lucky or, even, not *un*lucky seemed like a betrayal of my own sensory experience—or masochism. Printed on the first page of my pain diary was the saying "Once you learn to live with arthritis in a way that you see some good out of it, then you've begun to heal."

Was there a way to understand pain that was both positive and true—or at least not actively false?

FORTUNE

Wandering around a vast Home Depot one day, looking for a certain kind of nail, I bumped into a man in an orange customer-service apron and asked for help. He was in his twenties, and half of his face was disfigured, the skin mottled with scar tissue.

"I'll show you," he said. I followed him as he strode confidently through the labyrinth of aisles. "I'm legally blind, so I can't pick out the package for you," he said, stopping finally before one column, "but it should be right in this row here."

I saw that his brown eyes had a filmy look. I asked what had happened, and he told me that when he was seventeen, he had been the driver for a hunting party. A teenager in the backseat had been fooling around with a rifle and had shot him at point-blank range. But God had saved him, he said. He had been crazy then—drinking, knocking at death's door—but God gave him a second chance.

"I was very fortunate," he said earnestly. "The accident saved my life."

I stared at him to see if he was joking.

This is what people mean when they talk about the beauty of the human spirit, I thought: to put aside a million objections and mentally turn misfortune inside out. *God let me be shot* becomes *God diverted the bullet,* and *I lost half my face to a teenager's stupidity* becomes *the accident saved my life.*

If this were *Pilgrim's Progress,* this moment would be offering me the key to escape imprisonment in Doubting Castle. I didn't believe in divine intervention, but as with the hundred blessings, I knew that if the man believed the accident saved his life, and acted accordingly, then that belief became true. Could I invent such a narrative about my pain?

"We say God and the imagination are one," Wallace Stevens wrote. "How high that highest candle lights the dark."

A Positive Idea Conjured by the Power of Imagination rewrote my pain. An Inspirational Narrative saved me.

"I am very fortunate," the young man reiterated, smiling a crooked smile with the whole half of his face.

THE CRACK WHERE THE LIGHT COMES IN

I decided to reread *Kitchen Table Wisdom*, the book that the train conductor who lost three of his limbs had found so inspiring. The book is boldly subtitled *Stories That Heal*, but the first time I read it, I had felt distinctly excluded from the healing.

Rachel Naomi Remen is a physician who counsels patients facing life-threatening illness, as well as their caretakers, and she has been a pioneer in the holistic health movement. Although I could see that Remen—who has struggled with Crohn's disease since she was a young woman—is a heroine, her book irritated me. Its central idea is that illness can be a gift. Using Judaism, Christianity, and Buddhism, Remen transforms terrible stories of disease into heartwarming tales of auspicious coincidence and lessons learned (or—I found myself thinking—embroiders sentiment upon tragedy, in a way that belies the material).

The incident in the book that struck me the most concerned a handsome college baseball player whose leg had to be amputated above the knee when a tumor grew in it. He refused to return to school, and he began drinking, using drugs, and alienating his friends. His former coach called Dr. Remen and asked her to meet with him. "Filled with a sense of injustice and self-pity," she wrote, "he hated all the well people."

During their second session, she asked him to draw a picture of his body. He drew a picture of a vase with a crack in it, going over and over the crack with a black crayon. Dr. Remen worked with the young man for two years, during which time he became involved in counseling young people facing deforming illnesses and injuries. His attitude changed, from complainer to consoler. He cheered a young woman in the hospital who had just lost both her breasts to a preventive mastectomy, and eventually he married her. During their last session, Dr. Remen showed him his old drawing again.

"It's really not finished," he said. He took a crayon and drew yellow streaks radiating from the cracks. "This is where light comes through," he explained.

I continued pursuing pain treatment, and I waited for a sense of the light, if there is light, and wondered where it might come in.

ROMANTIC AND PHYSICAL PAIN

R omantic pain and physical pain have nothing to do with each other, unless you let them. Conflating the two in my relationship with Kurt long ago had kept me from seeing each of them—the romantic and the physical—for what they were. Yet whenever I tried to keep my pain diary, the two immediately began to interweave. The space in the pain diary for Symptoms was right next to the space for Feelings. In Symptoms, I'd complain about pain; in Feelings, I'd inevitably turn to my romantic discontents.

For a number of years, I periodically went to physical therapy. I would go three times a week for a few months and make progress, and then I'd stop and faithfully continue my exercises every day for six months or a year, telling myself that *physical therapy is the ticket.* But eventually the mantra would wear out, and I'd fall off the wagon. I'd miss a day and then a week, and of course, it would make no difference, so I'd slack off more, and then after a few months I'd realize I had deteriorated, and—filled with self-reproach and new resolutions of commitment—I'd start all over again. At first I'd make tangible progress, but after some months the progress would plateau and motivation wane. Yet when I'd stop, I'd have to face the frustrating fact that after a point, physical therapy didn't make my pain better, but not doing it made it worse.

When I was single, I'd often schedule physical therapy appointments at the end of the day and arrange to meet a date for a drink afterward, just as the pain was setting in from the exercise. Dating and physical therapy struck me as bleakly parallel: small, futile-feeling gestures that require faith to believe they will eventually lead you somewhere. The feeling of pain would set in at just about the same time as the feeling of disappointment in the date: the person across the table would come into focus, and I would see that despite the initial intrigue, he was not my type after all— not at all, again and again. And the rare occasions I imagined otherwise, the relationships turned out badly—physically as well as spiritually.

At times I had the illusion that there was a conspiracy of men to thwart my attempts to get better. I got into a silly teenage-type spat with my large, ursine father involving a car, and in trying to wrest the car keys from my hand, he accidentally twisted my bad arm, and the bruises lasted all summer, and I was too embarrassed to go to physical therapy. And when I recovered from that, my relationship with the man I was dating then kept setting me back.

I had dated many men whose problems as a partner I had concluded stemmed from a lack of sufficient maternal love—a lack for which the women in their lives were doomed to try to compensate, *forever*. Zach, however, had a lovely doting Jewish mother who treated him like a prince; I fell in love with him when I met his mother. Unfortunately, I discovered, his conviction of his princeliness seemed to free him from the burden of *behaving* like a prince.

My book bag, gym bag, and duffel bag at that time were a set made of a flowered Laura Ashley print. *"Laura Ashley?"* he'd say when I couldn't bear the weight and would try to hand any of them to him. I bought a bunch of black bags and suitcases. Carrying those would make him look like a refugee or a homeless man, he grumbled. "I'm not a *camel*." My therapist advised that I try acknowledging his feelings. "I don't want you to feel like a beast of burden," I would begin, "but . . ."

"But *what*?" he'd say. "How is your physical therapy going?"

"Very well."

"You always say that."

"It's always true."

Zach's family owned a vast western ranch. As it happened, none of the family members were outdoorsy. They all had a morbid fear of bears, and their preferred mode of exercise was to drive half an hour into town to walk around a track. But their place in the landscape was clear: the sage-covered hills as far as the eye could see were theirs, whereas my place—on their property and in their family—was uncertain. I was always uneasy that one day Zach's father would take his son aside and tactfully convey that I was a weak seed, unmeet to be a help meet.

One afternoon we went to help a neighboring rancher with his lambing. The experience was decidedly unenchanting: the baby lambs turned out to be evil, oversize creatures who thought nothing of wrenching my arms from their sockets when the rancher casually directed me to still them.

By the time we got home, I was dumb with pain. We were going out to dinner; I had a new, overpriced dress for the occasion that I had bought because Zach had said approvingly that it made me look like the girls with whom he had gone to boarding school. Should I put on a ThermaCare as well—an invalid's necklace? Should I take a Percocet and risk seeming glazed, while inexplicably refusing champagne? I opted for the champagne, which made me explicably glazed. Better to look like a heavy drinker than a sickly specimen, I decided. Plenty of ranchers were drinkers.

When Zach's New York apartment had been renovated, he had saved an old solid-oak door, propping it against the wall behind his bedroom door and sealing the arrangement with the doorstop. He kept it that way for years, always leaving his bedroom door open in order to hold the antique door behind it. He failed, however, to inform me of the arrangement during the two years we dated, so once, when he was talking loudly on the phone in the living room, I unstopped the bedroom door and started to close it behind me. The antique door crashed down and knocked me unconscious. I woke a minute later with excruciating neck pain.

At the hospital, Zach filled out forms as to the nature of the accident, chuckling at the question about whether it derived from physical "abuse" and declining a consultation with a counselor on my behalf.

The next time I went to his apartment, I discovered that he had once again precariously balanced the door behind his bedroom door in exactly the same way.

"Well, you wouldn't close the bedroom door twice, would you?" he said. "That would be pretty stupid."

I was oddly drawn to men who seemed to possess a store of specialized knowledge, like the ancient priest-physicians who knew the magic formulas that spoke to the healing gods. Without that, it was hard for me to feel seduced, the way some women felt about men who were shorter or slighter than they. The kind of knowledge that had always appealed to me was in the humanities: literature, art, philosophy, psychoanalysis, film. But when, on a vacation, I happened to meet a pain doctor, I realized the field of medicine now possessed that same allure.

I was seduced by the way the pain doctor seemed to understand my body. With most men at some point I'd have to say: *Please don't throw your leaden arms on my delicate shoulder,* or, YOU ARE MASHING MY NECK. I was careful not to ask him for medical advice, because I had noticed that doing so irritated my physician friends, but his hands instinctively found the pained places in the dark, and occasionally, at an idle moment, he would lightly adjust my head on my shoulders so that it settled better. Sitting at an outdoor café once, he analyzed the muscular-skeletal problems of a woman walking down the street who had, he declared, an "antalgic gait"—unconsciously favoring certain motions to avoid pain. I felt he was seeing humans in a different way, a way I craved learning.

Visiting him at his fishing cottage in Nova Scotia, I was taking a shower at night when I discovered a tick half burrowed in my abdomen. He seemed oddly alarmed.

"Can't you just take it out?" I asked.

"I don't know. I could hurt you."

"In an erotic way?" I teased, and then, "Oh, come *on.* Didn't you, like, do a surgery rotation?"

He tried heating it with a candle flame in hopes that the tick would withdraw. When it didn't, he sterilized a knife in the flame and, holding the candle for light, began to pry it out. I lay back on the couch, my shorts pulled down, and he knelt before me holding a candle. We joked about how someone walking by the windows might imagine they were glimpsing a sadomasochistic scene.

In bed that night, I asked him about the formation of the face. He named the fourteen bones of the face one by one, touching my face lightly each time as he said the word, like Adam naming the animals. *"Neck?"* I asked sleepily, falling asleep as he touched my first vertebrae.

In the morning I discovered him downstairs, slumped in a chair, looking haggard and disturbed, stroking his three skittish cats. He looked horrified to see me; the cats scattered and darted beneath the sofa. After I fell asleep, he confided, he had had a fantasy that terrified him—forcing him to get out of bed and sit up all night alone. In the fantasy he had the knife and the candle again and I was lying back on the couch while he carved open my abdomen.

When I met Michael, I waited to have the conversation about pain I had had with all the men I had dated. I'd adjust my voice to a patient register and explain that (although it was hard to imagine, as it is always hard to imagine being in another's body, especially when you are a large, exceptionally sturdy younger man, as Michael is) I truly couldn't carry those book bags or groceries or some ordinary thing. I feared that conversation would make him realize it was a drag to have a partner who wasn't—in the basic sense—*handy*. Naturally, there would be the modern part of him— the dominant part, I hoped—that loved me for my mind, but perhaps there would also be a Hunter who wanted a Gatherer.

I prepared to tell him that I hoped he wouldn't see it as symbolic: that I had seen it that way myself, but had rejected such an interpretation, and that my personal flaws are not connected to my physical ones and I hoped he would remain clear on that point. Of course, a certain type of man might find this symbolism *attractive*—the Pea that proves the Princess. But I knew Michael was healthfully unattracted to helpless princessness, and indeed placed great value on competence, and I liked that about him, although it also worried me.

But that conversation—that brief, dreadful exchange I had come to expect and would try to forgive, but which would mark for me the beginning of the end of the relationship—that conversation never happened. I could hand Michael my bags without explanation, or, I noticed, if I simply waited, he would automatically pick them up. Whenever he asked me to carry anything—to take his briefcase, for example, while he was dealing with getting the four heavy suitcases that contained an excessive number of books and outfits—he would say in a neutral tone, "Can you take this, or is it too heavy for you?" allowing for the possibility that it was and making that possibility sound reasonable. Because he used this formulation even when asking me to pick up something very light, I was frequently in the satisfying position of being able to declare that I could.

I didn't want to thank him, because I was afraid saying something would jinx it. When I finally did, he said, "Oh, I never thought of that— that someone could be annoyed by that."

Once, he told me, he was alone in the house when the heat stopped working. He left a message for the landlord and resumed crafting computer code while the temperature steadily dropped. He put a sweater on and made tea. He put a second sweater on. He tried to read, but found he was unable to concentrate because part of his brain had begun to panic. *Will it always be like this? Will it continue to get colder until I perish? How can I get back to that old, warm way of living? How could I have not appreciated warmth while I had it?*

"I was thinking," he said. "Is this what it's like for you to have pain?"

I caught my breath.

"I didn't know you ever tried to picture it," I said.

The first summer we were living together, he came home from Costco one day with the car filled with flats of boxes of ThermaCare. "They were a good price," he explained, and began stacking them in the garage. "What's wrong? I thought you said a person could never have too much ThermaCare." I had sublet my apartment in New York to try living with him in Portland, Oregon, for the summer. There were six weeks left in the summer and three hundred boxes of ThermaCare. *I would like to marry this person*, I thought.

When Cynthia and I went shopping for a wedding dress, my sole criterion was that the dress be long-sleeved and high-necked to conceal the hateful parts of my body. "You're Orthodox?" the saleswomen would ask when I explained what I wanted.

"Why do you want to cover your beautiful shoulders?" a saleswoman at Kleinfeld asked in her Long Island accent as I stood in front of the lighted mirror. She tugged the bodice lower. "You have a lovely, long neck, like a swan."

I woke on my wedding day in the way I always awoke, into consciousness that is consciousness of pain, like a bird smacking into a window. It was no different from any other day, but I realized that I had subliminally expected it to be: I wasn't changing my name, but I still hoped to relegate pain to my single self. Since I had dismissed the idea that romantic pain had anything to do with the origin of the pain, there was no reason that marriage would cure it, but (since nothing else had) part of me still hoped that somehow it might.

I couldn't help but idly fantasize about narrating to a friend one day, from a cosseted married vantage point, perhaps in a museum tea shop: *I don't believe in magic, of course, but it was the strangest thing—even though*

I had had it for so many years, when I got married, my pain sort of magically disappeared . . .

At the collapse of the fantasy I felt a prick of sad anxiety: Would my wedding day be imperfect? I had spent thousands of dollars on the sleeveless dress, but inside the sparkles would be my old body, secretly gnarled in pain.

It was a frigid day, cold yet snowless—a typical January day. The climate had failed to make an exception for our wedding and turn balmy, but we didn't need it to. We had determined to have a joyous winter wedding, a candlelit wedding. I would rejoice in my new life in my old body.

And that was what happened.

ONLY NOT SHOWING YOU MY
DEVOTION IS PAINFUL

We had been married a year, and everything was almost perfect, but I still wanted not to have pain. In the back of my mind was the irksome image of the Hindu pilgrims during the festival of Thaipusam merrily mortifying their flesh for the benefit of some god or other—dancing with weighted fishhooks jangling from their pectoral muscles while crushingly large altars were balanced on their heads.

By this point I understood something of the physiology of acute pain: I had read of the ways in which the brain can temporarily block pain in a state of trance, like the nineteenth-century mesmerists, or through the release of endorphins triggered by a threat to survival, like a soldier in a battle (the phenomenon termed *stress-induced descending analgesia*). But I didn't fully believe any of it. After all, if it were really true, why couldn't *my* brain block *my* pain? I felt the need to prove the pilgrims' serenity untrue: a parlor trick, perhaps, the way I had heard that coal walking could be done painlessly if the coals were covered with a layer of ash and the participant walked quickly and had callused soles. Or perhaps the pilgrims were masochistic or smoking opium—or—who knows? So, although I wanted to stay home and celebrate our first wedding anniversary (our paper anniversary!), I decided to go by myself to watch the festival in Kuala Lumpur, one of the places where the holiday draws a large number of celebrants.

The festival marks the birthday of the god Lord Murugan, the Emancipator, when he received a sacred spear that he used to vanquish a demon that had been tormenting mankind. This divine spear, representing the power of mind over matter, is the power that pilgrims are said to channel through the ritual piercings of their bodies during the festival.

Self-inflicted pain struck me as a curious way to celebrate liberation from a demon. Isn't pain the demon that is always tormenting us and from which we still need to be free?

"When a Hindu child is hurt," Shree—a Hindu guru who had participated in the festival—explained on my first day there, "they are not fussed over or encouraged to be afraid of pain, the way you are in the West." As a small child, he had handled a cactus that left hundreds of spiny needles in his hand. There was no remedy but to have them pulled out needle by needle. His mother gave him a statue of Lord Ganesha, Remover of Obstacles, to look at while she worked. During the hours of the extraction Shree focused on Ganesha's contemplative elephant face instead of the pain. "After that, I wasn't afraid of pain," he concluded.

The story made no sense to me. Pain usually causes more—not less—fear of pain.

"When you are in pain, you have lost yourself, and you start to cry, not because of the pain, but because you have lost yourself. Pain can be mastered and controlled by one's own self," he said.

"You think?"

He recalled a childhood biking accident in which he fell off his bike and discovered that his torn, bloody knee didn't hurt. "Subconsciously, I already believed I had conquered pain. I prayed to the gods, 'Thank you for letting me believe I have conquered pain.'" Another time, he said, a school friend unexpectedly stabbed Shree's hand with a skewer. Alarmed, he felt pain and started bleeding profusely, reinforcing his belief that controlling pain was a function of mental preparation. "You know about the placebo effect. For you, you have placebo, but placebo was invented by scientists. For us, we have belief, which comes from the gods."

He recalled how once, walking on coals in a temple in India, he came to the cooling pot of milk at the end of the walk in front of the statue of the god and he chose not to step in it, despite his sizzling soles, because "I wanted to show the god: *for me pain is nothing now.* For me, only not showing you my devotion is painful."

He had been to Thaipusam many times, he said, and none of the rituals had ever hurt him. The ability to master ritual pain makes the Indians (a minority subject to discrimination by the Malaysian government) feel more powerful. The least powerful members of society, the poor and uneducated, are most often the piercers. "If we control pain, don't think we can't control the government," he told me, narrowing his eyes.

KAVADI

Each year, just after midnight during the first full moon of the Tamil month of Thai, a bejeweled wooden chariot containing a statue of the god Murugan is taken from a temple in downtown Kuala Lumpur. Barefoot pilgrims carry the chariot eight miles to the sacred Batu Caves on the outskirts of town. They arrive at daybreak and carry the chariot up the 272 steps into the largest cave, where they place the statue among the ornate shrines to other deities.

Hundreds of other devotees flock to the cave carrying their own *kavadi* ("burdens") in the form of shiny pots of milk, piercings, or homemade altars that rest on their heads or shoulders. They believe that if they bring Murugan these *kavadi*, he will release them from the real burdens of their lives—poverty, illness, infertility, misfortune. The larger, more grotesque and spectacular the *kavadi*, the greater the relief it is believed to engender.

The homemade altars—huge canopies weighing more than thirty pounds and embroidered with peacock feathers and images of the god— are held by wooden bows carried on the devotees' shoulders and attached by hooks that pierce the chest. There are also *kavadi* in the form of ceremonial carts pulled by ropes hooked into the pilgrims' backs, like ones I had seen in photographs.

The first morning of the festival, devotees gathered at a nearby river for a ritual cleansing. Although it was early, the sun was eviscerating. The stagnant river looked as filthy as the dusty shores. The men climbed out of the water, their bodies gleaming, and readied themselves for the piercing and the placing of the *kavadi*. I tried to persuade my translator—a plump young Indian woman who worked for the local English-language newspaper—to translate the questions I wanted to ask them, but she didn't want to. She was hot and bored. "I need a Coke," she complained.

Next to us, an older, gray-haired man pierced his ruddy cheeks with a gray metal skewer that looked like it was intended for shish kabob. A wave of dizzy nausea came over me. His grown daughter explained to me in English that her father had been bitten by a snake as a teenager and his mother had vowed to Lord Murugan that if he healed her son, her son would pierce his cheeks each Thaipusam for the rest of his life. Another daughter chimed in that after years of marriage she had still been childless, so her father asked Murugan for a child, and by the next year, the wish was granted. That year, her father was requesting a second child for her. I asked the daughters if they would ever pierce themselves, and they laughed shyly and said no—their father's sacrifice served the whole family.

"Ask him if it hurts," I told my translator.

"It doesn't."

"Just ask."

"He says the god comes into him, and he feels no pain," she translated.

I remembered how Shree told me that he feels that many of the pilgrims' understanding of Hindu theology is unsophisticated. "They say the god comes into them, but in Hinduism everything is god," he complained. "I am god and you are god. How can something come into you that you already are?" Rather, Shree said, the true meaning of the festival is to remind people of their own innate powers. "When we pierce, we are using the divinity we always possess to control our consciousness," he said.

Nearby, a priest stitched a crochet-size needle through the tongue of an older woman in a scarlet sari as nonchalantly as if he were pinning a mannequin. The woman's eyes looked sorrowful, but she did not flinch. The long needle forced her pierced tongue to stick out, as the needle caught against her cheeks. Women do not pierce their backs or chests, because it would be unseemly, my translator explained, but piercing their tongues is considered befitting because female tongues are often loose. On top of their heads, women carry milk pots as *kavadi*.

A beautiful young man with a crown of dark curls climbed up the riverbank and sat astride a stool before a priest, as water dripped off the young man's bare chest. The priest gathered his materials to perform the piercing. When he was eleven, the man explained, government soldiers came to his house and destroyed it and beat his family and took their land. He recalled the sight of his mother bleeding and how the pain of his own injuries disappeared. "What is painful like seeing that?" he said. The pain of that sight is a pain he can never forget. Through piercing, he believes he is improving his own karma, while the government's bad karma will eventually cause it to fall. "Seeing the Indian people suffer—that's what causes me pain now," he said.

I told my translator to ask him about the pain of the fishhooks.

"He'll be in a trance," she said impatiently.

"Ask him to explain in his own words."

She rolled her eyes and spoke to him. "He says the pain no longer belongs to him. The god frees him from this pain."

"But will he be in pain?"

"Lord Murugan's lance, the *vel*, vanquishes the pain."

Others gathered around the pilgrim, chanting "*vel, vel*" and beating drums as the priest deftly began threading the hooks into his back. At the end of each hook the priest hung a lime. The pilgrim's eyes rolled back in his head, and his tongue—dyed bright red with a special paste to look like a god's tongue—lolled forward. As he stood, the limes trembled on his back like charms on a bracelet. He stomped his feet, tossed his head back, and bellowed—a huge, terrifying sound. Then he knelt, and the enormous *kavadi* was hoisted on his shoulders. As his followers cheered, he began to dance.

"See, I told you, he's in a trance," my translator said. "Normally, he could barely lift it, but now he can dance."

Tourists pushed their way through the circle of followers and snapped pictures of the moment the hooks pierced the skin, as if trying to document the dream world they stumbled into on their vacation: *Look, look— look at the way it looks like it doesn't hurt.* I half worried that the gawkers would break the spell and the devotee would suddenly be as agog—revolted or frightened—as we were and wake to the pain. But the worshippers seemed as indifferent to the tourists as if we were looking at them through a one-way mirror.

If I were in that sacred space, would I be free of pain? Despite every-thing around me, I could feel my pain decorating my body. If I asked the priest to thread the hooks through my skin, would my pain be transformed into an offering so I could ask the god for something in return?

How much would it hurt?

"What about infection?" I asked my translator.

"No one gets infected during Thaipusam."

"Just ask the priest."

"He says the god takes care of it," she said without asking him.

I decided that my pain could be my *kavadi*—invisible to others, but seen, perhaps, by the gods with their extra eyes. I bought a wreath of yel-low flowers from one of the stands that lined the way to the caves and car-ried it around my neck as I joined the crush of thousands of people processing up each side of the stone steps. Just ahead of me, a couple lugged a child in a saffron-colored sling hanging from sugarcane stems over their shoulders. Children conceived after a request to Murugan are tradition-ally brought back on Thaipusam to show the god his handiwork. In the center of the steps, roped off from the throng, the pilgrims bearing *kavadi* marched to drumbeats and flutes. On the jutting sides of the cliff, small long-tailed monkeys darted and screamed. My translator, holding hands with her boyfriend, lagged farther and farther behind.

The steps led up into a cave whose stone ceiling arched a hundred me-ters high. Its rock walls looked like the drips of a melted candle. Muru-gan's shrine was at the top of the cave, guarded by a priest. Pilgrims discarded their sandals and approached the god barefoot, single file, with offerings of milk and flowers and coconuts. I took off my sneakers, but the priest came over and stopped me, asking in a British Indian accent if I was menstruating.

I flushed, startled at being asked the intimate workings of my body by a strange man, and said (fortunately) no. I told him I had brought the wreath around my neck as an offering.

"You can't give that," he said shortly.

"Why not?" I asked timidly, expecting him to tell me that I wasn't a Hindu.

"It's *used*. You can't give the god something that you have already worn."

"Oh . . . I was just wearing it on the way . . . I see . . . Can I still ask for something?"

"You do not need to bribe the god," he scolded. "What do you want?"
I hesitated.

"Not to be burdened by pain. To be unburdened."

He snorted and threw up his hands, and then gestured toward the procession of devotees flooding into the caves.

I remembered how—as the enormous *kavadi* were first lifted onto the pilgrims' shoulders—the pilgrims' knees buckled slightly as they rose and took their first slow steps up toward the mountain. Then, as their followers cheered and chanted, they would begin to dance: limes jingling on their bodies, peacock feathers trembling over their heads, their burdens light.

V

TO CURE THE MIND:

Pain as Perception

WHAT IS PAIN?

What, finally, is pain?

Pain is an experience one is never in doubt about having. One might pause to wonder, *Am I in love?* but never, *Am I in pain?* Indeed, uncertainty in the face of this question answers it in the negative. As Wittgenstein observes, "if anyone said 'I do not know if what I have got is a pain or something else,' we should think something like, he does not know what the English word 'pain' means." Why, then—in light of this extraordinary clarity—is pain so difficult to define?

Is pain sensation, emotion, or idea? Is it a product of biology or culture? If it is primarily a biological phenomenon, then why does it seem to vary so much from person to person and from culture to culture? If it is primarily a cultural one, then why does it seem so universal? After all, there is a word for *headache* in every language, ancient and modern. When the ancient Babylonian describes the headache that envelops like a garment, we know exactly what he means.

Or do we? The Thaipusam devotees possess the same tongues as the tourists, sensitized by the same nerves, but they do not appear to feel what we would expect them to feel when those tongues are pierced. Nevertheless, members of one culture can confidently torture someone from another, relying on the so-called universal language of pain. Or can they? A martyr may experience such torture quite differently from another type of victim.

Defining pain tests our understanding of the relationship between the body and the mind. For Hippocrates, pain was a physical sensation that emerged from discernible physical phenomena; for Aristotle, pain was what today we might call an emotion—a visceral reaction of the mind to physical or metaphysical stimuli, but one that might be overcome through reason's dominance over all other functions of the mind and the body.

Neither definition suffices. If pain is simply a sensation, then why is it so upsetting? If it's an emotion, then why does it feel like it necessarily entails a physicality not entailed by any other unpleasant emotion? One can feel mental pain without physical pain (the "pain" of betrayal), but the reverse is not true. Physical pain seems to always conjure distress. (Indeed, the blurring of the two is reflected by the word for pain in most languages. For example, the French *douleur* means not only physical pain but also grief and distress, and it is derived from the Latin word *dolor*, which means pain, suffering, and grief.) Pain that conjures no negative emotions would seem not to be painful. (A masochist might "enjoy" the feeling of pain, but the frisson of its aversiveness is part of what is enjoyable.) Dictionaries are vexingly circular on the topic, defining pain as "suffering, or distress" and then defining distress, in turn, as "great pain, anxiety, or sorrow" and suffering as "pain or distress"!

In the seventeenth century, philosopher René Descartes proposed a theory of pain as a simple physical sensation that is triggered when fire or other threats to the body are registered by a "delicate internal thread" that sends a message to the brain, causing it to create pain, the way pulling a rope sounds a bell. Descartes illustrated his idea with a sketch of a comely man-child whose foot touches a ball of fire. Through the boy's transparent body, one can see a rope stretching from the foot to the brain, where it is ringing a bell in the pain center.

Even though one of Descartes' primary intellectual contributions was the model of the body as machine, he saw problems with using such a simple mechanistic model for pain. He wrote of the perplexing relationship between pain and emotion, noting that "we may sometimes suffer pains with joy, and receive titillating sensations which displease us." He was fascinated by phantom limb pain, which he felt demonstrated that perception "must sometimes be at fault and deceptive" and "the sense will be deceived."

He was struck by the case of a young girl whose gangrenous lower arm had been amputated without her knowledge. After the operation, the girl complained of pain in her fingers, the physical absence of which was concealed from her beneath bandages. "And this clearly shows that the pain of the hand is not felt by the mind insofar as it is in the hand, but insofar as it is in the brain," he concluded.

Although the part of Descartes' writings on pain that became best known was the metaphor of the rope and the bell, according to which the brain's role in registering pain is a passive one, his recognition that the pain of the hand actually exists only in the brain could be said to set the stage for the modern understanding of pain as a perception *actively generated* by the brain, like hunger or thirst.

The model of pain as a bell attached to ropes turns out to be wrong in many respects. There are no ropes directly connected to a bell in the brain that can reliably command pain. And, whereas a bell cannot determine how loudly it will ring, the brain *does* determine how neural signals are transformed into pain. While there are neural signals indicating tissue damage that come into the brain from the periphery, the brain may or may not pay any attention to them.

A more apt analogy might be that of a watchman in a tower who is charged with surveying the landscape of the body and sounding the alarm in the case of an attack. In theory, the watchman should sound the bell softly in the case of a small incursion or loudly in the case of an onslaught. But the watchman is far from an ideal employee. He is erratic, lazy, easily confused, fearful, a poor multitasker, and sometimes just deluded. Sometimes he responds to a threat helpfully, with a proportional pain alarm. But sometimes he's preoccupied with a higher-priority task and does not sound the alarm at all. Other times he imagines a threat that isn't there and rings the bell with no cause. And in the case of chronic pain, he rings the bell ever louder, driving everyone mad. Or in certain states of mind, such as during a religious rite, the watchman regards the incursion into the integrity of the body not as a threat but as a cause for celebration.

This is why the brain can generate an experience of pain without any nociception at all, or it can fail to generate pain when tissue damage has occurred. On the occasion of his 1981 shooting, Ronald Reagan was initially unaware that he had been shot through the chest. He was taken to the hospital because he was coughing up blood (his lung had been punctured), and that's where the bullet wound was discovered. "I had never been shot before, except in the movies," he commented later. "Then you always act as though it hurt. Now I know that does not always happen." Perhaps he had imagined it would feel like a *shooting* pain. (In fact, being shot is often described as feeling like a thud followed by a burning sensation.)

Yet, a man who believes he has been shot when bullets have in fact missed him may start to wrench in agony. Once volunteers are repeatedly shocked by a painful electrical stimulus, their brains start to generate pain when they expect the stimulus to be applied again but *before* it is actually applied. The anticipation of pain is pain.

Pain is now understood to be neither sensation nor emotion alone, but rather an experience that draws upon both: the elusive intersection of three overlapping circles—cognition, sensation, and emotion. When any of these elements is missing, there is no pain. There is no such thing as being in pain without knowing you are. There is no such thing as being in pain without feeling the sensation of pain. And there is no such thing as pain that does not cause a salient emotional reaction.

"Pain is whatever the experiencing person says it is, existing whenever the person says it does," declared Margo McCaffery, a leader in the field of pain-management nursing. Highlighting the radical subjectivity of pain, this definition (which has been widely used by clinicians in recent decades) suggests that trying to characterize the kind of thing a person refers to when he refers to his pain is futile. In 1979, the International Association for the Study of Pain came up with the definition of pain that is most accepted today: "An unpleasant sensory and emotional experience associated with actual or potential tissue damage or described in terms of such damage."

Among its virtues, this definition aptly expresses pain's complex relationship to tissue damage: pain is a feeling that can be distinguished from other types of emotions and sensations by the way in which—accurately or not—*it connects that feeling to a sense of tissue damage.* Yet the definition makes explicit that the connection of pain to tissue damage is only by "association." A note following the definition elaborates that "activity induced in the . . . nociceptive pathways by a noxious stimulus is not pain, which is always a psychological state." In short, pain is not nociception, faithfully informing the brain about damage in the body the way a seismometer informs a scientist of the motion of tectonic plates. The relationship between pain and tissue damage can be compared to that between love and sex: it may or may not exist.

Pain is an aspect of bodily consciousness involving activation of the areas of the brain that process sensory information and those involving culture, memory, emotion, and association (the limbic system). The thick overlap between the limbic system and the other parts of the human brain is thought to explain the most perplexing aspect of our pain—its remarkable fluidity of meaning, from the agony of torture to the ecstatic pain of a sacred rite.

The contemporary paradigm of pain reconciles the ancient concept of pain as a spiritual signifier with the nineteenth-century conception of it as a biological function; analogously, the current understanding of dreaming reconciles the concept of dreaming as deeply meaningful (as signals from the gods or signals from the unconscious) with that of dreaming as random brain activity. Both reconciliations follow from the understanding that the brain's activity draws upon its meaning-making parts.

The shift in paradigms of pain correlates with shifts in types of treatment. The rope/bell mechanical view of pain, according to which there are fixed pain pathways, rationalized the ineffective nineteenth- and early-twentieth-century practice of snipping nerves in order to destroy those pathways. The contemporary model can be described as a model in which pain is regarded as a perception shaped by biological, psychological, and sociological factors. This understanding has led to the invention of multidisciplinary pain programs and treatments that attempt to intervene in pain in all its aspects. The treatments of the future will focus on targeting the brain's perception and modulation of pain.

THE DEMON IN THE MACHINE

For many years, researchers sought the demon in the machine—the "pain center" in the brain—in order to exorcise it. But there turned out to be none. Unlike senses such as vision and hearing that depend on activation of clustered portions of the brain, pain is a complex, adaptive network of neurons (a neuromatrix) involving roughly half a dozen areas of the brain that transmit information back and forth. As pain is one of evolution's most important functions, it is distributed over many different areas, so that if one part of the brain is disabled through injury or disease, the system can continue to generate pain.

Each of these regions contributes to the experience of pain. The nociceptors that detect tissue damage send a pain signal up the spinal cord through two major pathways. Dull pain runs slowly along one track, and sharp pain runs quickly along the other. The signal continues through the brain stem, the primitive part of the brain that controls autonomic nervous and various homeostatic systems (such as those regulating breathing, heart rate, and sleeping), and activates norepinephrine to create a feeling of arousal and vigilance. It then feeds into the thalamus—a region in the brain that acts as a way station for other senses, such as hearing and vision. The thalamus relays pain signals to several areas: the limbic system, the somatosensory cortex, and the prefrontal cortex. The limbic system (the collective name for a group of areas in the brain associated with memory, emotion, and attention) produces feelings of sadness and unpleasantness; circuitry shared by the brain stem and the limbic system is activated to produce a sense of anxiety. The somatosensory cortex locates the pain; signals that originate from the foot, for example, are registered in the part of the homunculus (the brain's internal map of the body) that represents the foot. Finally, the prefrontal cortex (an area associated with consciousness and cognition) ascertains the cause of the pain and formulates a strategy to stop it.

Disease processes or damage can alter or interrupt the flow of information among the parts. People with lesions on their somatosensory cortices still experience pain, but they are no longer able to identify where it is coming from. Patients who had cingulotomies—a radical surgical treatment once used to treat pain or mental illness that severed nerves in part of the limbic system known as the rostral anterior cingulate cortex (rACC)—reported that they were still aware of pain but they didn't "mind" it as much. Their emotional response had receded, and so their pain was diminished. (This was also true of patients who had the older treatment of lobotomy, a similar though more extensive procedure in the prefrontal cortex.) Similarly, when a rat's rACC is lesioned, he will cease to avoid a painful stimulus; it no longer pains him. Cingulotomies are rarely, if ever, performed now because, among other reasons, over time people's brains tend to rewire the pain circuitry around the damaged part, and their pain returns.

Most of the time, damage to the pain circuitry results in greater pain. For example, one of the most intractable, terrible pain syndromes—phantom limb pain—arises from neural reorganization in the somatosensory cortex. In 1871, the Civil War surgeon Silas Weir Mitchell coined the phrase "phantom limb," noting "thousands of spirit limbs haunting as many good soldiers, and every now and then tormenting them." The great majority of amputees suffer from phantom limb sensations, and many of them are excruciating. The missing limb (or teeth, eyes, internal organs, or breasts) may feel as if it is clenched or crooked or cramped or—oddly—too short. (Most people's only experience of phantom sensation is "phantom lip"— the peculiar feeling caused by local anesthesia at the dentist that the lip is not only numb but has suddenly grown uncomfortably fat.)

Historically, phantom limb pain was believed to arise from neuromas— injured nerve fibers at the tip of the stump that grow back irregularly and begin sending aberrant messages that translate into pain. Yet when surgeons tried shortening the stump to remove the neuromas through a second amputation, pain only worsened. Cutting the sensory nerves where they attach to the spinal cord also failed to alleviate pain. Moreover, the neuroma theory failed to explain why some people who lack limbs owing to congenital birth defects also suffer from phantom limb pain. Even more tellingly, people who are paralyzed by spinal cord injuries that prevent any pain signals from crossing the spinal cord into the brain can suffer from phantom pain that they experience as coming from the bodies they can no longer feel.

In recent years, brain imaging has shown that although neuromas can contribute, the primary source of phantom pain derives from pathological changes in the representation of the body that forms the homunculus. When a body part is lost, the sensory information normally transmitted to its corresponding neural area in the homunculus abruptly ceases. Although it is not understood why this causes pain, it has been theorized that the neurons register alarm at the absence of normal input, and this alarm translates into pain.

Moreover, for unknown reasons, the neurons of adjacent areas of the homunculus grow into the area corresponding to the missing limb. For example, one of the quirks of the homunculus is that the arm and hand areas are adjacent to the face area. When a person loses her arm, the facial neurons of the homunculus begin to grow pathways into the adjacent arm area. Because of that, stroking the face (particularly the lips) of an amputee who has lost a hand may trigger the sensation of being stroked on the phantom hand. It is not known how this cross wiring causes pain, but the greater the degree of cross wiring in the homunculus, the more severe pain the amputee suffers.

PAIN PERCEPTION AND PAIN MODULATION

Most people still think of pain the way Descartes did—as rising from the body to the brain. Perhaps the most important revision of the Cartesian model in the contemporary understanding of pain is that pain pathways are *bidirectional*: ascending to *and* descending from the brain.

The network of pain areas in the brain includes two different pain systems—one of pain perception and one of pain modulation, which involve both distinct and overlapping brain structures. The pain-modulatory system interacts constantly with the pain-perception system and can inhibit its activity. Much chronic pain is thought to involve either an overactive pain-perception circuit or an underactive pain-modulation circuit.

The brain can send "on" signals that amplify nervous impulses in the spinal cord, so that more signals flood into the brain and become pain, or the brain can send "off" signals that arrest those impulses. For example, at the time of acute injury, signals traveling up the spinal cord to the brain stem and brain evoke *counter-signals* traveling downward that have an analgesic effect by inhibiting the incoming signals. After several hours, however, the brain releases neurotransmitters into the spinal cord that actually amplify the incoming signals, augmenting pain. Thus, acute injuries always hurt more later, a feature that serves the adaptive purpose of enabling flight at first and later enforcing rest.

Although acute injuries provoke some pain modulation, under certain circumstances the modulatory system is dramatically activated. There is no existing practical pharmacological analgesia that can match the brain's innate pain-control system. It is the secret spell that occasionally allows soldiers, athletes, martyrs, and pilgrims to engage in battles, competitions, or acts of devotion without being distracted by the pain of injury. Electrical stimulation of parts of the brain involved in the pain-modulatory system (the periaqueductal gray matter and raphe magnus nucleus) produces not simply some pain relief, but *complete* analgesia in both humans and animals.

The modulatory and perception circuits are activated by various cognitive and affective states, the two most important of which are *attention* and *expectation*. Although the brain is quite busy, as a matter of course, with input from multiple sensory systems, the limbic system stamps pain with a valence sufficiently negative to give it priority. The greater the attention the brain pays to pain, the more pain one feels (readers, beware!). Dread of impending pain (a state of mind involving both attention and expectation) augments the perception of pain. In studies at Oxford University, Dr. Irene Tracey has shown that *simply asking subjects to think about their chronic pain* increases activation of their pain-perception circuits.

Many rituals surrounding torture involve forcing the victim to examine instruments of torture. As one survivor put it, "Torture isn't having your leg bit off by a shark, torture is being slowly lowered into the pool." Different kinds of fear have opposite effects on pain: fear of pain itself generates pain (via expectation). But fear of any other threat *besides* pain can reduce pain (by distraction). One of the most robust activating signals for pain modulation is a threat to survival. A rat exposed to a cat will become analgesic, just as did Bethany Hamilton (the young surfer who felt no pain when her arm was bitten off by the shark).

Perhaps the quenching effect of fear on pain was the hidden neural mechanism that helped some of the accused pass trials by ordeal in ancient times. For example, when Queen Emma of Normandy walked over red-hot plowshares without realizing it, had her fear distracted her brain from registering pain as she watched the judges like prey eyeing a predator? Although the details of her case may be mythical, presumably if *none* of the accused ever passed an ordeal, faith in the system would not have endured for so long. Conversely, in a society with widespread belief in ordeals, one might speculate that the guilty among the accused would expect to feel pain during the ordeal and that expectation would lead them to experience greater pain.

Ordinary distraction can be an effective analgesic. When Dr. Tracey's subjects performed a demanding counting task while receiving a painful heat stimulus, many parts of the pain-perception matrix became less active, while the cognitive parts of the brain required for the counting task became more active. Music also helps; listening to tones while receiving a painfully hot stimulus actually decreases activity in the pain-perception circuit. Even smells influence pain; Dr. Catherine Bushnell at McGill University demonstrated that pleasant smells decrease pain perception and unpleasant odors enhance it.

The corollary is that expectation of pain relief creates pain relief—an example of the placebo effect. The brain can lull itself and won't bother to create pain if it expects that a god or a medication will dispense with that pain anyway. Placebo may have played a role in ordeals, as those who were falsely accused but believed in the ordeal system would be convinced that they would be divinely protected from pain during the trial—and the placebo effect could make that belief true.

Placebo is a Latin word meaning "I shall please." Stemming from the word used in the first line of the vespers for the dead ("I shall please the Lord in the land of the living"), the placebo effect is like a prayer that is granted if the beseecher has faith that it will be. Yet the etymology of the word reflects the sense of fraudulence with which the placebo effect is popularly—and wrongly—linked. Chaucer disparaged those who "sing placebo," referring to the sycophants who show up at funerals insincerely reciting vespers and faking grief for the dead in order to partake in the lavish feasts that followed. In *The Canterbury Tales*, he gave the name Placebo to a character prone to false flattery.

But placebo is not false. People once speculated that the placebo effect is psychological—patients want to please the doctor so much that they either feign feeling better or convince themselves that they feel better. Yet when patients believe they are getting an opioid but actually get a placebo, they not only report pain relief, they also unconsciously display the autonomic side effects of opioids, such as respiratory depression.

Placebo is popularly understood as requiring some kind of sham treatment, like a sugar pill. But because the placebo effect is a result of the power of belief, or positive expectation, it can be created through verbal assurances or healing rituals as powerfully as through sham pills or procedures. Neuroimaging studies show that a placebo activates the brain's pain-modulatory system in a way that is *neurochemically indistinguishable from treatment with an opioid analgesic.* For example, in a 2005 study led by Dr. Jon-Kar Zubieta at the University of Michigan Medical School, the brains of men were imaged after a stinging saltwater solution was injected into their jaws. The men were then each given a placebo and told that it would relieve their pain. The men immediately felt better, and the screen showed how: in the image, the parts of the brain that release their own opioid-like substances (endorphins, enkephalins, and dynorphins) lit up. In a sense, fake painkillers caused the brain to dispense real ones. Like a New Age dictum—the kind I used to scorn—faith had become chemistry; belief had become reality; the mind had overridden the body.

Even opiate medications require the placebo effect for part of their effectiveness. Studies have found that when morphine or other strong opioids are administered covertly (say, added to an IV), they don't work nearly as well as when subjects know they are receiving them. The use of a placebo increases morphine's efficacy by more than a third (with the placebo in this example being simply the positive expectations created by telling patients they have been given morphine and will soon feel great relief). This is also true of other drugs, such as ones that treat anxiety or Parkinson's disease. The Egyptian Ebers Papyrus was right: *magic is effective together with medicine, and medicine is literally more effective with magic.*

One medication requires the placebo effect for *all* of its effectiveness. An intriguing 1995 clinical trial proved an analgesic called proglumide to be a more effective pain reliever than a placebo when both groups were told they were being given an exciting new painkiller. But when subjects were slipped proglumide without their knowledge, thus ensuring they had no placebo effect, they felt no relief at all. None.

I was stumped by what I read about proglumide. When given solely, how could a drug *require* the placebo effect yet be more effective than placebo alone? Does the drug have any mechanism of action besides placebo? If it does, why doesn't it work like other drugs when given covertly? If it is only a placebo effect, how did it provide greater relief than a sugar pill? The answer seemed to be none of the above. It reminded me of the line in *The Phantom Tollbooth* about the car that went without saying. There had to be a trick to it—but what?

The secret lies in this fact: while the brain's own endorphins create the placebo effect, there is another substance in the brain (a hormone called cholecystokinin) that dampens that effect by inhibiting endorphins. Proglumide works by blocking the cholecystokinin receptors, thus allowing the brain to create a more vigorous placebo response than it ordinarily would. Proglumide raises the intriguing question of whether drugs should be designed specifically in order to enhance or create a placebo effect. Chronic pain patients often fail to respond to placebo, so drugs that pharmacologically generate a placebo response and activate their sluggish pain-modulation circuits might be of particular benefit to them.

Placebo has a nasty twin: *nocebo* (Latin for "I will harm"), the negative effects of expectation. The brain will generate pain or other adverse responses in people who believe they have been given a harmful substance, even if they haven't. A patient who is given a fake opiate may feel undesirable side effects, such as itchiness or sleepiness, along with pain relief. Nocebo can even be fatal, as when, for example, people do actually die of fright after being bitten by what turns out to be a harmless snake. Another example is the curious phenomenon, well documented by anthropologists, of death following a voodoo curse (in which those who believe they will die from a voodoo curse in fact perish within a few days). A negative medical prognosis can also cause a fatal nocebo, as in the syndrome of patients dying soon after being told they have terminal cancer but before the malignancy develops further.

EXPECTATION RIVALS NOCICEPTION

I am desperately trying to make a case for the meaningfulness of the scientific literature that shows that expectation can be as powerful as nociception," John Keltner said. "I just don't know how to make my patients believe it."

Dr. Keltner helped to design a study at UCSF that used brain imaging to examine the effects of expectation on pain-perception circuitry. In the study, the brains of healthy Berkeley students were scanned while they received a painful heat stimulus and saw color-coded cues that allegedly indicated whether the temperature of the stimulus was high or low. The pain-perception circuitry in the subjects' brains turned out to be *as influenced by the cues as by the pain information coming from their skin.*

Volunteers were told that the blue cues indicated a low temperature and the red ones indicated a high one. When subjects were shown a blue cue and given a low heat stimulus, their brains generated little pain. When subjects were shown a red cue, but the heat stimulus was actually low, they weren't fooled: their brain activation remained low. But when subjects were shown a blue cue while the heat stimulus was actually high, they were fooled: their brain activity remained as low as when the stimulus was actually low. In fact, these three different scenarios all produced roughly *the same amount of neural activation.*

"Astonishingly, it turned out we could interchange cue and stimulus and get the same result," Dr. Keltner said. It turned out "that reducing expectation can be as significant as reducing the pain stimulus itself."

Only one scenario created dramatically greater brain activation: when the high stimulus was cued with a red cue, it was experienced as much *worse* than when the high stimulus was cued with a blue cue, illustrating the power of nocebo—the "additive" power of negative expectation to augment pain. This last scenario is the one that is most similar to the actual experience of chronic pain, in which the negative experience of being in pain is augmented by negative expectations of pain—one's own internal cuing. If you expect to enjoy taking a walk but you find that your back hurts, you may notice mild pain (i.e., the blue cue with the high pain scenario), but it will hurt much less than if you have chronic pain and expect to feel pain (i.e., the high pain with the red cue scenario). Moreover, if you feel pain every time you walk, pretty soon your brain will start to generate pain when you take your first step.

In his struggle to bring the insights of the lab into practice, Dr. Keltner has tried explaining the experiment to his pain patients. "When hard-core chronic pain patients come in, I've shown them posters of my results, because they make the simple argument in an extremely tangible way," he said. "I say, 'Look at the brains of these volunteers. We have demonstrated that expectation can be as powerful as pain. I tell them, '*You do not have to flat-out succumb to pain.'*

"Clinical medicine hasn't had the opportunity to really figure out the benefits of the placebo effect. If you change people's expectations, their brain activity should be reduced, but turning basic science into clinical tools is very elusive."

How can the expectations of chronic pain patients be changed? Of course they expect to be in pain: their pain is chronic.

"That chapter has not been written," Dr. Keltner said. "We know from the literature that psychological tools can reduce the pain experience by roughly 50 percent in acute pain patients and 30 percent in chronic pain patients. It's pretty stunning for a therapeutic intervention to come up with a zapper that gets that kind of relief—comparable to the best medications. I'd like to say, 'I've got Zoloft, I've got Neurontin, I've got steroids, but I've also got these other tools, these psychological tools, so you don't have to be at the whim of pain.' I have hundreds of patients who are suffering; this is one more tool that could be brought to bear. And you may need that tool because you may have used up all the others."

How could he get patients to believe in placebo?

"The obvious way is through deception," he said—that is, assuring the patients that whatever treatment he uses with them is "one of the most

effective therapies" and involves "new discoveries" and bolstering his state-
ments with a bogus statistic such as "in most cases—in 90 to 95 percent of
cases—it gets real relief" because "if they believe it, it might be true."

Nevertheless, in his own practice he does not use deception. "It's a
pregnant irony that striving for the placebo effect is a frank contradiction
to what clinical practice is all about," he said. "It's frustrating that you
can't use this simple tool that works so well in experiments. But a relationship with a doctor is one of the most important human interactions. Doctors are priests! People are more intimate with doctors than they are with
anyone. And honesty—simple, straightforward honesty—is the foundation of that experience."

THE MAGIC TAKES PLACE IN YOUR HEAD

Techniques such as prayer, meditation, and hypnosis are designed to alter pain perception by manipulating either expectation or attention, or both. The placebo response is created by expectation, which activates the pain-modulatory system, but for people who don't respond to placebos, techniques of controlling attention can alter pain perception. Even for those who do respond to placebo, that response is often short-lived; over time, the brain often catches on and the placebo loses its power.

On the other hand, learning to control attention in order to change pain perception is a skill that can be developed. When Thomas Aquinas insists that "the contemplation of divine things suffices to reduce bodily pain," and Kant suggests contemplating Cicero, they are talking about a form of controlling attention. Hypnosis is an extreme form of controlling attention by which the brain is able to exclude from consciousness all unwanted external stimuli, including pain. The nineteenth-century practice of mesmerism seems to have been a form of hypnosis. With hypnosis, subjects enter a state of autosuggestion by which they willingly grant authority to the hypnotizer to direct their attention and perceive only what the hypnotizer tells them to perceive. When the hypnotizer instructs them to feel no pain, their brain ceases to generate an experience of pain, even—in the case of mesmerism—under the ultimate test of surgery.

In China today, surgeries are still sometimes performed using acupuncture alone, which in this context is theorized to function like hypnotism.

The British neuroscientist Patrick David Wall (who, along with his colleague Ronald Melzack, first developed the gate-control theory of pain) told the story of watching surgeries performed using acupuncture in the mid-1970s in China.

The patients at the hospital had been prepared for the surgery by a long course of training and had trusting personal relationships with the acupuncturist. And indeed, Dr. Wall could detect no signs of pain as the incisions were made. But when he noticed that the surgeon cut into one woman's thigh *before* the acupuncture needles had been inserted, he began to wonder if the mechanism of pain relief that was at work was actually akin to hypnosis. The woman, confident of not being hurt—and protected by that confidence—continued calmly chatting.

His theory was confirmed by a horrifying incident with another patient. In the midst of his surgery, the patient suddenly broke free of the trance. His chest had been opened in order to remove part of his lung. Although the operation required a major incision in a nerve-rich area, the patient betrayed no distress. But then, at the end of the operation, after the doctor removed a surgical drain from inside the chest, the patient screamed and struggled to get off the table. He was held down and continued screaming and crying.

What had gone wrong? Dr. Wall believed that prior to the surgery, the acupuncturist had carefully rehearsed each step of the surgery with the patient, assuring him that each of the steps would be painless. But the acupuncturist had neglected to mention removing the drain, so the patient had responded to the procedure as he ordinarily would—with alarm and agony.

Although the surgeries were performed only on patients who had passed the training, there were others for whom acupuncture failed to have any effect. Not everyone, it turns out, can learn to achieve a trance; only some people are "highly hypnotizable." The explanation for this has long remained elusive. Do such people simply have greater abilities to concentrate, to focus attention, to perceive only what they want to perceive?

Recently, neuroimaging has provided some clues toward an explanation, showing that the brains of the highly hypnotizable are actually different from those who are not. An area of the brain (known as the anterior corpus callosum) that is involved in attention is about a third larger in those who are highly hypnotizable. Moreover, highly hypnotizable people turn out to have above-average abilities, in general, to control pain, because they are better able to filter out unwanted stimuli.

When I began researching pain, I assumed that the patients who told me their pain could be alleviated by hypnosis, acupuncture, meditation, or any other alternative treatment must not be in real pain. I was wrong. Some of the patients with the most severe conditions were helped by these kinds of techniques. For example, one of the worst forms of pain is central pain: pain caused by pathology of the central nervous system itself, common to multiple sclerosis, spinal cord injuries, and certain types of brain tumors and strokes that affect the thalamus. Holly Wilson (who was paralyzed by a botched surgery) told me that the only time she is free from the burning pain of the spinal cord injury she refers to as her "shadow" is when she's under hypnosis. Lily—a sixteen-year-old dying of a rare genetic disease at a children's hospital—recalled the one time her pain momentarily disappeared. With her wasted body curled in a fetal position, hooked up to a cadre of machines, Lily had a chart a thousand pages long; she had spent much of the last six years living in the hospital. A team of renowned specialists consulted regularly on her case. I had thought she would want to tell me about the care she had received from the distinguished, compassionate head of the pediatric pain service whose practice I had been observing. But the memory that made her face light up was a woman who once worked for the hospital in a clerical capacity but then moved away. "She laid her hands on me," Lily said with great feeling.

"She didn't even touch her," Lily's mother explained with equal enthusiasm. "She simply held her hands above her!"

On assignments in Africa I had been baffled by the testaments to pain treatments that appeared to have nothing to do with medical science. In Rwanda, a man with a pattern of burn marks encircling his forehead told me that he had undergone a traditional treatment for migraines that had cured his chronic headaches.

"Didn't it hurt?" I asked, trying to keep the horror from my voice. I had had a series of migraines during that trip, and worryingly, I was down to my last pill of Zomig, my favorite migraine medicine. I suspected there was no Zomig for sale anywhere in Rwanda.

"The more the treatment hurts, the more powerful it is," my translator said. "The treatment only hurts once, whereas the headaches used to hurt him every day. You should try it. If that headache medicine you take worked, you wouldn't have to take it all the time."

"I don't take it all the time," I said peevishly. I'd *like* to take it all the time because my occipital neuralgia gives me continual migraines, but my insurance pays for only six tablets of Zomig a month, each of which costs twenty-nine dollars. At home, I hoard the pink tablets, each wrapped in its own foil, but once in a while I use them all up, and then, during the next headache, I have to stumble to the pharmacy to buy an extra one. I always feel vaguely ashamed on these occasions and pay cash and crumple the receipt.

In the context of Africa, a $29 headache is obscene—an obscene over-valuing of my pain and undervaluing of the pain all around me. Yet at times, when I encountered Africans—people missing shoes, teeth, limbs—it would strike me that many of them seemed less discontented than I. Perhaps they thought of pain as part of the fabric of life, whereas I expected my life to be physically painless, and I endlessly grieved that it wasn't. I needed a cure for my pain, or I needed a cure for my belief that my pain needed to be cured.

When I asked John Keltner which alternative treatment works best, he shrugged.

"In my Zen way," he said ironically, "I'd say you're asking the wrong question. They can all work equally well because the magic isn't in the technique; the magic takes place in your head."

It's because the magic takes place in your head that such disparate interventions as ritual scarification, Zomig, hypnosis, and opioids can have the same effects. The variety of alternative techniques might be thought of as the array of props in a religious rite: it is not the lighting of the candles, the pouring of the wine, or the recital of the blessing that makes the Sabbath sacred. Each may—or may not—lead the way into the sacred space, the place where magic happens.

Yet do the effects of magic moments endure? Aren't you the same pained person the minute you stop meditating?

Dr. Keltner paused.

"Every pain-free moment competes with the onslaught of the chronic pain experience," he said. "Pain is supposed to be the warning for something that is literally life-threatening. With chronic pain, every experience, every movement, every situation gets inappropriately stamped and experienced in the mind as life-threatening. We're not supposed to be exposed to danger all the time, and we're not supposed to be hearing an alarm bell all the time. You can see how pain has the potential to make someone go insane."

The devastation of chronic pain is the way in which, over time, it "spreads out and pollutes the brain." He drew an analogy to phantom limb pain: if you cut four fingers off a hand, the neural area in the brain (the homunculus) that represents the remaining finger tends to grow, expanding into the areas that used to represent the other four fingers. The homunculus's remaining finger eventually swells to encompass the space once occupied by all five digits.

In the same way, he said, "pain is such a persistent, relentless experience, it actually poisons and infects your brain. Pleasure and relaxation are at a disadvantage compared to pain because, while pain dominates and imprints on consciousness, they are typically quiet, subtle states. People need to find a way to have experiences that are not only pleasurable but are as important and riveting as pain. Religious experiences can be that powerful, but unfortunately, doctors can't prescribe religion. But by whatever technique—sex, intimate conversation, listening to music—people need to create moments when their attention is sufficiently drawn away from pain that they are almost pain-free, so that they can begin to recondition and reclaim their brains."

A LESS DIRE NARRATIVE

For some, simply knowing that the brain creates and controls pain provides that control. The writer Susan Cheever told me that when she developed back pain, her doctor diagnosed her with—in short—aging. She was in her early sixties, showing signs of arthritis and scoliosis. But she had always been outstandingly healthy, athletic, and youthful-looking, and she did not care for the idea of these things changing. She decided to consult with John Sarno. After examining her, Dr. Sarno authoritatively declared, "This pain is not being caused by your arthritis or scoliosis or any other mechanical problem. *It is being caused by your brain.*"

The truism struck her as a revelation. "I know all about being led astray by my brain," she said wryly. The next time she felt leg pain, she thought of Sarno's theory of TMS—how repressed negative emotions cause pain and muscle tension. She told herself that the pain was not caused by problems in the disks of her spine: "It's caused by my brain, distracting me from my unacknowledged grief and rage." She noticed that crying relieved her pain. She enrolled in his workshop and began the long project of "reeducating a certain part of my brain to think about another part of my brain in a different way." The day of a friend's memorial service, the pain vanished from her leg and reappeared in her upper back. "I thought, *Oh*, come on—*this is so obvious.*"

When she told Dr. Sarno how difficult her childhood had been as the daughter of the troubled writer John Cheever, he expressed surprise at how well she was doing and attributed it to the power of her imagination to transform emotional pain and loss into her own writing. He enjoined her to use that power to transform her experience of bodily pain.

She became aware of the way that each time she felt the sensation of pain, she began to embellish it into an ominous narrative. At the first pinch of a headache, she would begin to write an internal story whose opening scene was a cloudy afternoon in Central Park and whose end was her death by brain tumor. "I have an apocalyptic imagination," she said. "Sarno gave me a much less dire narrative. Instead of thinking, *Maybe this is the first sign of my death*, I started thinking, *Maybe this is nothing*. Maybe this is psychosomatic. And when I did, my pains vanished. Poof."

She opened her hands with the same gesture as the priest in the Batu Caves: as if pain were something one might, simply, let go of.

I felt very envious.

Even though I knew that one of the four types of pain is psychogenic pain, the simplicity of Susan's story surprised me. But I knew that although Dr. Sarno's model doesn't work for everyone, he wouldn't have become popular unless it worked for some. I've heard other doctors express skepticism about his doctrines, but since pain is a perception, there is no such thing as fraudulent pain relief.

I was half tempted to consult with Dr. Sarno myself, but a telling characteristic of TMS is that the location of the patient's pain continually shifts. My pain was nothing if not stable. The right side of my face and forehead always hurt; the left side felt fine. My neck was never fine. Sometimes I pictured myself in my coffin, the pain finally fled, and the image would both comfort and alarm me.

Pain Diary:

I Try to Change My Perception

My mood today was: **0 (GOOD)–5 (BAD)**
My level of pain today was: **0 (MILD)–5 (SEVERE)**

I could read about the workings of the pain-modulatory system all day, but I could not channel it. Thomas Aquinas, the pilgrims at Thaipusam, and Susan Cheever might be blessed with mastery over their perceptions and compliant modulatory systems, but the aspect of my pain I felt most certain about was that it was *not* voluntary—a belief that was reinforced every day I had pain, which was every day. My modulatory system was like a genie trapped in some fold of my brain, unresponsive to commands. If it had a password, it was not one I had forgotten, but one I had never known. It occasionally emerged of its own accord for an emergency, such as a broken bone (at least long enough to allow for a psychotherapy session), but it could not be summoned.

No one knows why some people's modulatory systems can be activated by placebo while others' cannot. One theory of placebo is that it is a function of personality—certain kinds of people invest authority in physicians and believe what their doctors tell them.

I myself don't care for authority figures, but I am extremely suggestible. I don't believe in spirits, but if someone tells me a place is haunted, I shiver. I love symbols and metaphors and the costly healing tin of tea I bought in Beijing, inscribed with words that seem powerful because I can't read them. I would have guessed I would be a model placebo responder.

But I made many attempts to treat my pain with alternative techniques, and none of them worked—and placebo failed to add even a smidgeon of magic. I tried hypnosis, meditation, and acupuncture (which most pain doctors I talked to believe is placebo, although they didn't want to be quoted as saying so). I found them all relaxing, but afterward, my pain seemed the same. I tried homeopathy, which all the pain doctors I interviewed agreed is placebo, because the medicinal substances are so diluted as to be pharmacologically inert. I didn't know that when I tried it, though, so I brought positive expectations to bear, and it still failed. Massage does help, but the effects don't last.

Disappointingly, the treatments that help me the most are the conventional ones: physical therapy, Botox injections, Celebrex (and long-lost Vioxx), and tramadol, a quirky painkiller whose mechanisms of action are not fully understood, but which acts on the brain in several ways, including on the serotonin and noradrenaline systems.

My pain diary asked me to rank my pain daily on a scale of 0 to 5. I used to rate it with 4s and 5s; after years of treatment, it was usually a 3. Sometimes it was a 4, and sometimes it was dreadful, but at other times it was a 2, and occasionally I could mentally stretch into a 1. I noticed that rating it as a 1 cheered me, but rating it as a 0 just felt like a lie. The fact that it was so clearly a lie embarrassed me, after all the pain research I had done (even though that research reiterated that *chronic pain is a chronic disease, like diabetes* and that reducing pain to a manageable level, as I had, *is* a positive outcome). Still, if Susan Cheever and Danielle Parker and lots of others could be more or less cured, why not me? What about the power of my mind? Aren't I imaginative?

Even my most beautiful days sometimes seemed to me like the Vermeer painting of the town of Delft on a summer afternoon, where, above the still spires and shimmering river, the clouds hang oppressively low, and gloom and mortality press.

Sean Mackey, the head of the Stanford pain service, was working on a study about the effects on pain of cognitive control, using guided imagery. He recalled how, when he started working with pain patients, he "realized how much of the treatment involved trying to reverse learned helplessness"—to rally them out of the despair ingrained by years of unremitting pain and to cajole their minds to offer up the analgesic that the minds themselves are capable of creating.

The theory of learned helplessness builds on the observation that if you give dogs inescapable electrical shocks, two-thirds of them will internalize the notion that they cannot avoid pain and victimization. Later—when put in a setting where they can escape the shocks simply by jumping over a low barrier—those dogs will not even try and will instead lie on the ground, flatten their ears, and whine.

I had always associated learned helplessness with whining dogs. But what about the one-third of dogs who leap away?

"This applies to people, too—in roughly the same proportions of resilience and resignation," he said. *Pain upsets and destroys the nature of the person who has it*—but not always. Like the electric shocks, chronic pain is a repetitive, punishing stimulus over which subjects don't have control, and it creates learned helplessness in most patients. "How do we undo this effect?" Dr. Mackey asked. "I want to show patients that their mind matters."

Did I have learned helplessness? Dr. Mackey pointed to three key criteria in the theory: the subject must perceive the negative stimulus as *personal*, *pervasive*, and *permanent*.

I long ago rejected the idea that my pain is personal, in the sense of a symptom or symbol of any kind. I tried to think and talk about it straightforwardly—as a fact, not a private sorrow. It did feel pervasive, though, since it was always there, and although I hoped it wasn't permanent, I feared it was. But perhaps it *is* permanent; being realistic shouldn't make me a whining dog. Then again, in researching pain, since I now knew that pain is a perception, did it therefore follow that the barrier was only as high as I perceived it to be?

I asked Dr. Mackey for a clinical demonstration of his study. He attached a metal probe, which heated up and cooled down at set intervals, to the back of my wrist. I was told that although the heat probe would feel uncomfortable, my skin would not be burned. (Indeed, an important limitation of pain research in humans is that researchers cannot cause subjects serious tissue damage.) During one exposure I was instructed to think of the pain as positively as possible; during another, to think of it as negatively as possible. After each exposure I was asked to rate my pain on a 0-to-10 scale, with 10 being the worst pain I could imagine.

Although I discovered that I could make the pain fluctuate according to whether I was imagining that I was immersed in a lovely Jacuzzi or was the victim of an inquisition, I still rated all the pain as low, ranging from a 1 to a 3. If 10 were being burned alive, I thought I should at least be begging for mercy to justify a rating of 5. So I insisted that Dr. Mackey turn up the dial. I was surprised at how hot it felt, given that it couldn't be burning me. But even when I was trying my hardest to imagine the pain as negatively as possible, Dr. Mackey's initial assurance kept it from really hurting—hurting, that is, the way a burn would.

Afterward my skin reddened and then began to pucker and blister. Dr. Mackey was more than a little dismayed, but I was thrilled. It was a second-degree burn that eventually darkened into a square mark like a brand. The study's protocol had been carefully established to avoid injuring anyone, yet in my case that protection had failed because of the very phenomenon under study: the effect of the mind on pain. By that point I had spent several weeks observing Dr. Mackey's pain clinic. I was so convinced that he would not burn me that my brain had not perceived the stimulus as a threat. I admired him, I trusted him, I was positive that he wouldn't hurt me. And ipso facto, through the power of the placebo effect, he didn't.

Only once before had my modulatory system been similarly deceived into dispensing with pain.

For Valentine's Day a few years before, I had received a huge pink heart-shaped bar of soap, the size of a small coconut, from my boyfriend Zach. It would nest only in a giant's hand, so perhaps it was intended to be purely decorative. In what I tried not to see as a metaphor for the relationship (although, like the door accident, it was), the first time I tried to use it in the shower, the soap-heart slipped from my grasp and smashed my toes. It was startlingly painful. I curled up in a ball for an hour, and then I called Zach. I couldn't reach him, and I wanted to talk to a boyfriend-type, so I called my former boyfriend, Luke.

"It's not broken," he pronounced cheerfully.

"Oh . . . Umm, how do you know?"

"It would hurt a lot."

"Well, it does hurt. That's why I'm calling . . ." I said, feeling less certain.

"It would hurt more," he said definitively.

Upon reflection, I decided that perhaps it didn't hurt as much as I had thought. For the next few hours he seemed to be right, but I still couldn't walk, and then—even as I lay there quietly—the pain grew. It was as if Luke's assurance had put the pain in a box called *not-even-broken* that contained it for a while, but then the pain welled up and began to seep through the walls of the construct.

I called him back.

"It doesn't hurt the way a break would," he said. His certainty reframed the sensation once again. By the time the pain overflowed again, Zach had come over. "Why didn't you go to the doctor?" he reproached me. "You are so star-crossed." I began to cry.

Two of the toes were fractured. I knew I would never be able to call Luke about a medical problem again. Indeed, at times in our friendship after that when I felt that Luke was dismissive of my chronic pain, the dismissal did not succeed in dismissing the pain. I just felt more alone with it. It was the Placebo Dilemma again. Expectation may rival nociception, but it's impossible to make use of that fact, because as soon as you know your relief is only placebo, your expectations collapse. The genie is ingenious; he never falls for the same trick twice.

THE ANESTHESIA OF BELIEF

At times, when my chronic pain was tormenting me, the sight of the scar from the pain toleration test—a slightly darkened square of skin beneath the round face of my watch—both reassured and reproached me. *Here*, I'd think, *is the ultimate proof that my mind can control pain.* Yet how to make it do so with my real pain, the pain that wasn't experimental? The scar continued to fade so that after a few years it was visible only in certain lights, and the testament to my modulatory system seemed like a relic in which my faith was waning.

I thought of a story I had read of a 1930s Thai Buddhist monk named Sao Man who had a disciple who was racked with pain from malaria. Sao Man declared that "instead of trying to relieve physical symptoms, monks should go to the root of distress and cure their minds" and "observe the pain without reacting, for thereby they would realize the truth of suffering."

Observing my pain is exactly what I want to do. I want to watch my mind at work as it generates pain, and then change it, the way a computer programmer can fix a glitch in the code or Vermeer might have painted over some of those clouds. I want to conduct the neurons of my brain as if they were an orchestra making discordant music. Those areas generating pain—*pianissimo!* Those areas that are supposed to be alleviating pain—*fortissimo!* Down-regulate pain-perception circuitry. Upregulate pain-modulation circuitry. *Pronto.*

For most of history, the idea of watching the mind at work was as fantastical as documenting a ghost. You could break into the haunted house—slice the brain open—but all you would find would be the house itself, the architecture of the brain rather than its invisible occupant. Photographing it with X-rays resulted only in pictures of the shell of the house, the skull. The invention of the CT scan and the MRI were great advances because they reveal tissue as well as bone—the wallpaper as well as the walls—but the ghost still didn't show up. The photographs they produce are static. Consciousness remained elusive.

A newer form of MRI, functional magnetic resonance imaging (fMRI)—as well as a related technology, positron emission tomography (PET) scans—used with increasingly sophisticated software, aspires to watch a living brain at work. The films show parts of the brain becoming active under various stimuli by detecting areas of increased blood flow connected with the faster firing of nerve cells. For the first time in history, one can give a subject a painful shock and observe the person's brain creating an experience of pain.

"There is an interesting irony to pain," Christopher deCharms, a neurophysiologist and pain researcher, told me. "Everyone is born with a system designed to turn off pain. There isn't an obvious mechanism to turn off other diseases, like Parkinson's. With pain, the system is there, but we don't have control over the dial."

Dr. deCharms has collaborated with Sean Mackey to develop a science fiction–like investigational technique whose goal is to teach people to control their own "dials": to activate their modulatory systems without the stress of fleeing a shark or the deception of a placebo. Usually, brain imaging involves subjects who are scanned and researchers who analyze the scan. But what if the functional imaging machine could be equipped with an internal screen so that the subjects themselves could watch a scan of their own brain activity in real time, as their brains respond to pain? Would seeing their pain-modulation circuits at work enable subjects to learn how to control them more effectively?

Using real-time functional neuroimaging (real-time fMRIs), Dr. deCharms and Dr. Mackey asked volunteers, over the course of six sessions, to try to increase and to decrease their pain while watching a screen that showed the activation of the part of their brains involved in pain perception and modulation. Traditional biofeedback has proved that individuals can be trained to control autonomic bodily functions—such as heart rate, skin temperature, and even rhythms of electrical activity in the brain previously considered beyond volition—by using measurements of those functions. But such measurements only indirectly reflect the brain's activity. By contrast, Dr. deCharms and Mackey's technique, which they term *neuroimaging therapy*, allows subjects to interact (in a sense) with the brain itself.

The hope of neuroimaging therapy is that regular practice will strengthen the ineffective modulatory system so as to eliminate chronic pain, the way long-term physical therapy can eliminate muscular weakness. The scan would actually *be* the treatment, the subject his or her own researcher.

In preparation for the scans, subjects are trained in three types of pain-control strategy: changing their attention to the pain (to focus on or away from the pain); changing their assessment of the pain (to perceive it as more or less intense); and changing their perception of the stimulus (as a neutral sensory experience instead of a damaging, frightening, and overwhelming experience).

Although functional imaging studies have shown that distraction reduces pain, Dr. deCharms believes that paradoxically, an alternative approach to relieving pain is to focus directly on it, which he believes can activate the pain-modulatory system. He personally feels that for chronic pain sufferers, "the technique of distraction may not provide much benefit, because it takes you away from your pain for a few moments, but as soon as you stop distracting yourself, the pain is there again—unchanged."

He had recently suffered from a bout of neck pain himself and decided to see if neuroimaging therapy could help. But when he tried to focus on the pain in the scanner, he found it curiously difficult to do. "Even though it felt like the pain in the scanner was all I thought about—and all I talked about—I wasn't really focusing on it. The mind will do anything to avoid focusing on pain." Yet, when he succeeded in focusing on it, he "could feel pain melt away. I perceived myself as upregulating the pain-control system. It was a feeling similar to a 'runner's high.'"

Dayna—a middle-aged woman who had been unable to work because of back pain for several years—told me how she discovered that trying to distract herself from her pain with positive imagery actually worsened her pain. "I would picture horseback riding and hiking and all the fun, fun things I used to do," she told me. "In the scanner, I could see that these things were causing an increase in my brain activity because I associate them with a sense of loss—with knowing I can't do them anymore. I realized I needed to think of some new things." She tried, instead, to focus on accepting and even embracing pain. "I had an image of myself dancing with the pain," she said, and as they began to dance, she felt her pain transform from a stalker to a partner.

Please let it work for me, I thought.

Distraction had always been the most successful pain relief technique for me. Once, when I first had pain, I curled up in bed and cried. I had often done this when a romantic relationship ended, and the indulgence always made me feel better. But this time, when I finished crying, the pain was not only not better—it was worse. "Pain is not dissolved by tears, it is watered by them," I wrote in my diary. After that, when I had too much pain to do anything productive, I went to a movie or walked to a bakery and bought a marshmallow Rice Krispies treat. But I had never tried to focus calmly on the pain itself.

In one sense, neuroimaging therapy is simply a high-tech way to learn the ancient religious technique of meditation—by trying to make the process more transparent. But as Dr. Mackey pointed out, "it takes Buddhist monks thirty years of sitting on a mountain to learn control of their brains through meditation. We're trying to jump-start that process."

I had looked at pain through the premodern lens of metaphor, religion, and magic; I had looked at pain through the modern lens of biology and disease. Both had proved inadequate. I wanted to understand pain through a new paradigm, a postmodern paradigm, as it were, that would use the magic of science to see the science of magic—and to find treatments that would draw upon that understanding.

Lying on my back in a large plastic fMRI machine in the Stanford University lab, I peer through 3-D goggles at a small screen. The machine makes a deep rattling sound, and an image flickers before me: my brain. Me. *I am looking at my own brain as it thinks my thoughts, including these thoughts.*

"It's the mind-body problem, right there on the screen," Christopher deCharms commented later. "We are doing something that people have wanted to do for thousands of years. Descartes said, 'I think, therefore I am.' Now we're watching that process as it unfolds."

The screen shows activation of the rACC—the part of the limbic system that gives pain its emotional valence. The pain of pain, as it were, is the way it's suffused with a particular unpleasantness—the sadness, anxiety, distress, and dislike that researchers refer to as *dysphoria*—a reaction so fierce that you are instantly compelled to try to make the stimulus cease, not in five minutes, not in five seconds, *now.* You can feel heat or cold or pressure, and note them simply as stimuli, but as soon as those stimuli exceed a certain intensity, the rACC activates, riveting your attention, filling you with dysphoria, and causing you to try desperately to put an end to it.

The rACC is represented by a 3-D image of a fire in which the height of the flames corresponds to the degree of rACC activation. Subjects undergo five thirteen-minute scanning runs, each consisting of five cycles of rest followed by intervals during which they try to increase rACC activation and then decrease it.

"Increase Your Pain," the screen commands as the first run begins. I try to recall the mental strategies in which I had been instructed for increasing pain: *Dwell on how hopeless, depressed, or lonely you felt when your pain was most severe. Imagine that the pain will never end. Sense that the pain is causing long-term damage.*

I picture the pain—soggy, moldy, or perhaps ashy, like smokers' lungs. "Pain spreads out and pollutes the brain," John Keltner had told me. "It actually poisons and infects your brain."

In three months, it would be ten years since the day I went swimming with Kurt and first acquired pain. What had it done to my brain? The Apkarian study suggested that 1.3 cubic centimeters of the gray matter of the brain is lost with each year of chronic pain. If I multiply that by ten . . . On the screen, the flames of my rACC explode. I feed the flames further by thinking of descriptions of the burning of heretics in *Foxe's Book of Martyrs.*

"Decrease Your Pain," the screen commands.

The suggested pain-reduction strategies do little to quell the flames. *Tell yourself it's just a completely harmless, short-term tactile sensation.* I try to suffocate the pain with banal positive imagery of "flowing water or honey" and to picture myself in a "favorite vacation spot such as the mountains or the beach."

"Every pain-free moment competes with the onslaught of the chronic pain experience," John Keltner had told me. "People need to create moments when their attention is sufficiently drawn away from pain that they are almost pain-free, so that they can begin to recondition and reclaim their brains." But my mind keeps slipping back to the auto-da-fé, and the rACC fire flares.

What if I *were* a martyr? I think of the story of Rabbi Akiva, who recited a prayer with a smile on his lips as the flesh was being combed from his bones for defying the Roman prohibition on Torah study. "All my life," he explained to the puzzled governor orchestrating his execution, "when I said the words, 'You shall love the Lord your God with all your heart, with all your soul, and with all your might,' I was saddened, for I thought, *When shall I be able to fulfill this command?* Now that I am giving my life and my resolution remains firm, should I not smile?"

"Fortunate are you, Rabbi Akiva, to be martyred for the sake of Torah," the Talmud cheerfully concludes.

During my next Decrease Pain interval, I focus on myself as a martyr. (Jewish? Christian? Witch?). *Fortunate are you,* I tell myself, *to have this opportunity to lucidly recite a prayer of some faith while being burned at the stake. Fortunate are you to be so persuaded of your faith to see this opportunity as fortunate . . .* My rACC activation respectfully subsides.

But there was a twist, I recall, in the case of witches. Witches were sometimes believed to have insensitive areas, called devil's marks, which could be discovered by sticking pins in them. A lack of pain could constitute proof of sorcery! As soon as I focus on the need to feel the pain of the pinpricks to establish my innocence, my rACC helpfully flares. Soon I have the strategy down. Heretic-martyr: rACC low. Heretic-witch: rACC high.

I try to recall theories of the physiological mechanisms thought to account for the belief-induced anesthesia of heretic-martyrs. Perhaps they are in a trance—a state of autosuggestion or self-hypnosis. Or perhaps they benefit from "counterpleasure": if their pain serves a higher psychological goal, they might experience it as strengthening, rather than damaging, their ego. In *Sacred Pain*, Ariel Glucklich theorizes that intense pain can cause both a massive release of beta-endorphins and a sense of disassociation, which frees one from the anxieties and desires that normally constitute the self. He terms the resulting euphoria "hyperstimulation analgesia."

One might expect the experience of pain to compel a unique focus of attention on the body. But religious devotees insist that during certain rites, this focus paradoxically metamorphoses into its opposite: a feeling of transcending or being freed from the body. Ascetics describe the moment during mortification when pain becomes no-pain—when, as a pilgrim put it, "Pain, having become so intense, began to disappear," or, as a mystic wrote, "At one moment everything is pain; but at the next moment, every-thing is love."

How does pain cause the brain to create this sense of dislocation from one's own body? The Canadian psychologist Ronald Melzack (the coau-thor of the McGill Pain Questionnaire) theorized that each person has a unique "neurosignature" (the neural relay of the thalamus, cortex, and limbic system that constitutes the neuromatrix). The neurosignature cre-ates what he calls a "body-self neuromatrix" that integrates the continu-ous flow of sensory input into a conscious awareness of oneself. Intense pain, he speculated, overwhelms the neuromatrix with an excess of sen-sory information, interrupting the neurosignature and arresting the body-self template. Although the sensation of pain continues to register, it can no longer be processed. One remains aware of the pain but ceases to experience that pain as belonging to oneself—or, indeed, ceases to experi-ence a self for pain to belong to. This phenomenon is "either terrifying or exhilarating," Ariel Glucklich writes, depending on whether it was sought or not.

I remember watching the impassive face of the devotee at Thaipusam as the priest threaded the fishhooks with the dangling limes through his back and how he had said the pain no longer belonged to him. The god freed him from pain.

Distracted by thinking about hyperstimulation analgesia—and then distracted by thinking about Tracey's theory of the modulating effects of distraction—I watch as my rACC activation dwindles to nothing.

COGNITIVE CONTROL OVER NEUROPLASTICITY

The results of my scan, Sean Mackey tells me a few days later, indicate that I have significant control of my brain activity. A week later I am scanned again, in the sleek office at Omneuron, a Menlo Park medical-technology company Christopher deCharms founded to develop clinical applications of real-time functional neuroimaging. This time, it feels easier to control my rACC with less reliance on elaborate fantasy; I am interacting more directly with my brain.

This learning effect was demonstrated by a study they published in the prestigious *Proceedings of the National Academy of Sciences*. The study showed that while looking at images of their own brains' activity, subjects can learn to control the activation in a way that significantly regulates their pain. The first phase of the study looked at thirty-six healthy subjects and twelve with chronic pain. In the scanner, the healthy ones tried to modulate their responses to a painful heat stimulus. The chronic pain patients, however, worked to reduce only the pain they already felt. The chronic pain patients who received neuroimaging training reported an average decrease of 64 percent in their pain rating by the end of the study. Moreover, the benefit of the study continued after it was over: a majority of the pain patients reported that they continued to experience a reduction of pain by 50 percent or more. Healthy subjects also reported a significant increase in their ability to control the pain during the study.

"One big concern we had," Dr. Mackey says, "was: Were we creating the world's most expensive placebo?" To make sure that wasn't the case, he trained a control group in pain-reduction techniques without using the scanner (as in his previous experiment) to see if that was as effective as employing a multimillion-dollar machine. He also tried scanning subjects without showing them their brain images—and he tried tricking subjects by feeding them images of irrelevant parts of their brains or feeding them someone else's brain images. "None of these worked," Dr. Mackey says, "or worked nearly as well." Traditional biofeedback also compared unfavorably: changes in pain ratings of subjects in the neuroimaging therapy group were three times as large as in the biofeedback control group.

Subsequent phases of the study will assess whether the technique offers long-term practical benefits to a larger group of chronic pain patients by fundamentally changing their modulatory systems so that they can reduce pain all the time without constantly and consciously trying to do so. If they can, then the technique would not merely provide shelter from the storm of pain; it would bring about climate change. Unpublished work found that repeated training over six weeks of subjects with chronic pain significantly reduced their pain.

"I believe the technique could make lasting changes because the brain is a machine designed to learn," Dr. deCharms says. The brain is plastic: whenever you learn something, new neural connections form, and old, unused ones wither away (a process known as *activity-dependent neuroplasticity*). Thus, engaging a certain brain region can alter it. (Neuroimaging has shown, for example, that the part of the brains of London cabdrivers that deals in spatial relations is larger than usual. More strikingly, after merely three months of training, learning to juggle creates visible changes in parts of the brain involved with motor coordination.)

Many diseases of the central nervous system involve inappropriate levels of activation in particular brain regions that change the way they operate. Some regions experience less activity, and other regions become hyperactive. (For example, epilepsy involves abnormal hyperactivity of cells; stroke, Parkinson's, and other diseases involve neurodegeneration.) In the case of chronic pain, new nerve cells, recruited for transmitting pain, create more pain pathways in the nervous system, while nerve cells that would normally inhibit or slow the signaling begin to decrease or function abnormally. Neuroimaging therapy may mitigate this harm by teaching people how to increase the efficacy of their healthy brain cells.

"It gives people a tool they didn't know they had," Dr. Mackey says. "Cognitive control over neuroplasticity."

THE PAIN CHRONICLES

The technique may offer a particular advantage over drug therapy. It is difficult to design drugs to change a disease process in a specific region of the brain, because drugs work by targeting receptors, and most receptors, such as opiate receptors, are present in multiple systems throughout the brain and body (one reason such drugs almost always have side effects). Neuroimaging therapy, by contrast, is anatomically specific, allowing for the possibility of targeted neuroplasticity, much as a muscle can be isolated and trained.

Neuroimaging therapy "provides tangible evidence that people can change their own brains, which can be very empowering," Dr. Mackey says. Much as people were once puzzled by Freud's talking cure (how could describing problems *solve* them?), the idea of a "looking cure," as it were, makes us wonder: How could one part of our brain control another, and why would *looking* at the process help to do so? Who, then, is the "me" controlling my brain? The technique seems to deepen—rather than resolve—the mind-body problem, widening the Cartesian divide by splitting the self into agent and object, mind and brain, ghost and machine.

"The decision-making parts of the brain are thought to be the prefrontal regions of the cortex," Dr. Mackey says. But as for how those brain parts *cause* the change in the rACC—"Heck if I know! How do we get the brain to do *anything*? We can map out the anatomical circuits involved and the general functions of those circuits, but we can't tell you the mechanism by which any cognitive decision—large or small—is translated into action."

Neuroimaging therapy as a treatment for disease is one of those novel ideas that seems obvious in retrospect, but no one thought to try before. Although some researchers have experimented with teaching subjects to control their brain activation to create a "brain-computer interface," the purpose of those experiments has been theoretical rather than therapeutic. In one such experiment, for example, subjects were taught to navigate a cursor through a maze on a screen using only their brains. Subjects completed a sequence of mental strategies. Each strategy activated a different part of the brain that automatically moved the cursor a different way. By observing how certain activations resulted in corresponding movements of the cursor, subjects were able to learn how to navigate the cursor through the maze.

Perhaps the best example of a "looking cure" is a novel treatment for phantom limb pain. The neurologist Vilayanur S. Ramachandran used a mirror box (a box with two mirrors in the center, one facing each way), in which patients put their actual limb in one side and their stump in the other. When patients move their actual limb, looking in one side of the mirror box, they appear to be moving both arms. Phantom limb pain typically involves the sensation that the phantom arm is stuck in an uncomfortable position. By straightening her existing arm in the mirror box, a patient can have the illusion of uncurling her phantom arm, and the cramping pain goes away. (More recently, scientists from the University of Manchester have had success using a computer-generated simulation to create a more realistic-looking illusion.)

Since patients know it is an illusion, why does the trick help? Through an unknown mechanism, the visual cortex communicates the image to the somatosensory cortex, which somehow decides to mimic the image in the mirror by making the phantom limb relax. Phantom limb pain is theorized to derive from the neural reorganization in the somatosensory cortex. Functional imaging has shown that repeated use of the mirror can reverse those changes and reduce pain. Although more extensive trials are needed, repeated training has shown long-term improvements in some patients.

TERRA INCOGNITA

One of the limitations of pain treatment today is that pain presents the same symptom regardless of how it is generated or what type of pain it is, yet different conditions require different treatment. Brain imaging might be used diagnostically for individual patients, to determine the nature of their pain. It might also spur the development of more targeted pain drugs.

Irene Tracey—who directs Oxford University's brain imaging center in England and is a rising star in the field—believes that brain imaging could also be useful in medical malpractice and disability court cases to document the reality of the pain of a plaintiff. These cases are currently hampered by the lack of an objective measure of pain, leaving juries at a loss how to distinguish between honest plaintiffs and malingerers.

The Gothic kingdom of Oxford seemed gloomy in the late November afternoon as I made my way to Dr. Tracey's office. But inside, everything began to seem brighter. Her cheeks flushed as she discussed the future of her research. "In five to ten years," she said definitively, "we will be able to put someone in a scanner and say, 'Your pain comes 10 percent from hypervigilance [paying too much attention to the pain], 20 percent from catastrophizing [excessive worry], 20 percent from peripheral input [from the original injury or disease], and 50 percent from brain circuit dysfunction.' We can already scan people and tell them far more about their pain than they can tell us," she concluded crisply.

Beneath her pale blouse, with its pattern of tiny flowers, the swell of her third child was just visible. I pictured the fetus's brain cells dividing into neural networks in a design that would one day be known. One day, too, would my pain be known because imaging would identify each of the elements of which it is composed? Would the mystery of pain, then, finally be unveiled?

Three years later I write to Dr. Tracey, asking her to update me on her work. Since so much time had elapsed, I expect her to tell me that we are much closer to achieving her vision of using brain imaging to identify different kinds of pain. But instead she is much more circumspect. "In five to ten years, we *might* be able to put someone in a scanner and say, 'Your pain comes from a combination of hypervigilance . . .'" she writes.

I object that the conditional makes the prediction meaningless (after all, anything "*might*" happen . . . aliens might bring us pain-scanning technology), to no avail. She also writes that the idea of assigning an actual percentage to the different kinds of pain in a sufferer's mind sounds "amateur" because "all these factors are interactive, you see . . ."

I recall how Ari (the Israeli artist who suffered from migraines and fibromyalgia) had asked me if I believed there would be a cure for chronic pain. "Oh yes," I'd said. There had been an inspiring update to the crushing study on chronic pain shrinking the gray matter of the brain. A German research group found that when patients who had suffered from chronic hip pain got a total hip replacement, their gray matter regenerated, suggesting that the shrinkage that had been observed did not stem from neuronal loss, which is irreversible, but merely from a change in the size of cells. So, perhaps the damage of all chronic pain syndromes could be reversed. Perhaps, too, one day, chronic pain would be controlled just as acute pain can be controlled through anesthesia, and anyway, no one would develop chronic pain in the future, because pain would be treated at its onset. I launched into my pet analogy of TB and how pain clinics would all fold up shop like the sanatoriums. As I talked, I had an image of the consumptives packing their suitcases on the magic mountain, the directors discussing whether to turn it into a museum.

"One day . . ." Ari drawled, "in the next millennium?"

I hesitated.

"Let me put it this way," he said. "If you were a venture capitalist, would you invest in a company whose mission was to find a cure for chronic pain?"

I recalled the catch in my optimistic analogy: the lag time—the half century between the discovery of the tuberculosis bacterium and the discovery of antibiotics. And pain is not a simple bacterium, visible under a microscope, but a complex aspect of consciousness. The tools to look at the brain have only just been invented, and the brain itself is still mainly terra incognita—more like the ancient maps of faraway lands than like Google Earth. Would the discoveries of pain-related genes lead to the development of effective drugs soon? For how many years will the critical breakthrough about pain remain five to ten years hence?

"Not if I wanted to get rich quickly," I conceded.

"How's your pain?" he asked.

I never knew how to respond to that question. Okay. Better than it used to be. Bearable, almost never unbearable. But still there—always. Since my arthritic condition is degenerative, presumably it has degenerated further over the years, but I do not have more pain now—I have less— and for that I am grateful and thrilled. It's so hard to know the best attitude to assume! On the one hand, I want to be satisfied with the progress I've made: to accept the balance of pain that remains and close the pages of my pain diary forever. On the other hand, to fully accept it feels as if I am settling for a pained life. I want to keep a candle in the window of my mind for my pathography to have something besides a philosophical ending.

In the three years I've been married, though, I've been surprised to discover that my wishes have changed. On my first birthday after our wedding, I wished to have a child and realized that I wanted that more than I wanted not to have pain, and that if the Wish Fairy would grant only one wish, I'd choose the child. (Of course, if my pain worsened, that could change, I hastened to let the Wish Fairy know, lest she think I had forgotten how compelling pain can be.)

The next birthday I wished for a baby again. But on my last birthday, I had a new wish: that the twins with whom—through the miracle of medical science—we were about to be twice blest would be healthy, that their new bodies would be gifted with the pain-protective gene variant and spared the pain-sensitivity gene variant, and that their lives would not be blighted by persistent pain.

A UNIVERSE OF HURT

I hope functional imaging will progress in my lifetime enough to have clinical input," comments John Keltner, who spent several years working with Irene Tracey in her center before deciding to begin new training as a psychiatrist. He points out that CT scanning and MRI technology were revolutionary technologies, with huge immediate clinical impact, because they created the first anatomically accurate pictures of the inside of a body. How much more revolutionary it seemed when, in the late 1980s, functional imaging produced the first 3-D movies of the working brain. But the films were and remain largely indecipherable. Researchers puzzle over the images like Columbus staring at the gray shoreline, thinking, *India?*

"We don't understand virtually anything about the human brain," Dr. Keltner says soberly. "Pain, sleep, memory, thinking, adding two and two—we don't understand any of that stuff. When I started doing functional imaging research on pain twenty years ago, I thought it would soon lead to a meaningful diagnostic tool. Now I hope that in the next forty years I will help come up with a test that will be able to answer a simple clinical question about a patient's pain, such as, Should we focus on treating your toe or your emotional state? That's such a basic question, and right now there isn't a single diagnostic test that can answer it.

"Brain function turns out to be so complicated. It would be a lot easier if there were a part of the brain associated with pain and only pain, but so far we haven't been able to find a single unique marker that would allow us to definitively identify a pain state. If you show me a brain scan and say, *Is this person in pain or thinking about running from a tiger?* I wouldn't be able to tell you." A brain scan of a person in a state of repose would look different, of course, but pain and fear are both salient experiences with strong activation in common brain regions.

"We had to start recognizing that the fundamental pillars of human experience—pain, fear, anxiety, sadness, joy—involve the whole brain, with dozens of areas switching on and off. And many of those parts also light up in scans that have nothing to do with pain. Of the countless possible brain states, perhaps only ten thousand happen if a person is in pain. But nobody has come up with a rich and complicated enough model to analyze the complexity of the distributed patterns of neural networks and deduce any underlying rules. The daunting aspect is that it's a bit like chess. Chess is eight spaces by eight spaces and you have thirty-two pieces, yet by the third move of any game, there are a thousand possibilities." But instead of thirty-two pieces, the brain has a hundred billion neurons that can form an unknown number of neural networks.

"The pictures are so complicated," he says for the fourth time. "If we change one parameter in an experiment—say, change a visual cue from blue to red or change from color to sound—we'd expect to see corresponding changes in the auditory and visual sections of the brain. But instead we see changes in a dozen areas.

"I'm not discouraged," he adds, sounding like a hiker who has realized that he can't figure out where he is on a map, but is reminding himself that he likes hiking and should trudge on. "We're literally grappling with the fundamental aspects of human beings. We naively believed that pain is simple—it hurts or it doesn't hurt—so there should be a single brain state we could see every time someone is in pain. But what we've stumbled into is the discovery that there's a relative *universe of hurt*—that hurting is an immense, rich, and varied human experience, associated with an unknown number of possible brain states. From a scientific position, we're overwhelmed at how large that universe is. We're still at the stage where each step forward makes us realize how far we have to go . . ."

"We're getting there faster than we thought possible," Sean Mackey responds. He and his Stanford colleagues recently made a significant encroachment in an experiment in which they were able to distinguish, with approximately 85 percent accuracy, brain scans of volunteers given a painfully hot stimulus from those given a non-painfully hot stimulus or no stimulus. A further step, he points out, would be to ask volunteers to simply *imagine* being given a thermal stimulus and to see if he could distinguish those scans from the scans of volunteers who actually had the heat stimulus (in other experiments, imagined pain has been shown to engage similar brain regions as physical pain).

Although Dr. Mackey believes that this kind of simple, acute pain probably has very little to do with the experience of chronic pain, he also feels that "we are rapidly moving to a point where we may be able to detect the subjective experience of pain and to find a separate signature for it that allows us to distinguish it from other affective states, such as depression or anxiety." He points to the amazing acceleration of certain kinds of technology, such as machine learning techniques and pattern classifiers— complex software algorithms that can be fed a set of known examples (scans of people experiencing thermal pain, or not) and then used to classify new, uncategorized scans.

He feels it is important, however, to understand that this technology is a long way from being able to recognize—let alone provide insight into—the state of chronic pain. He has great concerns about how this kind of technology will be used, because he thinks it is "ripe for abuse by the legal community and insurance companies to try to disprove that somebody is having chronic pain and deny care." He has already seen a lawsuit that relied on claims about using scanning to detect pain. The suit involved a worker who developed chronic pain after his arm was injured by molten tar. The worker's lawyer claimed that a cognitive neuropsychologist had validated the man's chronic pain by scanning his brain. The expert had, in fact, scanned the man doing various activities, such as squeezing a ball, with both his injured and his uninjured arm. Because the two brain scans were different and the scan of the injured side showed more brain activity, the expert inferred that the scans proved the patient had more pain on the injured side.

Yet, Dr. Mackey points out, there is no evidence that greater brain activity necessarily indicates greater pain. The difference could reflect the man squeezing the ball harder with one hand (or feeling more anxious while using the injured hand, or any number of other factors). As a physician, Dr. Mackey believed in the worker's pain, but he felt it was important to refute what he believed was specious methodology, which could as easily be used in other cases to falsely discredit patients' pain.

"What was remarkable is that the expert who was arguing for it is an internationally acclaimed researcher in cognitive systems," he recalls. "It showed me that even a really smart person can be naive in regard to pain and approach it as if it were this Cartesian experience"—as if increased brain activity was the bell in the brain that simply rang louder when there was more pain.

"The holy grail" of functional imaging, he says, "would be to be able to distinguish different patterns for different types of pain and to use that information to tailor specific treatments for a particular person. As you know, when I treat a person with pain, I go through a process of trial and error of different medications that is very laborious and frustrating for both the patient and me. I hope that one day we could use scanning, along with other information, as a predictive tool in which we could tell someone, *You have this genetic profile, this type of injury, and based on this imaging information, we believe you are going to respond to this particular therapy.*"

When asked if he thinks there will be a breakthrough in the treatment of chronic pain that is similar to that of anesthesia, he points out that a century and a half later, we don't know how anesthesia works, and although anesthesia allows us "to conquer pain, the person can't be conscious!" Moreover, turning off an entire system, the way anesthesia does, is going to be much simpler than trying to turn off only the pain system, because pain is so intricately woven throughout the brain, with so many networks available to reroute it if one is disabled.

At the moment, the pictures offered by the current technology are too primitive—the resolution of the images too coarse—to fathom pain. But "ultimately," he says, "if we believe that our experiences and beliefs and perceptions are made up of firing of neurons and flow of information in neural circuits, then each experience has to be characterized by a different pattern. The limitation in understanding those patterns is only technological, and technology continuously improves." By contrast, he says, "some people believe that consciousness is uniquely human and God-given: that it is inherently nondeterministic and cannot be defined or distilled down to the firing of neurons. I believe that it can, and I'm of the opinion that we're inching closer and closer."

It's easy to think of obstacles. Perhaps we need to see how the neurons are wired together to recognize pain, which the scans cannot show. Perhaps— even though the technology is improving—the gap between the coarse current technology and what we would really need will always be too great. Or perhaps each individual's pain is simply too individual. Even if perceptions are all composed of neurons firing in particular patterns in particular networks, it may be that these patterns differ sufficiently from person to person in ways that will make it perpetually difficult for us to interpret them, even when we have functional imaging scans with far higher resolutions than today's.

The neural networking patterns of pain might turn out to be like fingerprints—something that everyone has and that, in essence, serve the same purpose for everyone, but differ too much in random detail from person to person to be able to meaningfully categorize them. After all, one could say that just as thoughts all spring from neuronal patterns, all the wondrous qualities of a painting depend on arrangements of paint on canvas. But we cannot now and probably never will be able to teach a computer to be able to analyze a new painting and say whether it has any merit—whether it is interesting, pleasing, or stirring—by showing it examples of thousands of famous paintings and hoping it can discern an underlying, predictive pattern.

"I'm not saying that we're going to be able to see the ghost in the machine—the experience of pain itself," Dr. Mackey responds. "My hope is that we can get to the point where imaging can become a clinically useful tool, in the same way that we can use a cholesterol test as a biomarker for heart disease to guide us to choose an effective therapy. I don't think functional imaging will allow us to 'see' pain or suffering or love in the foreseeable future. But in the same way that pattern-classifying software might enable us to identify a painting as being from the Impressionist period, or possibly even as a Monet, I think it will be able to identify different types of pain. In regard to using functional imaging as a diagnostic tool, I believe the question is now a *when*, not an *if*."

"The idea of functional imaging as a pain meter is unrealistic," counters Scott Fishman, the head of pain services at UC Davis. "Humans are variable enough in our physiologies that doctors can't even agree on reading an EKG or on what a stroke means, which are much more clear-cut things. How are scans going to prove or disprove someone else's pain and suffering—or even illuminate its nature?"

Pain and suffering are properties of the mind, he points out, and he doesn't believe that "functional imaging is actually looking at the mind. The mind is like a virtual organ—it doesn't have a physical address that we know of. Right now, imaging is just looking at the brain." Imaging shows the level of activation of different parts of the brain, from which we can *extrapolate* something about the mind, but to understand pain, "what we really need to see is how the parts talk to each other—and the complex nuances of their language."

Functional imaging is able to show that, of the brain's hundred billion neurons, a few hundred million of them, in various areas, become more active during the time at which the subjects report an experience of pain. What it does not do is explain the *connection* between that experience and the activity of those neurons. Imagine watching a silent film of a concert. You would be able to discern patterns in which the players in the bass section become active at one moment, vigorously gesturing, and then the rest of the orchestra joins in, but you wouldn't hear the notes themselves or deduce how they form strands of melody and harmony and meld together to create the ethereal experience of listening to music.

"Pain is an aspect of consciousness, and consciousness is not neurons firing," agrees Daniel Carr, the physician in whose clinic I first began to understand pain as a disease. "The gears of a watch rotate and keep time, but the turning of the gears is not time. Functional imaging is *a picture of a mechanism associated with the experience of consciousness*, but it is not consciousness. Consciousness is a transcendent emergent epiphenomenon that depends on the firing of neurons in some distributed way that we don't understand and perhaps can't understand."

Do we need to understand consciousness itself in order to understand pain? What are the limits of that understanding? Could we ever become fully transparent to ourselves? "If a higher being told us how consciousness works," he muses, "could we understand the explanation?"

RIGHT NEXT DOOR

The eminent neurobiologist Allan Basbaum told me a story about a pain researcher and a vision expert. "You still don't know how pain works?" the vision guy asks the pain guy.

"You may know something about how vision works," the pain man replies, "how the retina's rods and cones receive light stimuli, how its nerve cells transmit them via the optic nerve to the brain, and so on. But tell me—in what part of the brain does beauty lie?"

The vision guy falls silent.

"Let me know when you find it," the pain man says, "because pain is right next door."

NOTES

INTRODUCTION: THE TELEGRAM

3   *warned colleagues against visiting patients who had advanced consumption*: See "History of Tuberculosis," *Respiration* 65 (1998): 5.

3   *German physician identified* Mycobacterium tuberculosis: Robert Koch presented his finding on March 24, 1882.

4   *diseases are understood metaphorically*: See Susan Sontag, *Illness as Metaphor and AIDS and Its Metaphors* (New York: Picador, 2001), 34.

4   *"Where does it hurt?"*: See Michel Foucault, *The Birth of the Clinic* (New York: Routledge, 2003), xxi.

4   *articulated but not popularized*: See "Infectious Disease During the Civil War: The Triumph of the Third Army," *Clinical Infectious Diseases* 16 (1993): 580–84.

4   *decades before anyone thought to employ them*: Nitrous oxide was discovered in 1772 but was not used as an anesthetic until 1844. Sulphuric ether was known to resemble nitrous oxide by the 1820s but was not used as an anesthetic until 1846.

5   *serious, widespread*: Estimates of Americans experiencing chronic pain vary considerably, from 19 million to as high as 130 million. The International Association for the Study of Pain, along with the European Federation of IASP Chapters, released the results of a comprehensive survey in 2004 that found that one in five adults claimed chronic pain, which was defined as pain that persists or recurs for more than three months. More than a third of households in Europe included a chronic pain sufferer, compared with almost half (46 percent) of homes in the United States.

5   *a 2009 report by the Mayday Fund*: See *A Call to Revolutionize Chronic Pain Care in America: An Opportunity in Health Care Reform*, the Mayday Fund, November 4, 2009.

5   *Another study in the United States*: See "Broad Experience with Pain Sparks a Search for Relief," ABC News/USA Today/Stanford University Medical Center Poll, May 9, 2005.

6   *most chronic pain patients*: 2000 survey commissioned by Partners Against Pain, an educational program sponsored by Purdue Pharma.

6   *"history of man is the history of pain"*: See Vladimir Nabokov, *Pnin* (New York: Random House, 2004), 126.

6   *"place of pain"*: See *Bhagavadgita*, Edwin Arnold, trans. (Mineola, N.Y.: Courier Dover, 1993), 41.

7   *"Thorns also and thistles"*: See Genesis 3:18 (King James Version).

7   *"against these satanic agencies"*: See American Dental Association, *Transactions of the American Dental Association* 11–12 (1872): 105.

9   *origin of toothache*: See also Benjamin R. Foster, *Before the Muses: An Anthology of Akkadian Literature* (Bethesda, Md.: CDL Press, 2005), 995.

I. THE VALE OF PAIN, THE VEIL OF PAIN: PAIN AS METAPHOR

I gratefully acknowledge the assistance of Sara Brumfield, a doctoral student at UCLA, for her expertise on ancient Mesopotamia as well as her translations of biblical, Babylonian, and Sumerian texts.

15 *"pain remains veiled"*: Martin Heidegger, *Poetry, Language, Thought*, Albert Hofstadter, trans. (New York: Harper Perennial, 2001), 94.

15 *"uncanny strangeness"*: David B. Morris, *The Culture of Pain* (Berkeley: University of California Press, 1993), 25.

15 *"most truthful way of regarding illness"*: Sontag, *Illness as Metaphor*, 3–4.

16 *bowing before the whirlwind*: God appears to Job out of the whirlwind in Job 38:1.

16 *"love is love of* x*"*: See Elaine Scarry, *The Body in Pain* (New York: Oxford University Press, 1985), 5.

17 *Dickinson tries to describe this great blank*: See *The Poems of Emily Dickinson* (Cambridge: Harvard University Press, 1998), 501–502.

17 *"Head pain has surged up upon me"*: Foster, *Before the Muses*, 400.

17 dolor dictat: See Alphonse Daudet, *In the Land of Pain*, Julian Barnes, trans. (New York: Knopf, 2003), 27. Daudet sources the phrase to Ovid, but I was unable to confirm that. He also writes of a similar phrase by Sithus Itlaius, *dolor verba aspera dictat* (pain dictates the words I now write).

17 *"fine explorer in Central Africa"*: Ibid., 8–9.

26 *two different types of nerve fibers*: See Ursula Wesselmann, "Chronic Nonmalignant Nociceptive Pain Syndromes," in *Surgical Management of Pain* (New York: Thieme, 2002), 365 ff.

27 *forces the creature to tend to its wound*: See, for example, Patrick David Wall, *Pain: The Science of Suffering* (New York: Columbia University Press, 2000), 2–3.

28 *not thought to cause the invertebrate pain*: See a summary of evidence presented by The Senate [of Canada] Standing Committee on Legal and Constitutional Affairs, "Do Invertebrates Feel Pain?" www.parl.gc.ca/37/2/parlbus/commbus/senate/Com-e/lega-e/witn-e/shelly-e.htm, accessed December 31, 2009. "Although it is impossible to know the subjective experience of another animal with certainty, the balance of the evidence suggests that most invertebrates do not feel pain. The evidence is most robust for insects, and, for these animals, the consensus is that they do not feel pain."

29 *reduced by opiate pain medication*: See, for example, Janicke Nordgreen et al., "Thermono-ciception in Fish: Effects of Two Different Doses of Morphine on Thermal Threshold and Post-test Behaviour in Goldfish (*Carassius auratus*)" *Applied Animal Behavior Science* 119 (June 2009): 101–107.

29 *lacks the complexity that is necessary for consciousness*. See James D. Rose, "The Neurobe-havioral Nature of Fishes and the Question of Awareness and Pain," *Fisheries Science* 10 (2002): 1–38.

29 *interoceptive cortex*: See A. D. (Bud) Craig, "Interoception: the Sense of the Physiological Condition of the Body," *Current Opinion in Neurobiology* 13 (2003): 500–505.

30 *'etsev*: Help with the Hebrew etymology was provided by Sara Brumfield of UCLA.

32 *malevolent and beneficent demons and deities*: See Walter Addison Jayne, *The Healing Gods of Ancient Civilizations* (New Hyde Park, N.Y.: University Books, 1962), 89–128.

32 *eyes, mouth, nostrils, and ears*: Ibid., 104.

33 *trepanation*: See Robert Arnott et al., *Trepanation: History, Discovery, Theory* (Netherlands: Swets & Zeitlinger, 2003) and Symeon Misseos, "Hippocrates, Galen, and Uses of Trepana-tion in the Ancient Classical World: Galen and the Teaching of Trepanation," *Neurosurgical Focus* 23 (November 11, 2007).

33 *"free me from all possible evil"*: See the Ebers Papyrus, "Prayer to Isis," cited in *Pacific Medical Journal* 59 (1916): 459.

33 *Arrows thrown by Rudra*: See *The Rig Veda: An Anthology* (New York: Penguin, 1981), 222.

33 *"Apollo-" or "sun-struck"*: Jayne, *Healing Gods*, 308.

33 *"Artemis-" or "moon-struck"*: Ibid., 311.

34 *"Oh Father, Headache"*: Translation provided by Sara Brumfield of UCLA.

34 *Asclepius*: See Gerald David Hart, *Asclepius, the God of Medicine* (London: Royal Society of Medicine Press, 2000).

35 *"first taught pain the writhing wretch"*: See Pindar, *The Odes of Pindar: Literally Translated into English Prose* (London: Bell & Daldy, 1872), 272.

35 *"What are a ripe fig and an apple to me?"*: See Foster, *Before the Muses*, 995.

35 *"Magic is effective"*: Cited in Wolfgang H. Vogel and Andreas Berke, *Brief History of Vision and Ocular Medicine* (Amsterdam: Kugler Publications/Wayenborgh Publishers), 46.

36 *Poem of the Righteous Sufferer*: Ibid., 392 ff.

38 *"willingly or unwillingly"*: Morris, *The Culture of Pain*, 24–25.

39 *"I have given a name to my pain"*: Friedrich Wilhelm Nietzsche, *Basic Writings of Nietzsche* (New York: Random House, 2000), 174.

39 *"Pain, while always new to you"*: Daudet, *In the Land of Pain*, xi.

46 *Bethany Hamilton*: See Bill Hemmer, "Brave Surfer, Heart of a Champion," *CNN American Morning*, November 5, 2003.

47 *A 1981 study of Boston runners*: See D. B. Carr et al., "Physical Conditioning Facilitates the Exercise-induced Secretion of Beta-Endorphin and Beta-Lipotropin in Women," *New England Journal of Medicine* 305 (September 3, 1981): 560–62. However, there has been some recent disagreement with the idea of a "runner's high" among scientists, some of whom say that it is not clear that the endorphins reach the brain.

47 *an action that needs to be taken*: See Wall, *Pain*, 146.

47   *soldiers who had lost limbs*: Wall, *Pain*, 5–7.

47   *between half and two-thirds of amputees*: See M. T. Schley et al., "Painful and Nonpainful Phantom and Stump Sensations in Acute Traumatic Amputees," *Journal of Trauma* 65 (October 2008): 858–64. This offers a figure of 44.6 percent. The higher figure of 62 percent comes from S. W. Wartan et al., "Phantom Pain and Sensation Among British Veteran Amputees," *British Journal of Anesthesiology* 78 (1997): 652–59.

48   *three ages*: *The Rig Veda* (New York: Penguin, 1981), 285.

48   *lulled pain and brought forgetfulness*: Padraic Colum, *The Adventures of Odysseus and the Tale of Troy* (Rockville, Md.: Arc Manor, 2007), 38.

48   *"the wounded Scythians"*: Cited in Thomas Dormandy, *The Worst of Evils: The Fight Against Pain* (New Haven: Yale University Press, 2006), 27.

48   *"induces deep slumber"*: Ibid., 21.

49   *"I possess a secret remedy"*: Martin Booth, *Opium: A History* (New York: St. Martin's Press, 1999), 24.

49   *"How divine this repose is"*: Cited in Jean Dubos, *The White Plague* (Piscataway, N.J.: Rutgers University Press, 1987), 64.

52   *"Illness is as much a failure as poverty"*: Cited in Daudet, *In the Land of Pain*, 33–34.

60   *"Pain upsets"*: Aristotle, *The Nicomachean Ethics*, William David Ross, trans. (New York: Oxford University Press, 1998), 76.

62   'itstsabown: Help with the Hebrew etymology was provided by Sara Brumfield of UCLA.

63   *"the eyes of them both were opened"*: See Genesis 3:7 (King James Version).

63   *"The Lord gave"*: See Genesis 1:21 (King James Version).

64   *"Where were you?"*: See Job 38:4 (King James Version).

67   *"was silent as one who experiences no pain"*: *The Gospel of St. Peter: Synoptical Tables, with Translation and Critical Apparatus*, trans. John Macpherson (T. & T. Clark, 1893), Book 3, Verse 11.

67   *human palm is not substantial enough*: See Frank T. Vertosick, Jr., *Why We Hurt: The Natural History of Pain* (Orlando: Harvest Books, 2001), 156.

67   *extant skeleton of a man crucified in that period*: See Gary R. Habermas, *The Historical Jesus* (Joplin, Mo.: College Press, 1996), 174.

67   *damage the median nerves that supply the hands*: See discussion in Vertosick, *Why We Hurt*, 159.

69   *"to suffer little things now"*: See Thomas à Kempis, *The Imitation of Christ* (Milwaukee: Dover, 2003), 24.

70   *"Allow me to be eaten by the beasts"*: William A. Jurgens, *Faith of the Early Fathers* (Collegeville, Minn.: Liturgical Press, 1970), 22.

70   *Cosmas and Damian*: See Sabine Baring-Gold, *Lives of the Saints* (London: Hodges, 1882), 397–401.

71   *"when he was black in the mouth"*: See John Foxe, *Foxe's Book of Martyrs* (Grand Rapids, Mich.: Zondervan, 1978), 212–15.

72   *"When the blazing fire does not burn"*: *The Law Code of Manu*, Patrick Olivelle, trans. (New York: Oxford University Press, 2009), 119.

73   *King Athelstan*: See Hunt Janin, *Medieval Justice* (Jefferson, N.C.: McFarland, 2004), 14–15 and also Katherine Fischer Drew, *Magna Carta* (Westport, Conn.: Greenwood, 2004), 163.

73   *Babylonian river ordeal*: See Gwendolyn Leick, *The Babylonians* (New York: Routledge, 2003), 163.

73   *ordeals finally gave way to trial by jury*: Robert Von Moschzisker, *Trial by Jury* (Philadelphia: Geo T. Bisel, 1922), 40. See also Daniel Friedmann, *To Kill and Take Possession: Law, Morality and Society in Biblical Stories* (Peabody, Mass.: Hendrickson, 2002), 21.

73   *"The witch is executed"*: See Ariel Glucklich, *Sacred Pain* (New York: Oxford University Press, 2001), 41.

74   *"What are you doing at the moment?"*: Daudet, *In the Land of Pain*, 1.

74   *"Pain strengthens the religious person's bond"*: See Glucklich, *Sacred Pain*, 6.

75   *"deciphers it with his wounds"*: See Franz Kafka, *The Metamorphosis, In the Penal Colony, and Other Stories*, Joachim Neugroschel, trans. (New York: Simon & Schuster, 2000), 205 ff.

76   *"When pain transgresses the limits"*: Cited in Glucklich, *Sacred Pain*, 23.

76   *"the sweetness of this greatest pain"*: Ibid., 206.

78   *"one's own physical pain"* and *"another person's physical pain"*: Scarry, *The Body in Pain*, 3 and 4.

II. THE SPELL OF SURGICAL SLEEP: PAIN AS HISTORY

87   *"WE HAVE CONQUERED PAIN"*: See John Saunders, *The People's Journal* 3 (London: People's Journal Office, 1847): 25.

87   *"nothing so horrible as toothache"*: Heinrich Heine, *Works*, Volume 4, trans. Charles Godfrey Leland (New York: Dutton, 1906), 141.

88   *pain required interpretation*: This is clear in many of the well-known texts of these religious traditions. For example, in Saint Augustine's *Confessions*, written in the fourth century c.e., he speaks of pain as sometimes physical and sometimes spiritual, but his metaphors often blend them. Speaking of his *spiritual* pain, he writes of his relationship to God as a *physical* cure: "Under the secret touch of your healing hand my swelling pride subsided, and day by day the pain I suffered brought me health, like an ointment which stung but cleared the confusion and darkness from the eye of my mind." See *Confessions* (New York: Penguin, 1961), 144.

89   *Brutality began to recede*: The beginning of the nineteenth century saw many such reforms. Britain ended its slave trade in 1807 and in the following decades, a series of legislative acts began to restrict child labor.

90   *Christianity itself was influenced*: For a more extensive discussion, see Lucy Bending's *The Representation of Bodily Pain in Late Nineteenth-Century English Culture* (New York: Oxford University Press, 2000).

90   *they die painlessly*: In *Jane Eyre*, Helen Burns, dying of consumption, tells Jane, "We must all die one day, and the illness which is removing me is not painful; it is gentle and gradual: my mind is at rest." Jane sleeps through the moment of her death, so it is not described. In Dickens's *Old Curiosity Shop*, he forgoes describing Little Nell's passing and gently lingers instead on her corpse: "No sleep so beautiful and calm, so free from trace of pain, so fair to look upon. She seemed a creature fresh from the hand of God, and waiting for the breath of life; not one who had lived and suffered death."

92   *"robbed of its terrors"*: René Fülöp-Miller, *Triumph Over Pain* (New York: Literary Guild of America, 1938), 150.

92   *How terrible surgery had been*: See discussion in Peter Stanley, *For Fear of Pain: British Surgery 1790–1840* (Amsterdam: Rodopi B.V., 2003), 317.

92   *"an armed savage who attempts to get that by force"*: John Hunter, "Lectures on the Principles of Surgery" in *The Works of John Hunter* (London: Longman, 1835), 210.

92   *body's integrity was so well guarded by pain*: See the discussion of development of surgery in Dormandy's *The Worst of Evils* and in Stanley's *For Fear of Pain*.

92   *"moving, bleeding flesh"*: Quoted in Stanley, *For Fear of Pain*, 190.

93   *"amputate a shoulder in the time"*: Quoted in S. A. Hoffman, *Under the Ether Dome* (New York: Charles Scribner and Sons, 1986), 266.

93   *"spoil a hatful of eyes"*: Robert Brudenell Carter, "Lectures on Operative Ophthalmic Surgery," *The Lancet* (April 13, 1872): 495.

93   *mortality owing to amputation at the thigh*: James Young Simpson, *Anesthesia, Hospitalism, Hemaphroditism, and a Proposal to Stamp Out Small-Pox and Other Contagious Diseases* (Boston: Adam and Charles Black, 1871), 95.

93   *"How often have I dreaded"*: Valentine Mott, *Pain and Anaesthetics: An Essay* (Government Printing Office, 1862), 11.

93   *surgeons were typically of the lower class*: See Francis Michael Longstreth Thompson, *The Cambridge Social History of Britain 1750–1950: Social Agencies and Institutions* (Cambridge: Cambridge University Press, 1993), 176–77.

93   *helped dissuade Charles Darwin*: Charles Darwin, *Autobiographies* (London: Penguin, 2002), 21.

93   *"resolute and merciless"*: Quoted in Ian Dawson, *Renaissance Medicine* (Brooklyn: Enchanted Lion Books, 2005), 43.

94   *"indications of the patient's state of mind"*: Cited in Dormandy, *The Worst of Evils*, 108.

94   *gangrene*: See Frank M. Freemon, *Gangrene and Glory* (Madison, N.J.: Fairleigh Dickinson University Press, 1998), 46–49, for a detailed account of the treatment of wounds during the Civil War.

94   *"during the operation"*: Jonathan Warren quoted in Glucklich, *Sacred Pain*, 181.

94   *"Oh no, for mammy has told me that I ought"*: John Abernethy, *The Hunterian Oration* (London: Longman Hurst, 1819), 62, as cited in Stanley, *For Fear of Pain*, 254.

95   *patient of Dr. Robert Keate's*: See Stanley, *For Fear of Pain*, 265.

95   *amputation of his foot in 1842*: Wilson describes his experience in a letter to anesthesia pioneer James Simpson, printed in *The Obstetric Memoirs and Contributions of James Y. Simpson*, ed. by W. O. Priestley and H. R. Storer (Philadelphia: J. B. Lippincott & Co., 1856), 712.

96   *1812 letter by the English novelist and memoirist Fanny Burney*: See Fanny Burney, *Journals and Letters* (New York: Penguin, 2001), 431–44. Although the letter is addressed to her sister, Fanny had both her husband and teenage son copy her draft over to make a clean version, so it seems to have been written partly to share her experience with them— knowledge she had kept from them at the time of the operation.

96   *doctors most likely did not actually* examine *her breast*: See Claire Harman, *Fanny Burney: A Biography* (New York: Alfred A. Knopf, 2001), 290.

98   *"no half-measures will answer"*: Quoted in Dormandy, *The Worst of Evils*, 172.

100   *punching him on the chin*: As Dr. Larrey tells it, upon coming to consciousness, the colonel sputtered that the doctor had not behaved as a gentleman, but had taken "cowardly advantage"

of his temporary incapacity. Dr. Larrey explained that he knew "the insult would temporarily distract," showed the colonel the bullet he had removed from his foot, and asked him to shake hands. See Dormandy, *The Worst of Evils*, 1.

100 *"refrigeration anesthesia"*: Also known as "cryoanalgesia." Garotting—another technique of the day—involved cutting off the head's blood supply by compressing the carotid artery until the patient fainted. Practiced aggressively, it could cause brain damage; practiced cautiously, it risked too short a spell of unconsciousness for a complete surgery.

100 *"cut and [he] will feel nothing"*: Arnold of Villanova, quoted in William John Bishop, *The Early History of Surgery* (New York: Barnes and Noble, 1995), 60. See also Henry Smith Williams and Edward Huntington Williams, *A History of Science: The Beginnings* (New York: Harper and Brothers, 1904), 35.

102 *Henbane and mandrake were too dangerous*: "Whoso useth more than four leaves shall be in danger to sleepe without waking," a medieval text cautioned of henbane. See Sidney Beisly, *Shakespeare's Garden, or the Plants and Flowers Named in His Works Described* (London: Longman, Green, Longman, Roberts & Green, 1864), 87.

102 *Opium is the oldest and most important medicinal substance*: See Booth, *Opium: A History*, 15.

102 *"Many a penny"*: Elizabeth Gaskell, *Mary Barton* (New York: Penguin, 1996), 58.

102 *Greek word for shapes*: See discussion in Dormandy, *The Worst of Evils*, 255.

103 *Diocles of Carystos*: Quoted in Ibid., 24. His name is also spelled Carystus.

103 *"God's own medicine"*: Sir William Osler quoted in Michael Bliss, *William Osler: A Life in Medicine* (New York: Oxford University Press, 1999), 365.

103 *"causeth deepe deadly sleapes"*: William Bullein, *Bullein's Bulwarke of Defence Against All Sickness Soarenesse and Woundes That Doe Dayly Assaulte Mankinde* (1579), quoted in Booth, *Opium: A History*, 26.

104 *higher survival rate after ancient Peruvian trepanations*: See discussion in Richard Rudgley, *Lost Civilizations of the Stone Age* (New York: Simon & Schuster, 2000), 131.

104 *compensate their slaves with more cocaine*: See Steven B. Karch, *A History of Cocaine* (London: Royal Society of Medicine Press, 2003), 17.

105 *"When anyone suffers from toothache"*: Cited in Donald Meichenbaum, *Cognitive-Behavior Modification* (New York: Springer, 1977), 170–71.

105 *"the blessed delight"*: Quoted in Fülöp-Miller, *Triumph Over Pain*, 19.

105 *"I was absent from that part"*: Dhan Gopal Mukerji, *My Brother's Face*, quoted in E. S. Ellis, *Ancient Anodynes: Primitive Anesthesia and Allied Conditions* (London: W. Heinemann, 1946), 18.

105 *"I soon had recourse"*: Immanuel Kant, *Religion and Rational Theology*, trans. Allen W. Wood, George Di Giovanni (Cambridge: Cambridge University Press, 2001), 320–21.

106 *mesmerism*: See Alison Winter, *Mesmerized: Powers of Mind in Victorian Britain* (Chicago: University of Chicago Press, 2000), and a briefer discussion in Dormandy's *The Worst of Evils*, 195–99.

107 *"This Yankee dodge"*: Quoted in Stanley, *For Fear of Pain*, 294.

108 *"There can be few"*: Ibid., 290.

108 *"These phenomena I know to be real . . . independent of imagination"*: Ibid., 289.

108 *"a ready abandonment of the will"*: See *Blackwood's Edinburgh Magazine* 70 (1851): 84–85.

108 *"immoral tendency"*: James Braid, *Neurypnology; or, The Rationale of Nervous Sleep, Con-*

sidered in Relation with Animal Magnetism (London: John Churchill, 1843), 75–76. Braid distinguishes his practice of hypnotism from that of mesmerists because his practice does not depend on the magnetic emanations—or any other power—of the hypnotist.

110 *E. M. Papper theorizes*: E. M. Papper, *Romance, Poetry, and Surgical Sleep: Literature Influences Medicine* (Westport, Conn.: Greenwood Press, 1995), 136.

110 *"necessary to our existence"*: Quoted in Stanley, *For Fear of Pain*, 283.

111 *"To escape pain in surgical operations"*: Quoted in "A History of the Gift of Painless Surgery" in *The Atlantic Monthly* 78 (1896): 679.

111 *"appears capable of destroying physical pain"*: Cited in Paul G. Barash, et al., *Clinical Anesthesia* (Philadelphia: Lippincott Williams & Wilkins, 2009), 5.

111 *"the air in heaven"*: See Martin S. Pernick, *A Calculus of Suffering* (New York: Columbia University Press, 1987), 64.

111 *Ether frolics became the rage*: Ibid., 64–65.

113 *"In science the credit goes"*: Cited in William Osler, *Counsels and Ideals from the Writings of William Osler* (Boston: Houghton Mifflin, 1921), 294.

113 *at least three Americans were experimenting*: For accounts of these experiments, see Dormandy, *The Worst of Evils*, 202–26.

113 *doctor from Georgia*: In 1842 Crawford Long, of Danielsville, Georgia, excised a cyst from a patient's neck using ether anesthesia.

115 *"the wonderful dream"*: Johann Friedrich Dieffenbach, quoted in "Pain Relief: Fact or Fancy?" by Prithvi Raj, *Regional Anesthesia and Pain Medicine* 15 (July/August, 1990): 157–69.

116 *"The discovery that the inhaling"*: Henry Jacob Bigelow, "Address at the Dedication of the Ether Monument," in *Surgical Anesthesia; Addresses, and Other Papers* (Boston: Little, Brown and Co., 1900), 101.

117 *"questionable attempt to abrogate"* and *"destruction of consciousness"*: These criticisms are from physicians' letters cited in *The Obstetric Memoirs and Contributions of James Y. Simpson*, 616. Simpson responds in defense of the benefits of anesthesia. See also general discussion in Pernick, *A Calculus of Suffering*.

117 *"this would not be worth the consideration"*: Cited in Betty MacQuitty, *Victory Over Pain: Morton's Discovery of Anesthesia* (New York: Taplinger, 1971), 42.

117 *"the insensibility of the patient"*: See *Military Medical and Surgical Essays: Prepared for the United States Sanitary Commission* (Philadelphia: J. B. Lippincott & Co., 1864), 393.

117 *"a mere operator"*: See Edward Lawrie, "The Teaching of Anesthetics" in *The Lancet* 157 (1901): 65.

117 *"a remedy of doubtful safety"*: Isaac Parish, "Annual Report on Surgery, read before the College of Physicians" (College of Physicians of Philadelphia, November 2, 1847).

117 *"Pain during operations"*: See "Injurious Effects of the Inhalation of Ether," *Edinburgh Medical and Surgical Journal* (July 1847): 258.

117 *"The shock of the knife"*: See Stanley, *For Fear of Pain*, 305.

117 *"slavery of etherization"*: Quoted in Glucklich, *Sacred Pain*, 188.

118 *Henry Bigelow himself soberly warned*: Henry Bigelow, "Insensibility During Surgical Operations Produced by Inhalation," in *Boston Medical and Surgical Journal* 35 (1846): 309–17.

118 *"perfect insensibility to pain"*: See "Etherization in Surgical Operations," *The Lancet* 49 (January 16, 1847): 75.

118 *Sir James Young Simpson pioneered the use of chloroform*: See Stanley, *For Fear of Pain*, 302.

118 *"if the patient has a very great dread"*: By the mid-1850s, Syme himself had become a proponent, insisting to other surgeons that pain "most injuriously exhausts the nervous energy of a weak patient." See Linda Stratmann, *Chloroform* (Stroud, United Kingdom: History Press, 2003), 100.

118 *"Pain is the mother's safety"*: See discussion of labor pains in Charles D. Meigs, *Obstetrics: The Science and the Art*, 5th Edition (Philadelphia: Henry C. Lea, 1856), 372–73.

118 *in "toil"*: See *The Obstetric Memoirs and Contributions of James Y. Simpson*, 549 and 551.

119 *"anesthesia à la Reine"*: See Hannah Pakula, *An Uncommon Woman* (New York: Simon and Schuster, 1997), 123.

119 *"I dressed him, God healed him"*: Quoted in Dormandy, *The Worst of Evils*, 104.

119 *"Pain never comes where it can serve no good purpose"*: Quoted in Bending, *Representation of Bodily Pain*, 65. For further discussion of the split between science and religion, see Bending, 5–81.

III. TERRIBLE ALCHEMY: PAIN AS DISEASE

127 *there are only 2,500*: See Brenda Bauer et al., "U.S. Board Certified Pain Physician Practices: Uniformity and Census Data of Their Locations," *The Journal of Pain* 8 (March 2007): 244–50.

127–28 *just 5 percent of chronic pain patients*: See Roxanne Nelson, "Few Chronic Pain Patients See a Specialist," *Internal Medicine News*, October 1, 2006.

128 *first comprehensive textbook*: Bonica's first edition was published in 1953, but it has subsequently been revised and updated twice. See John David Loeser, John J. Bonica et al., *Bonica's Management of Pain* (Philadelphia: Lippincott Williams & Wilkins, 2001).

130 *a $1.5 million judgment*: The case is *Bergman v. Chin*. For a good summary, see Bruce David White, *Drugs, Ethics and Quality of Life* (Binghamton, N.Y.: Haworth Press, 2007), 115–18.

133 *"If for some disease a great many different remedies are proposed"*: See Anton Chekhov, *The Cherry Orchard* (New York: Samuel French), 18.

133 *sleep poorly*: In a survey by the National Sleep Foundation, two-thirds of chronic pain sufferers reported unrefreshing or poor sleep.

133 *symptoms of mental illness*: See, for example, Emma Young, "Are Bad Sleeping Habits Driving Us Mad?" *The New Scientist*, February 18, 2009.

133 *deconditioning and guarding behavior*: For a good review of the mechanisms by which pain syndromes can cause deconditioning, see "Disuse and Physical Disconditioning in Lower Back Pain" in Gordon J. G. Asmundson et al., *Understanding and Treating Fear of Pain* (New York: Oxford University Press, 2004).

133 *no specific diagnosis*: See I. Abraham et al., "Lack of Evidence-Based Research for Idiopathic Low Back Pain: The Importance of a Specific Diagnosis," *Archives of Internal Medicine* 162 (2002): 1442–44.

133 *up to 85 percent of such cases*: Richard A. Deyo et al., "What Can the History and Physical Examination Tell Us About Low Back Pain?" *Journal of the American Medical Association* 268 (1992): 760–65.

135 *"Whatever pain achieves"*: See Scarry, *The Body in Pain*, 4.

135 *"no words for the shiver and the headache"*: See Virginia Woolf, "On Being Ill," in *Selected Essays* (New York: Oxford University Press, 2008), 102.

138 *set by evolution at a relatively fixed point*: For a good explanation of the nociceptive threshold, see Christine Brooks, *Nursing Adults: The Practice of Caring* (Philadelphia: Mosby, 2003), 112.

140 *a full one-third of damaged disks*: O. L. Osti, "MRI and Discography of Annular Tears and Intervertebral Disk Degeneration: A Prospective Clinical Comparison," *Journal of Bone and Joint Surgery* 74 (1992): 431–35.

140 *nearly half of patients*: Cited in James M. Cox, *Low Back Pain: Mechanism, Diagnosis and Treatment* (Baltimore: Williams & Wilkins, 1998), 407.

141–42 *attached a small device to the base of subjects' thumbnails*: Drs. Clauw and Gracely presented this evidence at an October 2002 meeting of the American College of Rheumatology. They have published their findings in separate papers, including R. H. Gracely et al., "Functional Magnetic Resonance Imaging Evidence of Augmented Pain Processing in Fibromyalgia," *Arthritis & Rheumatism* 46 (2002): 1333–43, and "Evidence of Augmented Central Pain Processing in Idiopathic Chronic Low Back Pain," *Arthritis & Rheumatism* 50 (2004): 613–23.

143 *pain four years after their surgery*: Esther Dajczman et al., "Long-Term Postthoracotomy Pain," *Chest* 99 (1991): 270–74.

144 *study by Dr. Anna Taddio*: See Anna Taddio et al., "Effect of Neonatal Circumcision on Pain Response During Subsequent Routine Vaccination," *The Lancet* 349 (March 1, 1997): 599–603.

146 *Botox*: See Andrew Blumenfeld et al., "The Emerging Role of Botulinum Toxin Type A in Headache Prevention," *Operative Techniques in Otolaryngology—Head and Neck Surgery* 15 (June 2004): 90–96.

146 *more troublesome side effects*: See I. M. Anderson, "Selective Serotonin Reuptake Inhibitors Versus Tricyclic Antidepressants; a Meta-analysis of Efficacy and Tolerability," *Journal of Affective Disorders* 58 (2000): 19–36.

147 *According to a 2002 study*: See George Ostapowicz et al., "Results of a Prospective Study of Acute Liver Failure at 17 Tertiary Care Centers in the United States," *Annals of Internal Medicine* 137 (December 2002): 947–54.

147 *as many as one-fourth of all patients*: See Jay L. Goldstein and Russell D. Brown, "NSAID-induced Ulcers," *Current Treatment Options in Gastroenterology* 3 (2000): 149–57.

147 *6,000 to 7,500 Americans die*: See A. Lanas et al., "A Nationwide Study of Mortality Associated with Hospital Admission Due to Severe Gastrointestinal Events and Those Associated with Nonsteroidal Anti-inflammatory Drug Use," *American Journal of Gastroenterology* (August 2005): 1685–93. These estimates were generated from Lanas's statistics suggesting that the death rate attributed to NSAID/aspirin use was between 21.0 and 24.8 cases per million people, and then multiplying by the U.S. population.

148 *Women report more frequent pain*: See L. LeReseche, "Gender Considerations in the Epidemiology of Chronic Pain," in *Epidemiology of Pain* (Seattle: IASP Press, 1999), 43–52, or A. M. Unruh, "Gender Variations in Clinical Pain Experience," *Pain* 65 (1996): 123–67. Also K. J. Berkley, "Sex Differences in Pain," *Behavioral Brain Science* 20 (1997): 371–80.

148 *2003 Norwegian study*: Anne Werner and Kirsti Malterud, "It's Hard Work Behaving as a Credible Patient: Encounters Between Women with Chronic Pain and Their Doctors," *Social Science & Medicine* 57 (2003): 1409–19.

152 *2005 Stanford University survey*: See "Broad Experience with Pain Sparks a Search for Relief," ABC News/USA Today/Stanford University Medical Center Poll, May 9, 2005.

152 *A 2008 survey*: See Charles B. Simone et al., "The Utilization of Pain Medications and the Attitudes of Breast Cancer Patients Toward Pain Intervention," 2009 Breast Cancer Symposium.

152 *"the paradox of patients' satisfaction"*: See Ree Dawson et al., "Probing the Paradox of Patients' Satisfaction with Inadequate Pain Management," *Journal of Pain Symptom Management* 23 (March 2002): 211–20.

152 *single most important factor*: L. M. McCracken et al., "Assessment of Satisfaction with Treatment for Chronic Pain," *Journal of Pain Symptom Management* 14 (1997): 292–99.

154 *2004 study at the University of Milan*: E. Vegni et al., "Stories from Doctors of Patients with Pain: A Qualitative Research of the Physicians' Perspective" *Support Care Cancer* 13 (2005): 18–25.

156 *one-third and one-half*: See Thorsten Giesecke et al., "The Relationship Between Depression, Clinical Pain, and Experimental Pain in a Chronic Pain Cohort," *Arthritis & Rheumatism* 52 (2005): 1577–84 and studies discussed in Jeffrey Dersh et al., "Chronic Pain and Psychopathology: Research Findings and Considerations," *Psychosomatic Medicine* 64 (2002): 773–86.

156 *Stanford University study of major depression*: Alan Schatzberg et al., "Using Chronic Pain to Predict Depressive Morbidity in the General Population," *Archives of General Psychiatry* 60 (2003): 39–47.

156 *review study led by Dr. David A. Fishbain*: See D. A. Fishbain et al., "Chronic Pain Associated Depression: Antecedent or Consequence of Chronic Pain? A Review," *Clinical Journal of Pain* 13 (1997): 116–37.

157 *a common genetic vulnerability*: See, for example, Dan Buskila, "Biology and Therapy of Fibromyalgia: Genetic Aspects of Fibromyalgia Syndrome," *Arthritis Research & Therapy* 8 (2006).

157 *Brain imaging scans reveal similar disturbances*: Thorsten Giesecke et al., "The Relationship Between Depression, Clinical Pain, and Experimental Pain in a Chronic Pain Cohort," *Arthritis & Rheumatism* 52 (2005): 1577–84.

157 *abnormalities in the neurotransmitters serotonin and norepinephrine*: See Matthew J. Bair, "Depression and Pain Comorbidity: A Literature Review," *Archives of Internal Medicine* 163 (2003): 2433–45.

157 *depleting serotonin increases their pain responses*: See L. D. Lytle et al., "Effects of Long-term Corn Consumption on Brain Serotonin and the Response to Electric Shock," *Science* 190 (November 14, 1975): 692–94.

159 *not above growing and selling*: See Jung Chang and Jon Halliday, *Mao: The Unknown Story* (New York: Knopf, 2005), 276.

160 *"prolific in caresses and betrayals"*: See Charles-Pierre Baudelaire, "The Double Room," in *Baudelaire in English* (New York: Penguin, 1998), 238.

160 *2003 study led by Dr. Kathleen Foley*: See Kathleen Foley, "Opioids and Chronic Neuropathic Pain," *New England Journal of Medicine* 348 (2003): 1279–81 and M. C. Rowbotham

et al., "Oral Opioid Therapy for Chronic Peripheral and Central Neuropathic Pain," *New England Journal of Medicine* 348 (2003): 1223–32.

160 *slightly above 3 percent*: D. A. Fishbain et al., "What Percentage of Chronic Nonmalignant Pain Patients Exposed to Chronic Opioid Analgesic Therapy Develop Abuse/Addiction and/or Aberrant Drug-related Behaviors? A Structured Evidence-based Review," *Pain Medicine* 9 (2008): 444–59.

160 *moral equivalent of inflicting pain*: See Morris, *The Culture of Pain*, 191. "The crucial point," he writes, "beyond showing how fears of pain can destroy a person as effectively as cancer, is that *not* relieving pain brushes dangerously close to the act of willfully inflicting it."

162 *higher than 80 mg*: See Table 2 in "Interagency Guideline on Opioid Dosing for Chronic Non-Cancer Pain," Washington State Agency Medical Directors' Group, March 2007.

162 *fifteen such specialists*: See "Pain Management Specialists Directory," Washington State Agency Medical Directors' Group, March 17, 2008.

163 *action plan on OxyContin*: See "Action Plan to Prevent the Diversion and Abuse of Oxycontin," Office of Diversion Control, U.S. Department of Justice, February 8, 2001.

164 *Tina Rosenberg*: See Rosenberg's excellent article, "When Is a Pain Doctor a Drug Pusher?" *New York Times Magazine*, June 17, 2007.

167 *women are given psychotropic medications*: Cited in Jeffrey F. Peipert, *Primary Care for Women*, 2nd Edition (Philadelphia: Lippincott Williams & Wilkins, 2004), 51.

168 *"drug-seeking behavior"*: See R. Payne, "Sickle Cell–Related Pain: Perceptions of Medical Practitioners," *Journal of Pain Symptom Management* 14 (1997): 168–74.

168 *2005 study*: See Ian Chen et al., "Racial Differences in Opioid Use for Chronic Nonmalignant Pain," *Journal of General Internal Medicine* 20 (July 2005): 593–98.

168 *blacks as less compliant*: Michelle van Ryn and Jane Burke, "The Effect of Patient Race and Socio-economic Status on Physicians' Perceptions of Patients," *Social Science and Medicine* 50 (March 2000): 813–26.

168 *invisible hierarchy of pain sensitivity*: Pernick, *A Calculus of Suffering*, 157. Pernick details how theories of pain sensitivity were used in the decades after anesthesia's discovery as a basis for prescribing appropriate doses.

169 *Greek physician Galen*: Galen attributed pain to two disparate causes: dissolution of continuity in tissues, such as cuts or burns, or violent commotion in the humors. Harmony of the humors could be achieved through drugs or bloodletting and purgation.

169 *"a subjective matter"*: Fülöp-Miller, *Triumph Over Pain*, 397.

169 *"The savage does not feel pain as we do"*: Silas Weir Mitchell, *Characteristics: A Novel* (New York: The Century, 1913), 13.

169 *Cesare Lombroso*: Cesare Lombroso, *Criminal Man*, ed. and trans. Mary Gibson, Nicole Hahn Rafter (Durham: Duke University Press, 2006), 63, 69.

170 *Slaves' animal natures dulled them to pain*: God supported the social structure, Reverend Thomas Morong argued in his 1858 treatise *The Beneficence of Pain*, by endowing pain sensitivity according to circumstances—mitigating slaves' lots with an extra capacity for endurance. See Pernick, *A Calculus of Suffering*, 156.

170 *"will bear cutting"*: See Dr. James Johnson in *The Medico-Chirurgical Review and Journal of Medical Science* 9 (Burgess and Hill, 1826): 620.

170 *"the Negro . . . has a greater insensibility to pain"*: A. P. Merrill, "An Essay on Some of the Distinctive Peculiarities of the Negro Race," *Southern Medical and Surgical Journal* 7 (1856). Merrill writes:

> But slaves are submissive, and effective laborers, under very different treatment [from being treated with a "spirit of kindness"]. They submit to and bear the infliction of the rod with a surprizing [*sic*] degree of resignation, and even cheerfulness; and indeed manifest in many cases a strong and unwavering attachment to the hand which inflicts the punishment, particularly if it be the hand of the owner, or some person who has the right to exercise government over them. They are a submissive and yielding race, wholly incapable of bearing malice on account of their degraded condition as slaves; and equally incapable of forming and maintaining, an effective and permanent organization among themselves, to assert their freedom, or to avenge their wrongs. They differ from their white masters in no one particular more than this. (pp. 35–56)

170 *James Paget*: James Paget, "Experiments on Animals," in *Selected Essays and Addresses* (New York: Longmans, Green, and Co., 1902), 338. This comment occurs in the context of a discussion of the justification of pain inflicted on animals based on utility to humans, evoking Pernick's notion of a hierarchy of pain sensitivity.

170 *Sims obtained several Alabama slaves*: See J. Marion Sims, *The Story of My Life* (New York: D. Appleton and Co., 1894), 222–46.

171 *White children were subject to similar debate*: Educational theorists such as Horace Mann prescribed vigorous physical education as an antidote. See Horace Mann, *Lectures on Education* (Boston: Ide & Dutton, 1855), 313–14; Herbert Spencer, *Education: Intellectual, Physical, and Moral* (New York: D. Appleton and Co., 1901), 39; and Pernick, *A Calculus of Suffering*, 152.

171 *"With her exalted spiritualism"*: John Gideon Millingen, *The Passions; or Mind and Matter* (London: J. & D. A. Darling, 1848), 157.

171 *"exceedingly painful"*: Pernick, *A Calculus of Suffering*, 153.

172 *variations of which are found in classical India*: See Antti Aarne, *The Types of the Folktale*, trans. Stith Thompson (Helsinki: Suomalainen Tiedeakatemia, 1964), 240.

172 *1835 Andersen version of "The Princess and the Pea"*: See Hans Christian Andersen, "The Princess and the Pea," in *The Annotated Classic Fairy Tales*, ed. Maria Tatar (New York: W. W. Norton, 2002), 284–87.

174 *well-known study of housewives in the late 1960s*: R. A. Sternbach, "Ethnic Differences Among Housewives in Psychophysical and Skin Potential Response to Electric Shock," *Psychophysiology* 1 (1965): 241–46.

174 *tolerance markedly increased for Jewish subjects*: See E. Poser, "Some Psychosocial Determinants of Pain Tolerance." Read at the sixteenth International Congress of Psychology, Washington, D.C., 1963.

174 *hold their hands in painfully icy water*: Richard Stephens et al., "Swearing as a Response to Pain," *NeuroReport* 20 (August 5, 2009): 1056–60.

174 *benchmark 1972 Stanford University study*: Kenneth M. Woodrow et al., "Pain Tolerance: Differences According to Age, Sex and Race," *Psychosomatic Medicine* 34 (1972): 548–56.

175 *blacks showed more tolerance than Asian Americans*: The Asian group mixed subjects of Japanese and Chinese descent.

175 *women are more responsive to kappa-receptor drugs*: See H. L. Fields et al., "Brainstem Pain Modulating Circuitry Is Sexually Dimorphic with Respect to Mu and Kappa Opioid Receptor Function," *Pain* 85 (2000): 153–59, and Jon D. Levine et al., "Kappa-Opioids Produce Significantly Greater Analgesia in Women Than in Men," *Nature Medicine* 2 (1996): 1248–50.

175 *drug had opposite effects on the two sexes*: See J. D. Levine et al., "The Kappa Opioid Nalbuphine Produces Gender- and Dose-Dependent Analgesia and Antianalgesia in Patients with Postoperative Pain," *Pain* 83 (1999): 339–45.

175 *MC1R*: See J. S. Mogil et al., "The Melanocortin-1 Receptor Gene Mediates Female-Specific Mechanisms of Analgesia in Mice and Humans," *Proceedings of the National Academy of Sciences* 100 (April 15, 2003): 4867–72.

175 *2003 study . . . of postsurgical pain following*: M. Soledad Cepeda and Daniel B. Carr, "Women Experience More Pain and Require More Morphine Than Men to Achieve a Similar Degree of Analgesia," *Anesthesia & Analgesia* 97 (2003): 1464–68.

176 *men receive more analgesic benefit*: See, for example, J. S. Walker, "Experimental Pain in Healthy Human Subjects: Gender Differences in Nociception and in Response to Ibuprofen," *Anesthesia & Analgesia* 86 (1998): 1257–62.

176 *20 percent more general anesthesia*: See E. B. Liem et al., "Anesthetic Requirement is Increased in Redheads," *Anesthesiology* 101 (August 2004): 279–83.

177 *2006 Ohio State University study*: See Lee Bowman, "Obese People More Sensitive to Pain, Study Finds," Scripps Howard News Service, March 1, 2006.

177 *little or inadequate anesthesia*: See Philip M. Boffey, "Infants' Sense of Pain Is Recognized, Finally," *New York Times*, November 24, 1987, and Helen Harrison, "Why Infant Surgery Without Anesthesia Went Unchallenged," *New York Times*, December 17, 1987.

177 *editorial in* The New England Journal of Medicine: See A. B. Fletcher, "Pain in the Neonate," *New England Journal of Medicine* 317 (November 19, 1987).

178 *study led by Dr. Robert R. Edwards*: Robert R. Edwards, "Individual Differences in Endogenous Pain Modulation as a Risk Factor for Chronic Pain," *Neurology* 65 (2005): 437–43.

179 *subgroup of African Americans*: See M. McNeilly, "Neuropeptide and Cardiovascular Responses to Intravenous Catheterization in Normotensive and Hypertensive Blacks and Whites," *Health Psychology* 8 (1989): 487–501.

179 *A 2005 study at the University of North Carolina*: M. Beth Mechlin et al., "African Americans Show Alterations in Endogenous Pain Regulatory Mechanisms and Reduced Pain Tolerance to Experimental Pain Procedures," *Psychosomatic Medicine* 67 (2005): 948–56.

179 *Ethiopian Jews have a gene variation*: H. R. Lou et al., "Polymorphisms of CYP2C19 and CYP2D6 in Israeli Ethnic Groups," *American Journal of Pharmacogenomics, Genomics-related Research in Drug Development and Clinical Practice* 4 (6:2004), 395–401.

180 *article by Dr. Robert R. Edwards*: Robert R. Edwards, "Individual Differences in Endogenous Pain Modulation as a Risk Factor for Chronic Pain," *Neurology* 65 (2005): 437–43.

181 *victims of childhood sexual abuse*: See E. Walker et al., "Relationship of Chronic Pelvic Pain to Psychiatric Diagnoses and Childhood Sexual Abuse," *American Journal of Psychiatry* 145 (1988): 75–80.

181 *2005 study published in* Human Molecular Genetics: See L. Diatchenko et al., "Genetic

Basis for Individual Variations in Pain Perception and the Development of a Chronic Pain Condition," *Human Molecular Genetics* 14 (2005): 135–43.

181 *Another recent study*: Frank Reimann et al., "Pain Perception Is Altered by a Nucleotide Polymorphism in *SCN9A*," *Proceedings of the National Academy of Sciences* 107 (March 16, 2010): 5148–53.

182 *Danish survey*: See E. Aasvang and H. Kehlet, "Chronic Postoperative Pain: The Case of Inguinal Herniorrhaphy," *British Journal of Anaesthesia* 95 (2005): 69–76.

182 *British study found that 30 percent*: A. S. Poobalan et al., "Chronic Pain and Quality of Life Following Open Inguinal Hernia Repair," *British Journal of Surgery* 88 (2001): 1122–26.

182 *One of Dr. Apkarian's studies*: See A. Vania Apkarian et al., "Chronic Back Pain Is Associated with Decreased Prefrontal and Thalamic Gray Matter Density," *Journal of Neuroscience* 24 (November 17, 2004): 10410–415.

186 *a quarter or more of Americans*: See "Health, United States, 2006: With Charts on Trends in the Health of Americans," Centers for Disease Control, p. 74.

186 *for a quarter of those*: Ibid., 86. "Overall, 28% of adults with low back pain said they had a limitation of activity caused by a chronic condition."

186 *The amount of gray matter*: See Richard J. Haier, "Structural Brain Variation and General Intelligence," *NeuroImage* 23 (September 2004): 425–33.

186 *losses amounting to between 5 and 11 percent*: See Apkarian et al., "Chronic Back Pain Is Associated with Decreased Prefrontal and Thalamic Gray Matter Density," *Journal of Neuroscience* 24 (November 17, 2004): 10410–415.

186 *1.3 cubic centimeters*: Ibid.

IV. FINDING A VOICE: PAIN AS NARRATIVE

195 *"Physical pain has no voice"*: Scarry, *The Body in Pain*, 3.

195 *treat the patient rather than the disease*: See Owsei Temkin, *The Double Face of Janus and Other Essays in the History of Medicine* (Baltimore: Johns Hopkins University Press, 2006), 454.

195 *"What is the matter with you?"*: Foucault, *The Birth of the Clinic*, xxi.

196 Kitchen Table Wisdom: See Rachel Naomi Remen, *Kitchen Table Wisdom: Stories That Heal* (New York: Riverhead, 1997).

199 *"the factors that convert"*: Eric J. Cassell, *The Nature of Suffering and the Goals of Medicine* (New York: Oxford University Press, 2004), 46.

201 *Chosen integrative pain*: For a discussion of integrative vs. disintegrative pain, see Glucklich's *Sacred Pain*, 33–34 and David Bakan's *Disease, Pain, and Sacrifice: Toward a Psychology of Suffering* (Chicago: University of Chicago Press, 1968), 31–38, 67–85.

202 *"One word frees us"*: See Sophocles, *The Oedipus Cycle* (Boston: Houghton Mifflin Harcourt, 2002), 165.

202 *recruited Stanford students*: Data taken from Jared Younger, Sean Mackey et al., "Passionate Love Reduces Pain Via Activation of Reward Systems." (Prepublication copy sent to author by Sean Mackey.)

203 *Researchers at Oxford University*: See "Pulling Together Increases Your Pain Threshold," University of Oxford press release, September 28, 2009.

203 telic centralizing: See Bakan, *Disease, Pain, and Sacrifice*, 31–38, 67–85.

203 *"whoever was tortured"*: Jean Améry, *At the Mind's Limits* (Bloomington, Ind.: Indiana University Press, 1998), 34.

203 *"no pain or actual harm whatsoever"*: See Jay S. Bybee, assistant attorney general, "Memorandum for John Rizzo, Acting General Counsel for the Central Intelligence Agency" (August 1, 2002), 11.

205 *2005 study led by Dr. M. Ojinga Harrison*: M. Ojinga Harrison et al., "Religiosity/Spirituality in Patients with Sickle Cell Disease," *The Journal of Nervous and Mental Disease* 193 (April 2005).

205 *Those who attended church once or more per week*: Ibid.

205 *people who attend religious services live longer*: W. J. Strawbridge et al., "Frequent Attendance at Religious Services and Mortality Over 28 Years," *American Journal of Public Health* 87 (1997): 957–61.

206 *nine-year analysis*: Robert A. Hummer et al., "Religious Involvement and U.S. Adult Mortality," *Demography* 36 (May 1999): 273–85. Robert Hummer and his coauthors indicate that the link they found between churchgoing and mortality is simply a statistical correlation. They don't go as far as to say that churchgoing in itself directly reduces mortality. They note, for instance, that people who are unhealthy already are less likely to go to church.

206 *"positive religious coping"*: See A. C. Sherman et al., "Religious Struggle and Religious Comfort in Response to Illness: Health Outcomes Among Stem Cell Transplant Patients," *Journal of Behavioral Medicine* 28 (August 2005): 359–67.

208 *"If suffering occurs"*: Cassell, *The Nature of Suffering*, 46.

212 *Her husband told a reporter*: Alicia Dennis, "This Man Chose to Be in a Coma," *People*, August 10, 2009.

212 *creating a feared-for self*: Stephen Morley et al., "Possible Selves in Chronic Pain: Self-Pain Enmeshment, Adjustment and Acceptance," *Pain* 115 (2005): 84–94.

214 *2005 Stanford University survey*: See "Broad Experience with Pain Sparks a Search for Relief," ABC News/USA Today/Stanford University Medical Center Poll, May 9, 2005.

218 *Angel of Anatomy*: Mary Lowenthal Felstiner, *Out of Joint: A Private and Public Story of Arthritis* (Lincoln: University of Nebraska Press, 2007), xiv and 201.

218 *baby before age twenty*: See U.S. Department of Health & Human Services, "Breast Cancer: Risk Factors and Prevention," http://www.womenshealth.gov/breast-cancer/risk-factors-prevention, accessed October 21, 2009.

221 *"Dealing with Difficult Patients"*: See Ajay D. Wasan et al., "Dealing with Difficult Patients in Your Pain Practice," *Regional Anesthesia and Pain Medicine* 30 (March/April 2005): 184–92.

221 *a large study at a primary care clinic*: The cited study is J. L. Jackson and K. Kroenke, "The Effect of Unmet Expectation Among Adults Presenting with Physical Symptoms," *Annals of Internal Medicine* 134 (2001): 889–97.

221 *30 to 50 percent of chronic pain patients*: Wasan, "Dealing with Difficult Patients," 188.

229 *same kind of pathological pain sensitivity*: See L. F. Chu et al., "Opioid-Induced Hyperalgesia in Humans: Molecular Mechanisms and Clinical Considerations," *Clinical Journal of Pain* 24 (July/August 2008): 479–96.

230 *patient's relationship with his or her doctor*: See, for example, John D. Piette et al., "The Role of Patient-Physician Trust in Moderating Medication Nonadherence Due to Cost Pressures," *Archives of Internal Medicine* 165 (2005): 1749–55.

241 *low rates of response to a placebo*: See Harriët Wittink and Theresa Hoskins Michel, *Chronic Pain Management for Physical Therapists* (Boston: Butterworth-Heinemann, 2002), 295. The authors say that reaction to a placebo is closely correlated to whether the patient expects positive outcomes.

243 *"Build . . . an illness narrative"*: Arthur Kleinman, *The Illness Narratives* (New York: Basic Books, 1988), 54.

245 *"Even comparatively well-adjusted patients"*: Wasan, "Dealing with Difficult Patients," 185.

250 At the Will of the Body: Arthur W. Frank, *At the Will of the Body: Reflections on Illness* (Boston: Houghton Mifflin Harcourt, 2002).

250 *higher rate of them on Vioxx*: See Robert S. Bresalier, "Cardiovascular Events Associated with Rofecoxib in a Colorectal Adenoma Chemoprevention Trial," *New England Journal of Medicine* 355 (March 17, 2005).

250 *poses some cardiovascular risks for the same population as Vioxx did*: Celebrex is a Cox-2 inhibitor like Vioxx, but "the literature concerning the [cardiovascular] risk with the use of celecoxib is more heterogeneous" than that of Vioxx. See "Cardiovascular Risk Associated with Celecoxib," *New England Journal of Medicine* 352 (June 23, 2005): 2648–50.

250 *reduced the risk of breast cancer by 71 percent*: Randall E. Harris et al., "Reduction in the Risk of Human Breast Cancer by Selective Cycloxygenase-2 (COX-2) Inhibitors," *BMC Cancer* 6 (2006).

256 *A 2005 study*: David W. Dodick et al., "Botulinum Toxin Type A for the Prophylaxis of Chronic Daily Headache: Subgroup Analysis of Patients Not Receiving Other Prophylactic Medications: A Randomized Double-Blind, Placebo-Controlled Study," *Headache* 45 (2005): 315–24.

260 *"How high that highest candle"*: This is from the Stevens poem "Final Soliloquy of the Interior Paramour." See Wallace Stevens, *The Collected Poems of Wallace Stevens* (New York: Knopf, 1954), 524.

261 *"Filled with a sense of injustice and self-pity"*: See Remen, *Kitchen Table Wisdom*, 115–18.

V. TO CURE THE MIND: PAIN AS PERCEPTION

281 *As Wittgenstein observes*: Ludwig Wittgenstein, *Philosophical Investigations: The German Text, with a Revised English Translation* (Oxford: Wiley-Blackwell, 2001), 84.

281 *For Hippocrates, pain was a physical sensation*: For Hippocrates, pain as a sensation is physical and overwhelming, while for Aristotle pain as an emotion is cerebral and thus controllable. Pain, for Aristotle, seems largely an internal or mental affair, that might be overcome with willpower or the dominance of reason over bodily functions. At times Aristotle writes of pain (and pleasure) as *perceptions* of emotions (which appear to be akin to sensations—the *aisteta* of emotions come from the verb *aistanomai*, "to perceive or apprehend with the senses"). Aristotle writes, "Let the emotions be all those things on account of which people change their minds and differ in regard to their judgments, *and upon which attend pain and pleasure*, for example anger, pity, fear, and all other such things and their opposites" (emphasis added). Cited in David Konstan, *The Emotions of the Ancient Greeks* (University of Toronto Press, 2006), 33.

282 *"we may sometimes suffer"*: René Descartes, *The Philosophical Writings of Descartes*, volume 1, ed. John Cottingham (Cambridge: Cambridge University Press, 1985), 361.

283 *"I had never been shot"*: See Wall, *Pain*, 7.

284 *"Pain is whatever"*: Margo McCaffery, *Nursing Practice Theories Related to Cognition, Bodily Pain, and Man-Environment Interactions* (Los Angeles: UCLA Press, 1968), 95.

284 *"An unpleasant sensory and emotional"*: See Chryssoula Lascaratou, *The Language of Pain: Expression or Description* (Amsterdam: John Benjamins, 2007), 15.

286 *Each of these regions*: For an excellent technical account of how pain works see Michael J. Cousins, Philip O. Bridenbaugh, Daniel B. Carr, and Terese T. Horlocker, eds., *Cousins & Bridenbaugh's Neural Blockade In Clinical Anesthesia and Management of Pain*, 4th ed. (Philadelphia: Lippincott Williams & Wilkins, 2009), 693–751. This is widely considered the most authoritative academic textbook on pain medicine for health professionals, edited by the leading figures in the field.

287 *"thousands of spirit limbs"*: Robert Fitridge, Matthew Thompson, *Mechanisms of Vascular Disease: A Textbook for Vascular Surgeons* (Cambridge: Cambridge University Press, 2007), 302.

290 *studies at Oxford University*: See Irene Tracey et al., "Imaging Attentional Modulation of Pain in the Periaqueductal Gray in Humans," *The Journal of Neuroscience* 22 (April 1, 2002): 2748–52.

291 *Ordinary distraction*: Susanna J. Bantick et al., "Imaging How Attention Modulates Pain in Humans Using Functional MRI," *Brain* 125 (February 1, 2002): 310–19.

291 *Even smells influence pain*: Chantal Villemure et al., "Effects of Odors on Pain Perception: Deciphering the Roles of Emotion and Attention," *Pain* 106 (November 2003): 101–8.

292 *the brains of men were imaged*: Jon-Kar Zubieta et al., "Placebo Effects Mediated by Endogenous Opioid Activity on µ-Opioid Receptors," *The Journal of Neuroscience* 25 (August 24, 2005): 7754–62.

297 *"the contemplation of divine things"*: Cited in Fülöp-Miller, *Triumph Over Pain*, 19.

298 *The patients at the hospital*: Wall, *Pain*, 71–72.

306 *The theory of learned helplessness*: See Martin Seligman and Steven Maier, "Failure to Escape Traumatic Shock," *Journal of Experimental Psychology* 74 (1967): 1–9.

309 *1930s Thai Buddhist monk*: Kamala Tiyavanich, *Forest Recollections: Wandering Monks in Twentieth Century Thailand* (Honolulu: University of Hawaii Press, 1997), 111. Also cited in Glucklich, *Sacred Pain*, 20.

314 *theorizes that intense pain*: Glucklich, *Sacred Pain*, 30.

315 *"neurosignature"*: Ronald Melzack, "Pain and the Neuromatrix in the Brain," *Journal of Dental Education* 65 (December 2001): 1378–82.

315 *"either terrifying or exhilarating"*: Glucklich, *Sacred Pain*, 60.

316 *This learning effect*: Christopher deCharms et al., "Control Over Brain Activation and Pain Learned by Using Real-time Functional MRI," *Proceedings of the National Academy of Sciences* 102 (December 20, 2005): 18626–31.

317 *London cabdrivers*: Eleanor Maguire et al., "Navigation-Related Structural Change in the Hippocampi of Taxi Drivers," *Proceedings of the National Academy of Sciences* 97 (April 11, 2000): 4398–4403.

317 *learning to juggle creates visible changes*: See Bogdan Draganski et al., "Neuroplasticity: Changes in Grey Matter Induced by Training," *Nature* 427 (January 22, 2004): 311–12.

ACKNOWLEDGMENTS

In the eight years I was working on this book, there were many helping hands.

I was honored to work with Eric Chinski, who has the three qualities an editor needs: keen insight, steady kindness, and extreme patience. Thanks to Eugenie Cha for invaluable assistance in the publication process, to Chris Peterson for copyediting, to Rebecca Saletan for her early support, and to Sarita Varma for publicity. My wonderful agent, Henry Dunow, came through for me at every stage.

Ilena Silverman at *The New York Times Magazine* not only worked with me on pain-related articles, but lent her talents to crafting the manuscript. Huge thanks to her. Thanks to Gerry Marzorati for giving me a journalistic home and to Dean Robinson, who first gave me an assignment to write about chronic pain. I cannot thank Charles Wilson enough for the scrupulous fact-checking and research assistance that rescued me from mortifying misconceptions and mistakes, both large and small. Sara Brumfield lent her expertise in Near Eastern languages and civilizations, as did Elisha Cohn with Victorian history, Joy Connolly and Ben Platt with ancient Greek and Roman civilization, and James Mickle with medical expertise.

I am blessed to have a circle of gifted and giving writerly friends who took time away from their own work to improve mine. Cynthia Baughman, Brian Hall, Julie Hilden, Tom Reiss, and Michael Ryan read multiple drafts and drew me a new map each time I was lost in the thicket of the subject. Deborah Baker, Jeff Dolven, Jascha Hoffman, Robert Klitzman, Dani Shapiro, and Joshua Wolf Shenk also offered valuable guidance and moral support along the way. Mark Woods meticulously polished countless sentences, and Kristin Thiel provided crucial assistance in the final stages. Thanks, too, to Kevin Baker, Max Berger, Susan Cheever, Nicholas Dawidoff, Richard Halpern, Oliver Hobert, Dan Kaufman, Bonnie Lee, David Lipsky, Amanda Robb, and David Shaffer.

In researching this book I had the opportunity to observe the practices of some extraordinary physicians. Through the years, conversations with and observations of the practices of Daniel Carr, Scott Fishman, John Keltner, and Sean Mackey stamped my understanding both of pain and of how good pain medicine can be. Scott Fishman lends his talents as president to a valuable pain-advocacy organization for patients, the American Pain Foundation, that has helped me as a patient as well as a researcher. I owe a profound intellectual debt to Daniel Carr, whose insights about pain are drawn on throughout this book.

While researching the book and pain-related articles, I was grateful to observe the practices of or interview many leading clinicians, researchers, and scholars, including Allan Basbaum, Pamela Bennett, Charles Berde, David Borsook, Bertie Bregman, William Breitbart, Kenneth Casey, Eric Cassell, Richard Chapman, Rita Charon, B. Eliot Cole, Ray D'amours, Christopher deCharms, Stuart Derbyshire, Richard Deyo, Steven Feinberg, Philip Fisher, Kathleen Foley, Arthur Frank, Rebecca Garden, Ariel Glucklich, Christine Greco, Geoffrey Hartman, Craig Irvine, Jean Jackson, Donald Kaminsky, Peter Koo, Lynda Krasenbaum, Paul Kreis, Kathryn Lasch, Sophie Laurent et Nuno de Sousa, Alyssa Lebel, J. K. Lilly, John Loeser, Alexander Mauskop, Michell Max, Patrick McGrath, Jacques Meynadier, Christine Miaskowski, David Morris, Jeffrey Ngeow, Richard Payne, Clint Phillips, Russell Portenoy, Joshua Prager, Ali Rezai, Daniel Rockers, Alain Serrie, Mark Sullivan, Irene Tracey, Dennis Turk, Vijay Vad, Frank Vertosick, Seth Waldman, and Clifford Woolf, among others. Apologies to anyone I may have omitted! I also benefited from observing the excellent Tufts University program in pain research, education, and policy, and from participating in a conference at the Rockefeller Foundation Bellagio Center in Italy, "Narrative, Pain, and Suffering," organized by Daniel Carr, John Loeser, and Davis Morris (writing from which is collected in the volume *Narrative, Pain, and Suffering*, published by IASP Press).

Few writers in history, apart from members of royal families, have been granted more pleasant circumstances in which to slave over an impossible subject than I was when Ellis Alden allowed me to live in his marvelous hotel, the Stanford Park, for several months while researching pain at Stanford University, and then went on to offer extensive comments on my draft. Myriad thanks to him and his wife, Karen. Crucial work on this book was also done at Yaddo, as well as the Writers Room and Paragraph. Thanks to Jeffrey and Rachel Selin for creating the Writers' Dojo in Portland, where I wrote the final draft of my book.

Thanks to all the patients in this book who allowed me to observe their appointments and shared their experiences with me over the years. Particular thanks to Danielle Parker and Holly Wilson, whose stories I hope the reader will find as inspiring as I do.

Finally, I am lucky to have an extended family who includes editing among their familial duties. Many thanks to my parents, Stephan and Abigail; my father-in-law, Jim; and my mother-in-law, Felicity, who showed forbearance when I continued to split infinitives. My deepest intellectual and emotional sustenance came from my husband, Michael Callahan. I knew he had read too many drafts when he looked up and commented, about a single sentence, "Why did you drop the eel image?" Love and thanks to him for not only improving my prose, but for giving my story a happy ending in the deepest sense of the word. I cannot imagine a better partner. I hope that by the time our children, Violet and Kieran, are old enough to read this book, they will find it antiquated, as we do conditions that afflicted earlier generations and which we no longer can—or wish to—fully imagine.

INDEX

A

abdominal pain, 148

acetaminophen, 147, 240; *see also* Tylenol

acupuncture, 56, 133, 159, 227, 232, 299, 305; surgery in China with, 297–98

acute pain, 5, 8, 16, 43–47, 160, 178, 180, 191, 241, 270, 295, 325

Adam, 7, 62–63, 65, 89, 117, 171

addiction, 159–62, 168, 202, 242; benzodiazepine, 242; chloroform, 115; cocaine, 104; opioid, 146, 152–53, 159–66, 202, 228, 232; pseudo-, 161–62; substance abuse, 221

adrenaline, 27, 46, 47, 179

Advil, 54, 146; *see also* ibuprofen

aerobic exercise, 47, 55, 226

Africa, 17, 18, 57, 83, 94, 159, 178, 299–300

African Americans, 174; pain sensitivity, 174, 175, 178–79; pain treatment, 168, 170; religion and, 205–206; slavery, 170, 179

AIDS, 16, 168

Akiva, Rabbi, 314

Akkadians, 32, 33

alcohol, 54, 90, 101, 102, 103, 112, 146, 159, 161, 240

Aleve, 54, 146, 147, 250

Alexander the Great, 34

allodynia, 139, 229

alternative medicine, 56–57, 208–209, 213, 226–27, 297–301; acupuncture, 57, 133, 159, 227, 232, 297–99, 304; biofeedback, 133, 310, 317; chiropractic, 11, 133, 227, 231, 232; homeopathy, 305; massage, 56, 133, 253, 305; meditation, 133, 226, 297, 299, 305, 312; *see also* herbal medicine

American Pain Foundation, 128

American Pain Society, 132, 152

American Revolution, 89

Améry, Jean, 123, 203

amputation, 47, 93, 107, 196, 261, 282, 290; phantom limb pain, 11, 47, 181, 196, 287–88, 318–19; wartime, 97; without anesthesia, 94–95

ancient world, 6–7, 9, 17, 32–37, 48–49, 72, 88, 285; medicinal substances, 35, 48–49, 101–104; pain and

H

G

N

U

T